What's New in Surgical Oncology

Andrea Valeri • Carlo Bergamini
Ferdinando Agresta • Jacopo Martellucci
Editors

What's New in Surgical Oncology

A Guide for Surgeons in Training and Medical/Radiation Oncologists

Springer

Editors

Andrea Valeri
General, Emergency and Minimally
Invasive Surgery
Careggi Hospital
Florence, Italy

Carlo Bergamini
General, Emergency and Minimally
Invasive Surgery
Careggi Hospital
Florence, Italy

Ferdinando Agresta
Local Healthcare Unit ULSS 19 – Veneto
Adria, Italy

Jacopo Martellucci
General, Emergency and Minimally
Invasive Surgery
Careggi Hospital
Florence, Italy

ISBN 978-88-470-3937-7 ISBN 978-88-470-5310-6 (eBook)
DOI 10.1007/978-88-470-5310-6

Springer Milan Dordrecht Heidelberg London New York

Softcover reprint of the hardcover 1st edition 2013

Cover design: Ikona S.r.l., Milan, Italy
Typesetting: Graphostudio, Milan, Italy

Springer-Verlag Italia S.r.l. – Via Decembrio 28 – I-20137 Milan
Springer is a part of Springer Science+Business Media (www.springer.com)

Preface

The idea for a volume covering those aspects of oncology most relevant to the general surgeon arose when the ACOI (Italian Association of Hospital Surgeons) assigned to me the presidency of the XXXIInd national congress.

This book therefore aims to identify and describe the treatment options for malignancies that are most frequently adopted in general surgery departments, with emphasis on the most innovative and efficient procedures. While, given the importance of financial constraints, issues of cost-effectiveness are not neglected, our main concern has been to approach the topic in a way that will enable new generations of surgeons to apply rapidly emerging techniques and technologies with confidence. Moreover, a multidisciplinary, integrated approach has been emphasized that also involves medical and radiation oncologists, radiologists, and other specialists.

This textbook has been made possible by the fruitful cooperation of leading Italian surgical teams who play a key role in the various fields of surgical oncology. All of them have demonstrated that they are able to follow a broad multidisciplinary approach in the treatment of cancer patients, which is a *sine qua non* for achievement of the best therapeutic outcome.

Our colleagues and friends have also participated enthusiastically in this project. We feel a deep gratitude for their efforts and their intense research. In addition, we would like to thank the staff of Springer Verlag, who have followed and assisted us in our work step by step with outstanding professionalism.

Personally, I wish to thank my coeditors, Ferdinando Agresta, Jacopo Martellucci, and, last but not least, Carlo Bergamini, who has again been a source of strength in bringing this latest project to successful fruition.

Florence, May 2013 Andrea Valeri

Contents

Esophageal Cancer

1

Riccardo Rosati, Giovanni Pallabazzer, Alessandra Melis, Biagio Solito, Maria Grazia Fabrini, Laura Ginocchi, and Stefano Santi

1.1 Introduction

The overall 5-year survival of patients with cancer of the esophagus submitted to resection is 15–34%. Most patients who undergo radical esophagectomy relapse during the course of their disease. In recent years, there has been a growing interest in neoadjuvant treatments, which have produced better results in comparison with adjuvant protocols. There is clear evidence supporting chemoradiotherapy (CRT) for cancers of the esophagus. CRT gives a high rate of complete response (CR), and some researchers have questioned the role of surgery in cases of CR. This has led to trials on definitive chemoradiotherapy (dCRT). These experiences have produced a growing indication for a very demanding procedure: salvage surgery.

Resection of esophageal cancers carries a high rate of morbidity. Efforts have been made in recent years to verify if the application of minimally invasive surgery in this field could be advantageous in reducing the rate of mor-

R. Rosati (✉)
General and Minimally Invasive Surgery, Humanitas Clinical and Research Center, Rozzano (Milan), Italy
e-mail: riccardo.rosati@humanitas.it

G. Pallabazzer · B. Solito · S. Santi
Esophageal Surgery, Azienda Ospedaliero-Universitaria Pisana, Pisa, Italy

A. Melis
Department of Surgery, University of Milan, Italy

M.G. Fabrini
Radiotherapy Unit, Azienda Ospedaliero-Universitaria Pisana, Pisa, Italy

L. Ginocchi
Oncology Unit, Azienda Ospedaliero-Universitaria Pisana, Pisa, Italy

A. Valeri et al. (eds.), *What's New in Surgical Oncology*,
DOI: 10.1007/978-88-470-5310-6_1, © Springer-Verlag Italia 2013

bidity (especially in terms of respiratory complications). Also, in recent years, increasing numbers of patients have been selected for endoscopic treatment for early cancers.

The aim of this chapter is to give on overview on these topics (neoadjuvant and adjuvant treatment, dCRT and salvage surgery, minimally invasive surgery and endoscopic resection) in the treatment of esophageal neoplasms.

1.2 Therapeutic Strategies in Esophageal Cancer

Surgery is considered the treatment of choice for patients with localized esophageal cancer in terms of locoregional control and long-term survival. However, 5-year survival in significantly influenced by nodal involvement: 5-year survival for patients who undego radical resection for N+ cancers is ≈25% [1]. Surgery alone is considered inadequate for patients with advanced cancers (T3, N+ and, according to some oncologists, also for T2 esophageal cancers). An increasing number of patients with esophagogastric cancer are treated with preoperative chemotherapy (CT) or CRT.

1.2.1 Neoadjuvant Treatment

The aim of neoadjuvant treatment is to increase the number of R0 resections, to eradicate micrometastases, and to decrease the dissemination of cancer cells during surgery without affecting postoperative morbidity and mortality [2]. In addition, the radio-sensitizing properties [3] of certain chemotherapeutic agents and the increased oxygenation of undisturbed tissue in the tumor bed enhance the effects of perioperative radiotherapy (RT) [4].

The standard option for patients with localized esophageal cancer, based on the results of several randomized trials, is CRT followed by surgery, A randomized trial [5] comparing preoperative CRT, based on cisplatin and 5-fluorouracil (5FU) *versus* surgery alone demonstrated an increase of survival in patients treated with neoadjuvant therapy (3-year overall survival (OS) 32% *versus* 6%). A similar result was obtained in the Cancer and Leukemia Group B (CALGB) 9781 study [6]. Even though the study was closed prematurely for poor accrual, the results demonstrated a survival advantage for patients treated with neoajuvant treatment. That is, a median survival of 4.48 *versus* 1.79 years in favor of CRT (exact stratified log-rank, p=0.002) with a 5-year survival of 39% for CRT followed by surgery *versus* 16% for surgery alone. The Preoperative Chemotherapy or Radiochemotherapy in Esophagogastric Adenocarcinoma Trial (POET) study [7] randomized patients with locally advanced adenocarcinoma of the gastro-esophageal junction (GEJ) to CT or CRT followed by surgery. Although the study was stopped early and statistical significance was not achieved, the results indicated a survival advantage for preoperative CRT (3-year OS 47.4% *versus* 27.7%, p=0.07). Moreover, patients in the CRT group had a significantly higher rate of pathologic CR (15.6% *vs* 2.0%) or tumor-free lymph nodes (LNs; 64.4% *versus* 37.7%); the rate of postoperative mortality was higher in this group of patients but the difference was not significant (10.2% *versus* 3.8%, p=0.26).

A recent phase-III trial [8] compared CRT (carboplatin and paclitaxel and radiotherapy) plus surgery (178 patients), with surgery alone (188 patients) in patients with squamous cell carcinoma (SCC) or adenocarcinoma of the esophagus. An R0 resection was achieved in 92% of patients in the CRT group comapared with 69% in the surgery group (p<0.001). The rate of pCR was 29%. OS was significantly better in these patients (hazard ratio (HR), 0.657 (0.495–0.871, p=0.003). Postoperative complications and deaths carried a similar rate in the two treatment groups. The most recent phase-III trials [9-11] demonstrated that cisplatin based neoadjuvant CT increased the number of R0 resections in patients with adenocarcinoma of the lower esophagus and GEJ compared with surgery alone. In the MRC Adjuvant Gastric Infusional Chemotherapy Trial (MAGIC) [9], gastric adenocarcinoma and GEJ adenocarcinoma were assigned randomly to three perioperative and three postoperative cycles of ECF (epirubicin, cisplatin and fluorouracil) CT (250 patients) or surgery alone (253 patients). With respect to the latter, the perioperative CT group had a higher likelihood of OS (HR, 0.75; 0.60–0.93, p=0.009) and 5-year survival (36% *versus* 23%). Moreover, the Fédérale Nationale des Centres de Lutte Contre Le Cancer (FNLCC) ACCORD 07/FFCD 9703 phase-III study [10] demonstrated that neoadjuvant CT with cisplatin and 5FU improves OS (HR, 0.69; 0.50–0.95, p=0.02), 5-year survival (38% *versus* 24%) and curative resection (84% *versus* 73%) in stomach adenocarcinoma and GEJ locally advanced adenocarcinoma. A similar benefit was also shown in the OEO2 Allum trial [11] with a HR of 0.84 (0.72–0.98, p=0.03) and a 5-year survival of 23% *versus* 17.1%, in the CT setting for adenocarcinoma and SCC. A recent meta-analysis [12] involving 9 trials for 1981 patients confirmed the benefit of neoadjuvant CT in terms of OS with a HR of 0.87 (0.79–0.96; p=0.005) compared with surgery alone. Four meta-analyses [3,13–15] provided strong evidence for a survival benefit of neoadjuvant CRT or CT over surgery alone. However, a clear demonstration of the advantage of one stratery compared with the other was lacking.

1.2.2 Adjuvant Treatment

Two trials in the 1980s demonstrated that adjuvant radiotherapy does not elicit any benefit in patients submitted to resection for cancer of the esophagus. Data on adjuvant CT or CRT are limited except for adenocarcinoma of the lower esophagus and GEJ. Although multiple clinical trials [16–20] did not show significantly longer OS, several meta-analysis [21–24] suggested a small relative (12–28%) reduction in the risk of death for esophageal and GEJ adenocarcinoma after adjuvant CT, with an absolute survival benefit of 3–7%. In the US Southwest Oncology Group/Intergroup (SWOG) 9008/INT 0116 trial

[25], 556 patients with resected gastric or GEJ (≈20%) adenocarcinoma were randomly assigned to surgery plus 5FU and leucovorin postoperative CRT or surgery alone. The median OS was longer after complementary CRT (36 months) than after surgery alone (27 months) with a HR for death of 1.35 (1.09–1.66, p=0.005) and a HR for relapse of 1.52 (1.23–1.86, p<0.001). Although the study by Macdonald et al. elicited positive results, ≈54% of patients underwent a less than D1 resection. Hence, adjuvant CRT could have compensated for insufficient surgery. Three phase-III trials [26–28] on SCC that compared adjuvant CT with surgery alone did not find any benefit in OS. The most recent study among them demonstrated an advantage for 5-year disease-free survival (DFS) for CT compared with surgery alone (55% *versus* 45%, p=0.037), but did not demonstrate any significant difference in OS (61% *versus* 52%, p=0.13). Five-year survival in patients with LN-positive disease was 52% *versus* 38% (p=0.041). It appears that adjuvant CT should be reserved for patients with lymph-node metastases.

In conclusion, there is evidence of an advantage for preoperative CT for esophageal cancer independent from histology. However, this evidence is stronger for adenocarcinoma, which should be treated with preoperative and postoperative CT. Although a meta-analysis and a recent phase-III trial suggested that preoperative CRT confers survival benefit, it is not clear which patients (based on stage, tumor location, histology) will benefit most this treatment. Moreover, the rate of postoperative mortality seems to be increased after this treatment. Data on adjuvant CT/CRT are limited, except for lower esophageal/GEJ adenocarcinoma treated with limited surgery (LN dissection D1 and less) [29].

1.2.3 dCRT

The postoperative rate of mortality for radical esophagectomy is high, ranging from 5.7% to 14%, except in high-volume and dedicated treatment centers. CRT gives a rate of CR of 25–40% depending on tumor stage. Therefore, dCRT has gained interest among oncologists: dCRT is a treatment protocol of combined chemotherapy (mainly consisting of cisplatin and 5-FU) and a radiation total dose of 50–60 Gys, whereas the radiation dose in a neoadjuvant setting is ≈40–45 Gys.

Traditionally, dCRT has been used in patients with cancer of the cervical esophagus (where surgery includes laryngectomy and loss of phonation), in advanced cancers of the thoracic esophagus (either with extended involvement of the LNs) or with non-resectable disease (T4b)) or in patients who are unfit for surgery.

Phase-II trials that investigated the results of CRT alone demonstrated a rate of local control of 40–75%, with a median OS of 12.5–40 months and 3-year survival of 13–37% [30]. More than 70% of patients with a CR after CRT have a complete pathological response, so whether all patients who undergo CRT should also undergo surgery is controversial.

Two randomized studies have been published comparing dCRT with neoadjuvant CRT, and one further study has addressed the comparison between dCRT and surgery alone [1, 7, 29, 31]. dCRT did not give improved survival in comparison with individuals who had undergone resection. However, the rate of morbidity of these treatments was significantly higher for patients undergoing dCRT, even though the mortality (which was mainly postoperative) was significantly higher in resected patients.

The multicenter trial reported by Bedenne and coworkers demonstrated that the addition of surgery to CRT for locally advanced SCC of the esophagus may give mainly improved local control at the expense of a higher post-treatment rate of mortality [32].

However, a study on a series of patients submitted to esophagectomy for ypT0N0M0R0 in high-quality centers demonstrated that survival and local control were better in patients submitted to surgery, which raised the question of the "quality control" of surgery [33]. Quality of life (QoL) also seems to be improved in in patients treated with surgery compared with patients receiving dCRT [34].

We know that it is very difficult to be sure that a complete clinical response equals a complete pathological response, and accurate predictors of post-treatment response are, at the moment, lacking.

It has also been demonstrated that the pure costs of a therapeutic treatment for cancer of the esophagus (surgery, multimodal therapy or dCRT) are influenced significantly by post-treatment complications, which increase costs by between 9% and 25% [35]. Limiting the rate of treatment-related morbidity is clearly a major factor in controlling costs.

In the absence of level-I evidence to base the decision for the treatment of cancer of the esophagus, it appears that the results of different therapeutic approaches for this cancer are influenced significantly by the postoperative rate of mortality and morbidity in terms of clinical results (survival) and costs.

Therefore, it is crucial that these patients have the treatment and care delivery of their choice in centers that can offer a low rate of morbidity and mortality. Several studies have shown that one parameter that appears to be related to postoperative mortality is hospital volume.

In conclusion, it is thought that patients with resectable tumors (apart those with early neoplasms) should receive neoadjuvant CRT. Elderly or surgical high-risk patients who have achieved a complete clinical response might be considered for dCRT and be submitted to intensive observation.

1.2.4 Salvage Esophagectomy

It is estimated that 40–60% of patients submitted to dCRT will manifest persistent or recurrent neoplasms within 1 year. Salvage esophagectomy is carried out after concurrent dCRT (with a protocol that involves >50 Gy) and is selectively indicated for isolated local failures and recurrences, or for treatment-related complications. Salvage surgery is usually taken into consideration for patients with cancer of the cervical esophagus or for subcarinal cancers. For cancers of the upper thoracic esophagus, the likelihood of direct invasion to neighboring organs is very high and radical resection is seldom possible (Table 1.1)

Surgery after dCRT results in a high rate of morbidity and mortality. Table 1.1 reports the results of some Japanese works comparing the results of salvage surgery with trimodal therapy or surgery alone [36–38].

Salvage surgery results in a high rate of postoperative respiratory and anastomotic complications. The postoperative rate of mortality is significantly higher compared with other treatment strategies. One multivariate analysis has shown that dCRT is an independent factor associated with these complications. The main reasons for postoperative mortality are graft necrosis, anastomotic leaks, perioperative hemorrhage, acute distress respiratory syndrome, and tracheobronchial necrosis.

It has been demonstrated that the rate of morbidity and mortality for salvage surgery is increased significantly if patients receive a total radiation dose >55 Gy. In the series reported by D'Journo et al., [39] hospital mortality increased from 14% to 30% in patients receiving more than this radiation dose, and surgical complications increased from 28% to 60%.

The dose and quality of radiotherapy, therefore, influence significantly the results of salvage surgery.

Radiotherapy also influences the rate of anastomotic leaks. Previously, irradiated tissues may have a compromised the blood supply, which would not promote good anastomotic healing.

Other factors that seem to be associated with the high rate of complications for salvage surgery are malnutrition and immunosuppression. Preoperative treatments seem to induce a significant reduction of immunological parameters such as the activity of natural killer cells and total lymphocyte count. Frequently, patients who are candidates for salvage surgery are malnourished with high preoperative weight loss and low albumin levels. Both factors can lead to a high rate of complications. The role of immunonutrition in patients undergoing multimodal treatment to counteract these negative parameters needs to be evaluated.

When dealing with salvage surgery, there are some technical aspects that might act as protective measures for ischemic tracheobronchial lesions and for pulmonary complications during esophagectomy. Care should be taken to preserve the right posterior bronchial artery whenever possible; dissection around the airways should be very carefully managed; and neck dissection should be minimized as much as possible to preserve the blood supply from the inferior thyroidal artery to the trachea [40].

Median survival after salvage esophagectomy has been reported to vary between 7 months and 25 months, with 5-year survival between 0% and 37% [38]. Some parameters appear to influence survival after salvage surgery. The most important is prediction of R0 resection: in case of R1–2 salvage surgery, no survival is reported beyond 13 months. In this respect, Triboulet et al. [41] report-

Table 1.1 Results of some Japaneses work comparing the results of salvage surgery with trimodal therapy or surgery alone [9–11]

		n.	Compl	Pulm	Anast	M
Morita [36]	Surgery alone	253	24,5%	9,9%	13%	2,4%
	Preoperative CRT	197	40,1%	14,7%	23,4%	2,0%
	Salvage surgery	27	**59,3%**	**29,6%**	**37%**	**7,4%**
Miyata [37]	Preoperative CRT	112		22%	22%	4%
	Salvage surgery	33		**33%**	**39%**	**12%**
Tachimori [38]	No/Preoperative	553		20%	25%	2%
	Salvage surgery	59		**32%**	**31%**	**8%**

Compl, complications; *Pulm*, pulmonary complications; *Anast*, anastomosis; *M*, mortality.

ed that criteria for R0 prediction are tumor length <5 cm and limited aortic coverage. Other parameters that favorably influence survival are recurrent instead of persistent disease and a longer free interval compared with earlier relapse.

In conclusion, it appears that salvage esophagectomy is technically feasible but at the expense of a high rate of morbidity and mortality. However, it may be the only established treatment strategy that offers any chance of long-term survival. Due to the high rate of complications and results in terms of survival, it should be attempted only if R0 resection is deemed possible. The selection of patients for salvage esophagectomy should be very meticulous. Among selected patients, 5-year survival of ≤25% can be achieved. The selection and treatment of patients forf salvage surgery should be undertaken only in referral centers.

1.2.5 Minimally Invasive Esophagectomy (MIE)

R0 surgery represents the "gold standard" multimodal treatment of tumors of the esophagus because it offers the best chance of cure even though esophagectomy (despite the significant technical improvements and advances in surgical technique and perioperative management) is associated with significant morbidity and mortality. Minimally invasive surgery has been developed to reduce the complications related to esophagectomy, especially respiratory diseases (which represent the main cause of mortality). Although minimally invasive surgery for esophageal cancer started in the early 1990s, debate continues regarding its safety, efficacy, and benefits (contrary to the situation, for example, with colorectal surgery). Thus, in recent years, minimally invasive surgery for esophageal cancer has spread worldwide. However, this spread has been slower compared with other laparoscopic and thoracoscopic procedures, mainly due to the technical difficulties that this surgery entails and the lack of consensus in the literature. The reason for this is multifactorial and based on the relative rarity of esophageal tumors (which limits randomized studies) and the great variety of minimally invasive surgical approaches more or less associated with traditional surgery. A recent international survey involving 269 surgeons indicated that 78% of them continued to favor open approaches, 14% indicated a preference for minimally invasive resection, and 8% had no preference [42]. What emerges from numerous studies is that MIE is definitely a time-consuming process, as confirmed by the meta-analyses of Butler et al. [43] and Watanabe et al., [44] with a steep learning curve, but with a significant reduction in blood loss. In these studies, the percentage of conversion differs widely and is closely dependent on the experience of the surgeon, so in high-volume centers the rate of conversion is 0–7.3% [45–48], whereas in low-volume centers it is 10–36% [43,49,50]. In the meta-analysis of Butler et al., [43] the median mortality in total minimally invasive transthoracic esophagectomy was 1% (range, 0–6.5%), and in minimally invasive transhiatal esophagectomy (THE) it was 0% (range, 0–4.6%). The rate of mortality of MIE was similar to that for open surgery in the meta-analysis of Nagpal et al. [51] ($p = 0.26$) and in the meta-analysis of Uttley et al. [52], in which mortality was 2.4% for MIE and 3.8% for open surgery. The possible role of MIE in the reduction of morbidity in general and for respiratory complications in particular has been investigated by many retrospective and prospective studies as well as meta-analyses (Table 1.1). In particular, the meta-analysis of Nagpal et al. [51], which took into account 12 studies involving 672 patients (MIE and hybrid mininvasive esophagectomy [hMIE]) compared with 612 patients (open esophagectomy [OE]), showed a reduction of morbidity, including respiratory complications ($p = 0.04$). However, the same authors pointed out that there may be a bias in the analysis related to the inclusion of studies involving THE. Conversely, in the meta-analysis of Watanabe et al. [44], 10 of the 17 retrospective cohort studies did not show substantial differences in respiratory complications. Many authors [46,53–55] believe that the prone position (PP) could reduce pulmonary complications and have technical and physiological advantages. Regarding the former, certainly the visualization of anatomical structures is better because the lungs do not obscure the surgical field, even with one-lung ventilation. Moreover, the esophagous does not lie in the most declivous portion of the chest and is not obscured by overlying blood. Trauma to the lung is also reduced because it does not need to be retracted; the surgeon operates in a plane parallel to the camera with a similar view to that enabled by abdominal laparoscopic surgery. Finally, mobilization of the esophagus and lymphadenectomy become easier, especially at the level of the aortopulmonary window and close to the recurrent nerve, also on the left side. The undoubted physiological advantage in the prone position is the ability to operate without the excluded lung or a partially desufflated lung, thereby avoiding the pulmonary insufflation and desufflation that causes the release of mediators of inflammation and, even if not clinically tested [56], could be responsible for respiratory complications. The limits of the PP are an increase in operating time, and the difficulty in conversion to thoracotomy in case of massive bleeding. Only one randomized trial between MIE carried out in the PP and open surgery has been published, by Biere et al. [57]. They studied 115 patients randomized to an open esophagectomy or total MIE in the PP and esophagogastric anastomosis in the neck. Pulmonary infections in the first 2 weeks were 29% in the open group and 9% in the minimally invasive group (p = 0.005%). The rate of anastomotic leaks and re-operation was greater for minimally invasive surgery (7% *vs*. 4%, p = 0.390 and 14% *vs*. 11%, p = 0.641 respectively), whereas the rate of vocal-cord paralysis was higher in the open group (14% *vs*. 2%, p = 0.012). The duration of hospital stay was shorter in the MIE group compared with the open group (14% *vs*. 11 days, p = 0.044).

The goal of surgery is to obtain an R0 resection. Since the advent of minimally invasive surgery there has been a debate as to whether this approach could be similar for open surgery for oncological outcomes. Some studies have focused on the margins of resection, lymph-node retrieval as well as short- and long-term survival. In the meta-analysis of Butler et al., [43] the positive resection margins have been reported in 0–14% of cases. Martin et al. [58] reported that 13.9% (5/36 patients) of patients, who underwent a transthoracic three-stage esophagectomy had involved margins. In the study of Smithers et al., [53] there was no difference in the resection margins between open, total minimally invasive, and hMIE (19%, 14% and 20%, respectively); however in patients referred to surgery alone, the lateral margin involvement was greater in the open group compared with the assisted thoracoscopic group (15% *vs*. 8%).

LN retrieval during esophagectomy correlates directly with long-term survival, and several studies have confirmed this aspect [59–60] with a possible cutoff of 23 LNs [60]. Case series studies show no differences between open, MIE and hMIE in terms of LN retrieval (MIE *vs*. open, p = 0.83 and hMIE *vs*. open p = 0.62) [53]. In the meta-analysis of Dantoc et al., [61] the median (range) number of LNs found in the open group, MIE and hMIE groups was 10 (3–32.8) 16 (5.7–33.9) and 17 (17–17.15) respectively. There was a significant difference between the MIE and open groups (p = 0.032) but not between MIE and hMIE (p = 0.25). The explanation provided by several authors is that the increased visualization of LNs by thoracoscopic methods has led to a greater yield of LNs [54,62]. Despite numerous retrospective studies and meta-analyses, few authors have also evaluated the prognosis of patients who underwent MIE and if this technique gives the same oncological outcomes compared with open surgery. In the study of Dantoc et al., [61] there are no significant differences in survival to 5 years between MIE *vs*. OE and hMIE *vs*. OE (p = 0.33 and 0.41, respectively). Thus, based on this meta-analysis, minimally invasive surgery seems to have no advantage or disadvantage in terms of long-term survival. Similar results were reported by Osugi et al. [63] who compared 77 patients who underwent video-assisted thoracoscopic (VATS) esophagectomy *vs* 72 OE patients who underwent three-stage esophagectomy. Survival at 3 years and 5 years showed no significant differences (70% and 55% and 60% and 57%, respectively).

One of the major technical difficulties of minimally invasive esophageal surgery is intra-thoracic anastomoses, which may explain (at least in part) the choice of some authors to carry out three-stage esophagectomy and anastomosis in the neck even in patients with tumors of the distal esophagus and cardia. It is hard to compare the different studies in the literature with regard to the location (thoracic or cervical) and type of anastomoses (manual or mechanical and end-to-end, side-to-side, end-to-side). Maas et al. [64] conducted a review of 12 studies reporting on total minimally invasive Ivor Lewis esophagectomy in which the anastomotic leaks ranged from 0% to 10% and anastomotic stenoses from 0% to 27.5% (Table 1.2). Anastomotic stenoses were more common with the transoral technique. Based on these data, we believe that minimally invasive intrathoracic anastomoses should be undertaken only in controlled trials.

In conclusion, although >20 years have passed since the first MIE, and despite numerous studies, there are many unresolved issues. First, the multiple studies in the literature are, for the most part, retrospective and case series, with a limited number of patients, and are hard to compare with each other with respect to stage of disease, surgical technique, and adjuvant treatments. In addition, most studies have methodological limitations that reduce the statistical significance (e.g., authors at the beginning of their surgical experience may have selected patients with early-stage disease or with a better performance status). For these reasons, MIE, although achieving similar results in terms of oncological outcomes, has not demonstrated a clear advantage with respect to traditional surgery and, even if it is a safe alternative, it cannot be considered the procedure of choice. Second, it is very difficult to carry out randomized trials because, in most cases, it is preferable to choose a tailored surgery centered on patient need and not on a surgical technique that some authors consider better than another. Third, minimally invasive surgery should be totally consistent with the open approach (including surgical indications), so tumors of the cardia and distal esophagus should be approached using the Ivor Lewis procedure. In fact, it is well known that anastomoses in the neck have a higher percentage of fistulas and a greater number of recurrent nerve injuries. Moreover, in esophageal adenocarcinoma, laparoscopy may change the management strategy for up to 20% of patients with occult peritoneal or hepatic metastases. For this reason, carrying out the thoracoscopic stage first could make surgery become palliative. Robotic technology, in which three-dimensional vision and articulated arms facilitate surgical dissection, could have, especially in anatomically confined spaces, an important role in this very challenging type of surgery. We must emphasize that MIE is an advanced procedure requiring knowledge of advanced laparoscopic and thoracoscopic techniques and experience in conventional esophageal surgery. Therefore, it should be undertaken only in centers with vast experience in esophageal surgery.

Table 1.2 Pulmonary complications

Study	Number of cases	Pulmonary morbidity
Nguyen [47]	MIE 18 OE 16 THE 20	11% NA 19% 15%
Osugi [63]	TE 77 OE 72	15,6% NS 19,4%
Smithers [53]	tMIE 23 hMIE 309 OE 114	30% NS 26%
Fabian [70]	MIE 22 OE 56	5% p = 0.002 23%
Zingg [71]	MIE 56 OE 98	3.6% NS 4.7%
Parameswaren [72]	MIE 50 OE 30	8% p = 0.05 23%
Pham [54]	MIE 44 ILE 46	25% NS 15%
Schoppmann [62]	MIE 31 OE 31	9.7% p = 0.008 38.7%
Gao [73]	MIE 96 OE 78	13.5% NS 14.1%
Berger [74]	MIE 65 OE 53	7.7% NS 18%
Kinjo [75]	tMIE 72 hMIE 34 OE 79	7% NA 29% 9%
Sundaram [76]	MIE 47 TTE 26 THE 31	10.6% NS 34.6% 32.3%
Mamidanna [77]	MIE 1155 OE 6347	30% NS 31.4%

MIE, minimally invasive esophagectomy; *OE*, open esophagectomy; *THE*, transhiatal esophagectomy; *tMIE*, total minimally invasive esophagectomy; *hMIE*, hybrid minimally invasive esophagectomy; *ILE*, Ivor–Lewis esophagectomy; *TTE*, transthoracic esophagectomy; *NS* not significant; *NA*, not assessed; *a*, frequency of pneumonia.

1.2.6 Endoscopic Therapies for High-grade Dysplasia and Early Esophageal Cancer

In the last decade, the incidence of superficial esophageal cancer (carcinoma in situ (T*is*) and T1 lesions) has increased as a result of advances in endoscopic techniques that can be used to detect high-grade dysplasia and early esophageal carcinoma [65]. Early esophageal cancer is a localized lesion with a low risk

Table 1.3 Minimally invasive intrathoracic anastomosis

Study	Number of patients	Anastomotic leaks	Anastomotic stenosis	Surgical approach	Anastomotic technique	Type of anastomosis
Watson [78]	2	0	0	Transthoracic	End-to-side	Handsewn
Cadiere [79]	1	0	0	Transthoracic	Side-to-end	Handsewn
Lee [80]	8	0	1 (12.5%)	Transhiatal and transthoracic	End-to-side	Circular stapled
Nguyen [81]	1	0	0	Transthoracic	End-to-side	Circular stapled
Misawa [82]	5	0	0	Transthoracic	End-to-side	Circular stapled
Bizekis [83]	50	3 (6%)	6 (12%)	Transthoracic	End-to-side	Circular stapled
Thairu [84]	18	0	NR	Transthoracic	End-to-side	Circular stapled
Sutton [85]	10	1 (10%)	NR	Transhiatal	End-to-side	Transorally circular stapled
Nguyen [86]	51	5 (9.8%)	14 (27.5%)	Transthoracic	End-to-side	Transorally circular stapled
Campos [87]	37	1 (2.7%)	5 (13.5%)	Transthoracic	End-to-side	Transorally circular stapled
Ben-David [88]	6	NR	0	Transthoracic	Side-to-side	Linear stapled
Gorenstein [89]	31	1 (3.2%)	NR	Transthoracic	Side-to-side	Linear stapled

NR, not reported.

of LN metastasis and a high potential for cure after complete resection.

T*is* is the earliest stage; T1 lesions can be subdivided into T1m (tumor invading lamina propria) and T1sm (tumor invading submucosa). Mucosal lesions are subdivided into three groups: m1, carcinoma limited to the epithelium; m2, carcinoma with invasion into the lamina propria; and m3, carcinoma with invasion into but not through the muscularis mucosa.

Submucosal lesions are also subdivided into three groups, sm1, sm2, sm3, i.e., lesions with invasion into the superficial one-third of the submucosa (<200 μm), intermediate, or deepest one-third of the submucosa, respectively. Traditionally, surgery is the treatment of choice for patients with early-stage esophageal cancer and is highly curative. However, resection of the esophagus is an invasive procedure associated with significant morbidity and mortality. Many patients with esophageal cancer are elderly and often have multiple medical comorbidities: surgery is not the best option in these high-risk patients. Endoscopic therapy might be the "golden middle" between intensive biopsy follow-up and surgery. High-resolution endoscopy, endoscopic ultrasound (EUS), and high-frequency probe ultrasonography may be helpful in helping to differentiate between T1m (see below) and T1sm tumors and in selecting patients for potentially curative endoscopic therapeutic procedures.

There are different possibilities for the endoscopic management of high-grade dysplasia (HGD) and early esophageal cancer (EEC). Endoscopic mucosal resection (EMR) [66], endoscopic submucosal dissection (ESD) and endoscopic ablative therapies have been shown to be safe and effective alternative treatments in patients with early-stage cancer and significant comorbidity.

Endoscopic management offers the chance of eradication of the lesion with less morbidity and mortality than esophagectomy. Multiple local endoscopic ablation techniques exist or are under investigation, and the optimal method of ablation has yet to be determined. The opportunity for histologic examination of the resected specimen represents the major advantage of EMR over endoscopic ablative therapies. These include laser therapy (Nd-YAG-laser), argon-plasma coagulation (APC), and mono- or multipolar electrocoagulation and cryoablation as thermal destructive methods. Radiofrequency ablation (RFA) [67] and photodynamic therapy (PDT) [68,69] are non-thermal treatment approaches, as is EMR. Endoscopic management include patients with T1 disease confined to the mucosa (T1m/T1a), well-differentiated histopathology, no lymphovascular invasion, with a tumor size <2 cm and no suspicious adenopathy. Suspicious nodes should be sampled *via* EUS-guided fine-needle aspiration biopsy, if possible. Patients who do not meet these criteria should be treated by surgery or referred for neoadjuvant therapy protocols.

If EMR is carried out, the histological preparation of the resection specimen provides information on the true stage of neoplasia, the correctness of prior staging procedures, and if the resection was within healthy margins.The use of these techniques is limited to mucosal tumors because of the high risk of stage N1 in early tumors invading into the submucosa. LN metastasis is closely related to the degree of invasion into the esophageal wall. Esophageal lesions confined to *m1* and *m2* layers do not present LN metastasis. As the lesion becomes deeper, the rate of metastasis is: *m3* (9.1%), *Sm1* (15.4%), *Sm2* (40.0%), and *Sm3* (44.1%). The most commonly employed modalities of EMR are strip biopsy, double-snare polypectomy, resection with combined use of highly concentrated saline and epinephrine, and resection using a cap. We carry out EMR with use of a clear cap and pre-looped snare inside the cap. After insertion, the lesion borders are marked with a coagulator; 15–20 mL of saline are injected into the submucosal layer to swell the area containing the lesion. The cap is then placed on the lesion and the mucosa containing the lesion is drawn up inside the cap by aspiration. The mucosa is caught by the snare and strangulated, and finally resected by electrocautery. This is called the "lift, suck and cut" technique. The resected specimen is retrieved and submitted for microscopic examination for determination of the depth of tumor invasion, resection margin and possible vascular involvement. The resulting "ulcer" heals within 3 weeks. The major complications of endoscopic mucosal resection include postoperative bleeding, perforation and stricture formation. The rate of complications is 0–50% and recurrence is 0–8%.

PDT is a minimally invasive treatment of solid tumors employing a photosensitizing drug and laser light. Photosensitizers accumulated in malignant tissues remain inactive until exposed to a specific wavelength (665 nm) of visible, non-thermal red light.

In the USA, PDT has been approved to treat early-stage esophageal cancers, and HGD associated with Barrett's esophagus. The generally accepted mechanism of action of PDT is the generation of singlet oxygen, which causes irreversible oxidation of essential cellular components. In addition to the destruction of tumor cells, vascular disruption and activation of anti-tumor immunity aid in the anti-tumor activity of PDT. The advantage of PDT in early esophageal cancer, as reported by many authors, seems to be an overall rate of cure of >80% cure. Although there is still a role for PDT in certain situations, it appears that RFA is at least as effective as PDT and results in fewer complications. However, there has not been a randomized trial comparing the two modalities.

RFA is a new minimally invasive modality for the treatment of Barrett's esophagus and dysplasia. Endoscopic resection of esophageal mucosal irregularities and nodules that are dysplastic or which contain carcinoma combined with subsequent RFA of the remaining flat Barrett's esophagus and dysplasia can effectively and safely eradicate the disease.

Furthermore, a recent multicenter randomized control trial found that in patients with Barrett's esophagus containing nodules or mucosal irregularities which contained high-grade dysplasia or cancer, subsequent RFA resulted not only in eradication of Barrett's esophagus and dysplasia, but also significantly less esophageal stricture compared with patients who had circumferential endoscopic mucosal resection for their disease. RFA has an efficacy of 80–90% or greater with respect to complete clearance of Barrett's esophagus and dysplasia, with durability up to 5 years and a favorable safety profile. In patients with dysplastic Barrett's esophagus, RFA is associated with a high rate of complete eradication of dysplasia and intestinal metaplasia as well as a reduced risk of disease progression.

In general, the prognosis of esophageal cancer is quite poor because most patients present with advanced disease. The overall 5-year survival is ≈15–20%, with most patients dying within the first year of the diagnosis. Individualized prognosis is dependent largely upon stage. Those with cancer restricted entirely to the esophageal mucosa have an overall 5-year survival of ≈80%, but submucosal involvement brings this down to <50%.

The evolution of endoscopic resection methods has expanded the range of indications for endoscopic resections. However, such procedures are not indicated in cases with Sm2 and Sm3 invasion detected by EUS endoscopic ultrasound.

Whereas endoscopy has been used mainly to diagnose cancers, new technologies such as PDT, RFA and endoscopic mucosal resection have provided endoscopic treatments with the potential for curing early-stage tumors of the esophagus.

References

1. Stahl M, Budach W, Meyer HJ et al (2010) Esophageal cancer: Clinical Practice Guidelines for diagnosis, treatment and follow up. Ann Oncol 21 (Supplement 5):v46-49
2. Mariette C, Piessen G, Triboulet JP (2007) Therapeutic strategies in oesophageal carcinoma: role of surgery and other modalities. Lancet Oncol 8:545-553
3. Fiorica F, Di Bona D, Schepis F et al (2004) Preoperative chemoradiotherapy for oesophageal cancer. A systematic review and meta-analysis. Gut 53:625-630
4. Lim L, Michael M, Mann GB (2005) Adjuvant therapy in gastric cancer. J Clin Oncol 23:6220-6232
5. Walsh T, Noonan N, Hollywood D et al (1996) A comparison of multimodal therapy and surgery for esophageal adenocarcinoma. N Engl J Med 335:462-467
6. Tepper J, Krasna M, Niedzwiecki D et al (2008) Phase III trial of trimodality therapy with cisplatin, fluorouracil, radiotherapy, and surgery compared with surgery alone for esophageal cancer: CALGB 9781. J Clin Oncol 26:1086-1092
7. Stahl M, Walz M, Stuschke M et al (2009) Phase III comparison of preoperative chemotherapy compared with chemoradiotherapy in patients with locally advanced adenocarcinoma of the esophagogastric junction. J Clin Oncol 27:851-856
8. Van Hagen P, Hulshof M, van Lanschot JJ et al (2012) Preoperative chemotherapy for esophageal or junctional cancer. N Engl J Med 366:2074-2084
9. Cunningham D, Allum W, Stenning SP et al (2006) Perioperative chemotherapy versus surgery alone for resectable gastroesophageal cancer. N Engl J Med 355:11-20
10. Ychou M, Boige V, Pignon JP et al (2011) Perioperative chemotherapy compared with surgery alone for resectable gastroesophageal adenocarcinoma: an FNCLCC and FFCD multicenter phase III trial. J Clin Oncol 29:1715-1721
11. Allum W, Stenning S, Bancewicz J et al (2009) Long-term results of a randomized trial of surgery with or without preoperative chemotherapy in esophageal cancer. J Clin Oncol 27:5062-5067
12. Sjoquist K, Burmeister B, Smithers BM et al (2011) Survival after neoadjuvant chemotherapy or chemoradiotherapy for resectable oesophageal carcinoma: an updated meta-analysis. Lancet Oncol 12:681-692

13. Gebski V, Burmeister B, Smithers BM et al (2007) Survival benefit from neoadjuvant chemoradiotherapy or chemotherapy in esophageal carcinoma: a meta-analysis. Lancet Oncol 8:226-234
14. Ronellenfitsch U, Schwarzbach M, Hofheinz M et al (2010) Meta-analysis of preoperative chemotherapy (CTX) versus primary surgery for locoregionally advanced adenocarcinoma of the stomach, gastroesophageal junction, and lower esophagus (GE adenocarcinoma). 2010 ASCO Annual Meeting
15. Sjoquist K, Burmeister B, Smithers BM et al (2011) Survival after neoadjuvant chemotherapy or chemoradiotherapy for resectable oesophageal carcinoma: an updated meta-analysis. Lancet Oncol 12(7):681-692
16. Bouche O, Ychou M, Burtin P et al (2005) Adjuvant chemotherapy with 5-fluorouracil and cisplatin compared with surgery alone for gastric cancer: 7-year results of the FFCD randomized phase III trial (8801). Ann Oncol 16:1488-1497
17. Nitti D, Wils J, Dos Santos JG et al (2006) Randomized phase III trial of FAMTX or FEMTX compared with surgery alone in resected gastric cancer. A combined analysis of the EORTC GI Group and ICCG. Ann Oncol 17: 262-269
18. De Vita F, Giuliani F, Orditura M et al (2007) Adjuvant chemotherapy with epirubicin, leucovorin, 5-fluorouracil and etoposide regimen in resected gastric cancer patients: a randomized phase III trial by the Gruppo Oncologico Italia Meridionale (GOIM 9602 Study). Ann Oncol 18:1354-1358
19. Di Costanzo F, Gasperoni S, Manzione L et al (2008) Adjuvant Chemotherapy in Completely Resected Gastric Cancer: A Randomized Phase III Trial Conducted by GOIRC. J Natl Cancer Inst 100:388-398
20. Cascinu S, Labianca R, Barone C et al (2007) Adjuvant Treatment of High-Risk, Radically Resected Gastric Cancer Patients With 5-Fluorouracil, Leucovorin, Cisplatin, and Epidoxorubicin in a .Randomized Controlled Trial. J Natl Cancer Inst 99:601-607
21. Mari E, Floriani I, Tinazzi A et al (2000) Efficacy of adjuvant chemotherapy after curative resection for gastric cancer: A meta-analysis of published randomised trials: A study of the GISCAD (Gruppo Italiano per lo Studio dei Carcinomi dell'Apparato Digerente). Ann Oncol 11:837-835
22. Panzini I, Gianni L, Fattori PP et al (2002) Adjuvant chemotherapy in gastric cancer: a meta-analysis of randomized trials and comparison with previous meta-analysis. Tumori 88(1):21-27
23. Janunger K, Hafström L, Glimelius B (2002) Chemotherapy in gastric cancer: a review and updated meta-analysis. Eur J Surg 168(11):597-608
24. Pignon J, Rougier P, Sakamoto J et al (2010) Benefit of adjuvant chemotherapy for resectable gastric cancer: a meta-analysis. JAMA 303(17):1729-1737
25. Macdonald J, Smalley S, Benedetti J et al (2001) Chemoradiotherapy after surgery compared with surgery alone for adenocarcinoma of the stomach or gastroesophageal junction. N Engl J Med 345:725-730
26. Ando N, Iizuka T, Kakegawa T et al (1997) A randomized trial of surgery with and without chemotherapy for localized squamous carcinoma of the thoracic esophagus: the Japan Clinical Oncology Group Study. J Thorac Cardiovasc Surg 114:205-209
27. Pouliquen X, Levard H, Hay JM et al (1996) 5-Fluorouracil and cisplatin therapy after palliative surgical resection of squamous cell carcinoma of the esophagus. A multicenter randomized trial. French Associations for Surgical Research. Ann Surg 223:127-133
28. Ando N, Iizuka T, Ide H et al (2003) Surgery plus chemotherapy compared with surgery alone for localized squamous cell carcinoma of the thoracic esophagus: a Japan Clinical Oncology Group Study-JCOG9204. J Clin Oncol 21:4592-4596
29. Stahl M, Budach W, Meyer HJ et al (2010) Esophageal cancer: clinical practice guidelines for diagnosis, treatment and follow up. Clinical practice guidelines. Ann Oncol 21:v46-v49
30. Herskovic, Russell W, Liptay M et al (2012) Esophageal carcinoma advances in treatment results for locally advanced disease: review Ann Oncol 23(5)1095-1103
31. Chiu PW, Chan AC, Leung SF et al (2005) Multicenter prospective randomized trial comparing standard esophagectomy with chemoradiotherapy for treatment of squamous esophageal cancer: early results from the Chinese University Research Group fro Esophageal Cancer

(CURE). J Gastrointest Surg 9:794-802
32. Bedenne L, Michel P, Bouche O et al (2007) Chemoradiation followed by surgery compared with chemoradiation alone in squamous cancer of the esophagus: FFCD 9102. J Clin Oncol 25:1160–68
33. Vallböhmer D, Hölscher AH, DeMeester S et al (2010) A multicenter study of survival after neoadjuvant radiotherapy/chemotherapy and esophagectomy for ypT0N0M0R0 esophageal cancer. Ann Surg 252(5):744-749
34. Bonnetain F, Bouché O, Michel P et al (2006) A comparative longitudinal quality of life study using the Spitzer quality of life index in a randomized multicenter phase III trial (FFCD 9102): chemoradiation followed by surgery compared with chemoradiation alone in locally advanced squamous resectable thoracic esophageal cancer. Ann Oncol 17(5):827-834
35. Kuppusamy M, Sylvester J, Low DE (2011) In an era of health reform: defining cost differences in current esophageal cancer management strategies and assessing the cost of complications. J Thorac Cardiovasc Surg 141:16-21
36. Morita M, Kumashiro R, Hisamatsu Y et al (2011) Clinical significance of salvage esophagectomy for remnant or recurrent cancer following definitive chemoradiotherapy. J Gastroenterol 46(11):1284-1291
37. Miyata H, Yamasaki M, Takiguchi S (2009) Salvage esophagectomy after definitive chemoradiotherapy for thoracic esophageal cancer. J Surg Oncol 100(6):442-446
38. Tachimori Y (2009) Role of salvage esophagectomy after definitive chemoradiotherapy. Gen Thorac Cardiovasc Surg 57(2):71-78
39. D'Journo XB, Michelet P, Dahan L et al (2008) Indications and outcome of salvage surgery for oesophageal cancer. Eur J Cardiothorac Surg 33:1117-1123
40. Watanabe M, Yoshida N, Karashima R et al (2009) Transcervical Superior Mediastinal Lymph Node Dissection Combined with Transhiatal Lower Esophageal Dissection before Transthoracic Esophagectomy: A Safe Approach for Salvage Esophagectomy. JACS 208(4):e7-e9
41. Triboulet JO (2011) Salvage surgery: cancer of the esophagus. Bull Cancer 98:73-78
42. Boone J, Livestro DP, Elias SG et al (2009) International survey on esophageal cancer: part I surgical techniques. Dis Esophagus 22:195-202
43. Butler N, Collins S, Memon MB et al (2011) Minimally invasive oesophagectomy: current status and future direction. Surg Endosc 25:2071–2083
44. Watanabe M, Baba Y, Nagai Y et al (2012) Minimally invasive esophagectomy for esophageal cancer: an updated review. Surg Today [Epub ahead of print]
45. Luketick JD, Pennathur A, Awais O et al (2012) Outcomes after minimally invasive esophagectomy: review of over 1000 patients. Ann Surg 256:95-103
46. Palanivelu C, Prakash A, Senthilkumar R et al (2006) Minimally invasive esophagectomy: thoracoscopic mobilization of the esophagus and mediastinal lymphadenectomy in prone position - experience of 130 patients. JACS 203:7-16
47. Nguyen NT, Roberts P, Follette DM et al (2003) Thoracoscopic and laparoscopic esophagectomy for benign and malignant disease: lessons learned from 46 consecutive procedures. JACS 197:902-913
48. Berrisford RG, Wajed SA, Sanders D et al (2008) Short-term outcomes following total minimally invasive oesophagectomy. Br J Surg 95:602-610
49. Robertson GS, Lloyd DM, Wicks AC et al (1996) No obvious advantages for thoracoscopic two-stage oesophagectomy. Br J Surg 83:675-678
50. Van den Broek WT, Makay O, Berends FJ et al (2004) Laparoscopically assisted transhiatal resection for malignancies of the distal esophagous. Surg Endosc 18:812-817
51. Nagpal K, Ahmed K, Vats A et al (2010) Is minimally invasive surgery beneficial in the management of esophageal cancer? A meta-analysis. Surg Endosc 24:1621–1629
52. Uttley L, Campbell F, Rhodes M et al (2012) Minimally invasive oesophagectomy versus open surgery: is there an advantage? Surg Endosc. 2012 Oct [Epub ahead of print]
53. Smithers BM, Gotley DC, Martin I et al (2007) Comparison of the outcomes between open and minimally invasive esophagectomy. Ann Surg 245:232–240
54. Pham TH, Perry KA, Dolan JP et al (2010) Comparison of perioperative outcomes after com-

bined thoracoscopic-laparoscopic esophagectomy and open Ivor-Lewis esophagectomy. Am J Surg 199:594–598
55. Kuwabara S, Katayanagi N (2010) Comparison of three different operative methods of video-assisted thoracoscopic esophagectomy. Esophagus 7:23–29
56. Funakoshi T, Ishibe Y, Okazaki N et al (2004) Effect of re-expansion after short-period lung collapse on pulmonary capillary permeability and pro-inflammatory cytokine gene expression in isolated rabbit lungs. Br J Anaesth 92:558–563
57. Biere SS, van Berge Henegouwen MI, Maas KW et al (2012) Minimally invasive versus open oesophagectomy for patients with oesophageal cancer: a multicentre, open label, randomised controlled trial. Lancet 379:1887-1892
58. Martin DJ, Bessell JR, Chew A et al (2005) Thoracoscopic and laparoscopic esophagectomy: initial experience and outcomes. Surg Endosc 19:1597-1601
59. Rizk N, Ishwaran H, Rice T et al (2010) Optimum lymphadenectomy for esophageal cancer. Ann Surg 251(1):46
60. Peyre C, Hagen J, DeMeester S et al (2008) The number of lymph nodes removed predicts survival in esophageal cancer: an international study on the impact of extent of surgical resection. Ann Surg 248(4):549
61. Dantoc MM, Cox MR, Eslick GD (2012) Does minimally invasive esophagectomy (MIE) provide for comparable oncologic outcomes to open techniques? A systematic review. Gastrointest Surg 16:486–494
62. Schoppmann SF, Prager G, Langer FB et al (2010) Open versus minimally invasive esophagectomy: a single-center case controlled study. Surg Endosc 24:3044–3053
63. Osugi H, Takemura M, Higashino M et al (2003) A comparison of video-assisted thoracoscopic oesophagectomy and radical lymph node dissection for squamous cell cancer of the oesophagus with open operation. Br J Surg 90:108-113
64. Maas KW, Biere SS, Scheepers JJ et al (2012) Minimally invasive intrathoracic anastomosis after Ivor Lewis esophagectomy for cancer: a review of transoral or transthoracic use of staplers. Surg Endosc 26:1795-1802
65. Tan A, Douglas O, Faigel (2009) Role of endoscopic ultrasound in superficial esophageal cancer. Dis Esophagus 22:104-112
66. Pech O, Ell C (2005) Endoscopic Resection for High-Grade Dysplasia in Barrett's Esophagus. Tech Gastrointest Endosc 7:66-68
67. Shaheen NJ, Sharma P, Bergein F et al (2009) Radiofrequency Ablation in Barrett's Esophagus with Dysplasia. N Engl J Med 360:2277-2288
68. Overholt BF, Panjehpour M, Halberg DL (2003) Photodynamic therapy for Barrett's esophagus with dysplasia and/or early stage carcinoma: long-term results. Gastrointest Endosc 58:183-188
69. Wang KK (2005) Combined Endoscopic Mucosal Resection and Photodynamic Therapy for High-Grade Dysplasia and Early Cancer in Barrett's Esophagus. Tech Gastrointest Endosc 7:69-72
70. Fabian T, Martin JT, McKelvey AA et al (2008) Minimally invasive esophagectomy: a teaching hospital's first year experience. Dis Esophagus 21:220–5
71. Zingg U, McQuinn A, DiValentino D et al (2009) Minimally invasive versus open esophagectomy for patients with esophageal cancer. Ann Thorac Surg 87:911–93
72. Parameswaren R, Veeramootoo D, Krishnadas R et al (2009) Comparative experience of open and minimally invasive esophagogastric resection. World J Surg 33:1868–75
73. Gao Y, Wang Y, Chen L, Zhao Y (2011) Comparison of open three-field and minimally-invasive esophagectomy for esophageal cancer. Intract Cardiovasc Thorac Surg 12:366–9
74. Berger AC, Bloommenthal A, Weksler B et al (2011) Oncologic efficacy is not compromised, and may be improved with minimally invasive esophagectomy. J Am Coll Surg 212:560–8
75. Kinjo Y, Kurita N, Nakamura F et al (2012) Effectiveness of combined thoracoscopic-laparoscopic esophagectomy: comparison of postoperative complication and midterm oncological outcomes in patients with esophageal cancer. Surg Endosc 26:381–90

76. Sundaram A, Geronimo JC, Willer BL et al (2012) Survival and quality of life after minimally invasive esophagectomy: a single-surgeon experience. Surg Endosc 26:168–76
77. Mamidanna R, Bottle A, Aylin P et al (2012) Short-term outcomes following open versus minimally invasive esophagectomy for cancer in England: a population-based national study. Ann Surg 255:197-203
78. Watson DI, Davies N, Jamieson GG (1999) Totally endoscopic Ivor Lewis esophagectomy. Surg Endosc 13(3):293-7
79. Cadière GB, Dapri G, Himpens J, Rajan A (2011) Thoracoscopic esophagectomy in prone position. Ann Surg Oncol 18(3):838
80. Lee KW, Leung KF, Wong KK et al (1997) One-stage thoracoscopic oesophagectomy: ligature intrathoracic stapled anastomosis. Aust N Z J Surg 67(2-3):131-2
81. Nguyen NT, Follette DM, Lemoine PH et al (2001) Minimally invasive Ivor Lewis esophagectomy. Ann Thorac Surg 72(2):593-6
82. Misawa K, Hachisuka T, Kuno Y et al (2005) New procedure for purse-string suture in thoracoscopic esophagectomy with intrathoracic anastomosis. Surg Endosc 19(1):40-2
83. Bizekis C, Kent MS, Luketich JD et al (2006) Initial experience with minimally invasive Ivor Lewis esophagectomy. Ann Thorac Surg 82(2):402-6; discussion 406-7
84. Thairu N, Biswas S, Abdulaal Y (2007) A new method for intrathoracic anastomosis in laparoscopic esophagectomy. Surg Endosc 21(10):1887-90
85. Sutton CD, White SA, Marshall LJ et al (2002) Endoscopic-assisted intrathoracic oesophagogastrostomy without thoracotomy for tumours of the lower oesophagus and cardia. Eur J Surg Oncol 28(1):46-8
86. Nguyen NT, Hinojosa MW, Smith BR et al (2008) Minimally invasive esophagectomy: lessons learned from 104 operations. Ann Surg 248(6):1081-91
87. Campos GM, Jablons D, Brown LM et al (2010) A safe and reproducible anastomotic technique for minimally invasive Ivor Lewis oesophagectomy: the circular-stapled anastomosis with the trans-oral anvil. Eur J Cardiothorac Surg 37(6):1421-6
88. Ben-David K, Sarosi GA, Cendan JC et al (2010) Technique of minimally invasive Ivor Lewis esophagogastrectomy with intrathoracic stapled side-to-side anastomosis. J Gastrointest Surg 14(10):1613-8
89. Gorenstein LA, Bessler M, Sonett JR (2011) Intrathoracic linear stapled esophagogastric anastomosis: an alternative to the end to end anastomosis. Ann Thorac Surg 91(1):314-6

2 Gastric Malignancies

Domenico Garcea, Andrea Rinnovati and Paolo Morgagni

2.1 Introduction

The incidence of gastric cancer (GC) has been decreasing in recent years. However, the increasing age of populations worldwide makes its detection still frequent. Even if GC treatment has been tailored according to disease stage, endoscopic or surgical resection must be always undertaken to guarantee a good outcome. Moreover, there is no hope of survival after incomplete surgery.

Optimal preoperative staging and a multimodal approach can lead to differentiated treatment, allowing also more specific results on complications, reducing morbidity and mortality. This therapeutic approach enables consideration of the hospital type and hospital-specific disease volume, considered as an important parameter for good results. Indeed, many studies have been done showing that morbidity and mortality improves in patients with esophageal cancer treated at high-volume hospitals, but few studies have described the same good results for GC, even if decreasing morbidity and mortality have been reported. A reason for this finding could be the lack of very-high-volume centers in western countries, which does not allow comparisons of different situations. However, we should probably also consider other variables, such as the availability of an experienced surgical team in medium-sized hospitals. In this regard, a study by Jensen et al. in 2010 showed results after the centralization of GC patients in a high-volume hospital in Denmark. The decrease from 37 to 5 departments after centralization resulted in an improvement in the mortality rate from 8.2% to 2.4% [1].

D. Garcea · P. Morgagni (✉)
Department of General Surgery, "G.B. Morgagni-L. Pierantoni" General Hospital, Forlì, Italy
e-mail: p.morgagni@ausl.fo.it

A. Rinnovati
General Surgery Unit, Ospedale del Casentino, Arezzo, Italy

A. Valeri et al. (eds.), *What's New in Surgical Oncology*,
DOI: 10.1007/978-88-470-5310-6_2, © Springer-Verlag Italia 2013

2.2 Endoscopic Approach

In recent years, the endoscopic approach for high-grade dysplasia and for a subset of early gastric cancer (EGC) not requiring lymphadenectomy has changed the quality of life of patients. Several studies and Japanese guidelines defined these subsets [2], i.e., mucosal differentiated cancer of diameter <2 cm without ulceration can be treated by endoscopic mucosal resection (EMR) or with endoscopic submucosal dissection (ESD). Not all mucosal cancer, differentiated tumors or small cancers, but only a subset of EGC with well-defined and associated characteristics did not present lymphatic spread; this subset should be considered for local endoscopic resection. If endoscopic treatment can cure patients considered to be N0, surgery must be proposed for all other patients suspected to have lymphatic diffusion.

2.3 Lymphadenectomy

The second-level lymphadenectomy (D2) proposed by Japanese surgeons can improve survival also in specialized western centers where morbidity and mortality is not significantly increased [3, 4]. A recent meta-analysis referring to old trials suggested that D1 is the better dissection, but revised studies also on the Dutch trial confirmed that D2 dissection improves survival if morbidity and perioperative mortality is low [5]. The McDonald study based in America added radiotherapy on perigastric areas that are submitted to insufficient lymphadenectomy, and revealed better long-term survival in relation to surgery alone [30]; radiotherapy could be considered in those patients as a sort of "radio-lymphadenectomy". Limited lymphadenectomy is, in general, proposed by Japanese guidelines for EGC patients. Even if correct, considering the eastern preoperative accuracy in diagnosis, such limited indications are not always applicable in western centers. In our opinion, surgically treated patients should be submitted to D2 lymphatic dissection because of the following reasons:

- TNM classification requires 16 dissected lymph nodes and only <45% of D1 dissections can be properly classified [4];
- Accurate dissection allows better staging of the disease owing to an higher number of lymph nodes retrieved;
- If the pathological report does not confirm an endoscopic diagnosis of EGC and an advanced cancer is diagnosed, surgeon dissection could be uncorrected;
- Wide lymphatic dissection in low cancer stage also improves survival in patients considered to be N0, as referred by the Japanese Clinical Oncology Group (GCOG) trial [6];
- Morbidity and mortality are not higher for D2 dissection also in western centers [3, 4].

2.4 Definition of D2 Dissection

In 2010, the Japanese Gastric Cancer Association presented a new D2 definition related not to the site of the cancer but to the type of gastrectomy, with the definition being different for subtotal or total gastrectomy [2]. Looking at lymphatic dissection, differences from previous definitions focused principally on gastric artery station 7 now being considered as D1 and mesenteric vein station (n14) being not dissected further in the new D2 definition and only being suggested in pylorus cancer. After subtotal gastrectomy, D2 lymphadenectomy requires dissection of 1, 3, 4sb, 4d, 5, 6, 7, 8a, 9, 11p and 12a node stations. Total gastrectomy requires dissection of 1, 2, 3, 4, 5, 6, 7, 8a, 9, 10, 11p, 11d, and 12a node stations [2].

2.5 Extended Lymphadenectomy D3

More extended lymphadenectomy D3 is now not recommended as prophylactic treatment in Japan after the JCOG 9501 trial [6]. This trial did not find any improvement for patients submitted to para-aortic dissection (PAND). In western centers (especially in Italy), this option is not completely excluded because 5-year survival rates of 17% have been reported after surgical dissection for patients with positive para-aortic nodes. Even if these patients are considered to be M1, their survival is better than that for other metastatic sites. In Japan, even if prophylactic PAND is not recommended, if the involvement of the para-aortic nodes is suspected, these patients are submitted to neoadjuvant treatment, and then to D3 dissection. [6, 7]. D3 dissection involves removal of the posterior lymph nodes of the hepatic artery (8p), hepatoduodenal ligament (12p), retro-pancreatic segments (13), and peri-aortic segments (16). Morbidity is improved, but has been reported to be 28%; mortality (2.1%) is quite similar in selected centers [7]. Western centers are looking for selective criteria to identify patients with suspected involvement of the para-aortic lymph nodes [8].

2.6 En block Resection and Retrieval of Lymph Node Stations

An interesting study based in Korea in 2011 confirmed that free cancer cells can be released from lymphovascular pedicles opened during surgery for GC, especially in advanced-stage disease. The authors found that this could be prevented by using an energy-based device [9]. The intraoperative use of devices makes *en block* dissection a secondary endpoint, whereas distant stations (e.g., 12a in the hepatoduodenal ligament or 9 at the splenic hilus) could be better dissected alone. An interesting question is who should dissect the lymphatic stations after surgery in the surgical specimen. Quarrels have arisen between pathologists and surgeons if a low number of lymph nodes are sampled. Lymphatic dissection on fresh specimens immediately after resection permits better collection of lymph nodes, and different stations are better recognized by surgeons (mainly if nearby stations have not been dissected intraoperatively). Dissection by surgeons in theatre immediately after resection must be suggested and stressed.

2.7 R0 Resection

The type of patient who could be considered for radical resection is an open question. The old Japanese definition of R0 was: no residual disease with a high probability of cure. This condition was achieved by a distance of 10-cm margin from the cancer and resection lines in T1/T2 tumors with a D lymphadenectomy level more than (N) lymphatic stage [10]. A recent R0 definition from the International Union against Cancer/American Joint Committee on Cancer (UICC/AJCC) stated "complete resection of the primary cancer without macroscopic or microscopic residual" [11]. The high prevalence of relapse after suspected R0 resection makes this definition inadequate, and perhaps the concept of circumferential/ lateral resection margin must be added [12]. The seventh tumor/node/metastasis (TNM) classification now necessitates cytology upon peritoneal lavage to avoid peritoneal cancer cells causing peritoneal relapse; positive cytological lavage has been added as M1 in the new TNM classification [11] and must be performed to define a R0 resection.

2.8 Neoadjuvant Treatment

The MRC Adjuvant Gastric Infusional Chemotherapy Trial (MAGIC) in England and FFCD 9703 trial (France) described significant survival improvement if perioperative chemotherapy was followed by surgery. In these clinical trials, several questions have been asked (for example: the number of patients recruited with cancer of the gastric cardia or early lesions, and surgical results) but a statistically robust solid improvement was observed. Unfortunately, a more selective trial with good preoperative staging, the European Organization for the Research and Treatment of Cancer (EORTC) trial, failed to find statistical power for the low number of patients recruited even if downstaging had been frequently observed. No information is available on survival in the Swiss Group for Clinical Cancer Research (SAKK) trial. Five trials on neoadjuvant treatment are ongoing: MAGIC B (England); Chemoradiotherapy after Induction chemotherapy in Cancer of the Stomach (CRITICS; the Netherlands); JCOG 0501 (Japan); Intergroup Trial of Adjuvant Chemotherapy in Adenocarcinoma of the Stomach (ITACA 2) and Istituto Scientifico Romagnolo per lo Studio e la Cura dei Tumori (IRST 151) (both Italy). These trials using neoadjuvant treatment involve different drugs and, sometimes, combination with radiotherapy and biological therapy. The importance of preoperative staging must be stressed to avoid irrelevant treatment in early lesions or delayed specific treatment in metastatic disease. Moreover, collaboration with oncologists in this new approach should be improved.

2.9 Minimally Invasive Surgery

Laparoscopic staging is accurate and allows collection of peritoneal fluid for cytology. Laparoscopic surgery for early lesions (T1 and T2) is proposed also in Japanese guidelines with modified limited lymphadenectomy. Doubt regarding the treatment of advanced forms has been wiped away due to a meta-analysis reporting less lymph-node dissection and difficult dissection of some stations with laparoscopic access [13]. In this regard, some trials are ongoing (JCOG 0912 and Korean Laparoscopic Gastrointestinal Surgery Study Group (KLASS)) and results are awaited but, at the moment, robotic surgery may offer a better and easier dissection compared with laparoscopy.

2.10 Splenectomy

The new Japanese guidelines for D2 dissection have confirmed that the splenic hilus station (n10) must be dissected after total gastrectomy, but evidence-based information on splenectomy is not available. To ascertain if splenectomy has a statistically solid prognostic value, we should wait for the conclusions of the JCOG 0110 trial in Japan [14]. Presently, splenectomy may worsen morbidity and mortality and must be indicated only for cancers sited on the great curvature, or if suspicious lymph nodes are detected at station 10 and from there are not easily removable.

2.11 Bursectomy

Tumors penetrating the serosa of the posterior gastric wall (T3 and T4a) are strongly associated with posterior peritoneal seeding. In these patients, bursectomy (removal of the inner peritoneal surface of the bursa omentalis) presented a survival improvement in a recent small randomized trial [15]. This technique, which is generally undertaken in eastern centers without worsening morbidity, is carried out only in selected western institutions. A new, geographically wider multicenter trial looking at this matter (JCOG 1001 is ongoing.

2.12 Resection Margin and Distance From Cancer

Infiltrated surgical margins are a significant negative prognostic factor [16], If certain eastern endoscopists propose new endoscopic treatments for positive lateral margins after ESD, all positive deep margins after endoscopic treatment and all surgical patients apparently treated by radical procedures except for resection lines should be submitted for a new resection. To avoid infiltration of the resection margin, a distance of 2 cm from EGC and ≥5 cm from undifferentiated lesions should be requested (German guidelines require 8 cm for Lauren histotype (diffuse) carcinoma). Moreover, all cancer classified by macroscopically infiltrated Borrmann type 4 require total gastrectomy. Frozen sections at resection-line specimens could be useful but may be insufficient (mainly for diffuse-type carcinoma when immunostaining is requested).

2.13 Peritonectomy and Hyperthermic Intraperitoneal Chemotherapy (HIPEC)

Current indications for peritonectomy and HIPEC are highly selective, and few patients can achieve good results. The indication for HIPEC is after complete cytoreductive surgery and 5-year survival rates of 19–25% have been reported. Indeed, it can be an interesting option in T4 cancer if only positive cytology has been observed in a previous laparoscopic peritoneal lavage. In the future, expression of the CXCL12 receptor in peritoneal washings may serve as useful molecular marker to identify a subset of GC patients at very high risk of peritoneal recurrence [17].

2.14 Reconstruction

In general, Roux-en-Y reconstruction is undertaken after total gastrectomy. Several techniques and pouches have been proposed, but none of the types has been widely accepted. Also, after subtotal gastrectomy, Roux-en-Y is currently used in western centres. In eastern countries, the Billroth-1 reconstruction is frequently carried out if small well-differentiated cancer is diagnosed in the distal third of the stomach. The Billroth-2 reconstruction is still proposed by several authors.

2.15 Cardia Carcinoma and the New TNM Classification

Carcinoma of the gastro-esophageal junction (GEJ) is a particular subset of carcinoma now considered by the new TNM classification to be esophageal cancer. This classification does not provide any clinical information for the surgical approach, and several authors propose a change. One of the most used classifications by surgeons is the Siewert classification, which differentiates three cancer sites. Siewert 1 cancer require thoracotomy and Siewert 3 laparotomy. However, there is considerable debate regarding Siewert 2 (an area situated 1-cm above and 2-cm below the anatomic GEJ). Differences in lymphatic spread and survival rates described by some authors justify different approaches. A trial in Japan [18] did not show significant advantages for left thoracotomy in patients with esophagus involvement of <3 cm, but higher morbidity. The authors suggested an abdominal approach for such patients. Different options may be debated on this type of cancer, but there are few doubts that in Siewert types 1 and 2 necessitate preoperative radiotherapy.

2.16 Liver Metastases

Liver metastases have been considered so far the limit for curative resection. In recent years, many authors have reported good results with reasonable 5-year survival for subsets of patients. Though indicated initially only for radical resection patients (T1, T2) and for methacronous metastasis, single or multiple resections are now also proposed for synchronous lesions if radical surgery associated with D2 dissection can be carried out [20]. Some prognostic scores have been proposed. Nevertheless, a clear indication for liver resection is lacking. Single or multiple resections (carrying out more than one resection influences survival) on the same lobe without extra diffusion in the liver after D2 dissection have been reported as resection criteria. Several authors have reported that 0.2–37.9% of all cases with liver metastasis are eligible for hepatic resection, and 1-year survival rates of 15–77%, and 0–42% at 5 years, have been documented [21,22]. Early detection of liver metastases is crucial and a close follow-up can be useful. Discussions by the multidisciplinary team considering surgery alongside other options could give hope to patients with a poor prognosis.

2.17 Follow-up

No studies have conclusively reported prognostic improvement based on follow-up. If relapse of liver metastases or the gastric stump can be treated, and new drugs can be developed (such as S1 in eastern countries), studies, based on data from follow-up could be of great interest. Recently, a new approach to follow-up in GC has been proposed by researchers on GC based in Italy: Gruppo Italiano di Ricerca sul Cancro Gastrico (GIRCG). Follow-up could be differentiated on the basis of a prognostic score, with a more intense program for patients treated radically and who are at a high risk of relapsing disease [19].

2.18 Frontiers in Molecular Medicine

Families with a highly penetrating inherited predisposition for the development of GC are rare. However, several kindred from various ethnic backgrounds showing diffuse, poorly differentiated GC harboring a germline E-cadherin (a transmembrane calcium ion-dependent adhesion molecule) alteration have been documented [23, 24]. GC developments can be associated with hereditary nonpolyposis colon cancer [25]. Genetic abnormalities of mismatch repair genes underlying this disease have been disclosed, and include potential tumor development in various tissue types [26]. Such gastric carcinomas are of the intestinal type, without infection by *Helicobacter pylori* and most exhibit microsatellite instability. GC has been reported in the kindred of Li–Fraumeni syndrome with an underlying *p53* germline alteration. Overall, GC is rare in these settings, and the exact contribution of the polyposis and underlying germline alterations of the APC gene and LKB1/STK11 to the development of gastric adenocarcinoma is not clear.

Of course, in the study of the molecular biology of GC we cannot have an overview about host and environmental factors. For instance, *H. pylori* infection appears to lead to a five-to-sixfold increase in the risk of gastric malignancies [27]. GC does not always develop in most of those infected with this microorganism. The importance of the interaction between the bacterial virulence, environmental, and host factors involved in the clinical outcome of this infection are important issues. Allelic variants of polymorphisms in pro-inflammatory cytokines such as interleukin-1β (a potent inhibitor of acid secretion) have been associated with GC, having been shown to be important determinants in the infection–host response. Microsatellite instability and associated alterations of transforming growth factor have been found in subsets of GCs [28]. Even if most GCs show significant aneuploidy, microsatellite instability has been found in 13–44%) of sporadic GCs. The degree of genome-wide instability varies with the high degree of microsatellite instability. Somatic alterations have been described at the molecular level in GCs. In most instances, the significance of these changes in gastric tumorigenesis remains unclear. In most GCs, the *p53* gene is altered. The effort to detect excessive expression of *p53* is an indirect means to identify mutations of this gene. The prognostic value in GC appears to be consistent. Many sporadic diffuse GCs display altered levels of E-cadherin (which is important in interactions with epithelial cells); when decreased in expression, it is associated with tumor invasiveness. Evidence of a tumour suppressor gene on chromosome 3p has been noted in several studies, including those focusing on allelic loss at 3p in primary GCs and homozygous deletion of 3p in GC cell lines. Alteration of other gene products (including those involved in regulation of the cell cycle, signalling of growth factors, telomerase activity, angiogenesis, and the structure of the extracellular matrix) has been described in basic science research. Study of the inhibition of apoptosis, the co-operativity of oncogenes and tumor suppressor genes as well as the epigenetics of cancer are the new frontiers in the molecular biology of cancer. In this sense, the use of genomic technologies has helped cancer researchers to make significant progress in the identification of the "molecular signatures" of cancer, mainly to understand the variable performances of therapy. From this viewpoint, DNA microarrays have been used to ascertain the molecular phenotypes of GCs. Integration of clinical genomics with clinical proteomic technologies [29] could enable the development of "personalized" methods for the diagnosis of treatment of cancer.

References

1. Jensen LS, Nielsen H, Mortensen PB et al (2010) Enforcing centralization for gastric cancer in Denmark. Eur J Surg Oncol Sep 36 Suppl 1:S50-54
2. Japanese gastric cancer treatment guidelines 2010 (ver. 3) (2011) Japanese Gastric Cancer Association. Gastric Cancer 14:113-123
3. Roviello F, Marrelli D, Morgagni P et al (2002) Italian Research Group for Gastric Cancer. Survival benefit of extended D2 lymphadenectomy in gastric cancer with involvement of second level lymph nodes: a longitudinal multicenter study. Ann Surg Oncol 9:894–900
4. Verlato G, Roviello F, Marchet A et al (2009) Indexes of surgical quality in gastric cancer surgery: experience of an Italian network. Ann Surg Oncol 16:594-602
5. Hartgrink HH, van de Velde CJ, Putter H et al (2004) Extended lymph node dissection for gastric cancer: who may benefit? Final results of the randomized Dutch gastric cancer group trial. J Clin Oncol 22:2069-2077
6. Sasako M, Sano T, Yamamoto S et al (2008) Japan Clinical Oncology Group (JCOG). D2 lymphadenectomy alone or with para-aortic nodal dissection for gastric cancer. N Engl J Med 359:453–462
7. 7) Roviello F, Pedrazzani C, Marrelli D et al (2010) Super-extended (D3) lymphadenectomy in advanced gastric cancer. Eur J Surg Oncol 36:439-446
8. de Manzoni G, Di Leo A, Roviello , et al (2011) Tumor site and perigastric nodal status are the most important predictors of para-aortic nodal involvement in advanced gastric cancer. Ann Surg Oncol 18:2273-2280
9. Han TS, Kong SH, Lee HJ et al (2011) Dissemination of Free Cancer Cells from the Gastric Lumen and from Perigastric Lymphovascular Pedicles during Radical Gastric Cancer Surgery. Ann Surg Oncol 18:2818–2825
10. Japanese Research Society for Gastric Cancer (1995) Japanese Classification of Gastric Carcinoma. Kaneara & Co Ltd, Tokyo
11. Sobin LH, Gospodarowicz MK, Wittekind C (2010) TNM classification of malignant tumours, 7th edition. Wiley
12. Biondi A, Persiani R, Cananzi F et al (2010) R0 resection in the treatment of gastric cancer: room for improvement.World J Gastroenterol 16:3358-3370
13. Kodera Y, Fujiwara M, Ohashi N et al (2010) Laparoscopic Surgery for Gastric Cancer: A Collective Review with Meta-Analysis of Randomized Trials. J Am Coll Surg 211:677-686
14. Sano T, Yamamoto S, Sasako M (2002) Randomized controlled trial to evaluate splenectomy in total gastrectomy for proximal gastric carcinoma: Japan Clinical Oncology Group study JCOG 0110-MF. Jpn J Clin Oncol 32:363–364
15. Fujita J, Kurokawa Y, Sugimoto T et al (2012) Survival benefit of bursectomy in patients with resectable gastric cancer: interim analysis results of a randomized controlled trial. Gastric Cancer 15:42-48
16. Morgagni P, Garcea D, Marrelli D et al (2008) Resection Line Involvement After Gastric Cancer Surgery: Clinical Outcome in Nonsurgically Retreated Patients. World J Surg 32:2661-2667
17. Mura G, Federici O, Garofalo A (2011) Hyperthermic Intraperitoneal Chemotherapy in Gastric Cancer: Indications and Technical Notes. In: de Manzoni G, Roviello F, Siquini W (eds) Surgery in the Multimodal Management of Gastric Cancer. Springer-Verlag, Milan
18. Sasako M, Sano T, Yamamoto S et al, for the Japan Clinical Oncology Group (JCOG9502) (2006) Left thoracoabdominal approach versus abdominal-transhiatal approach for gastric cancer of the cardia or subcardia: a randomised controlled trial. Lancet Oncol 7:644-651
19. Marrelli D, Caruso S, Roviello F (2011) Prognostic Factors and Score Systems in Gastric Cancer. In: de Manzoni G, Roviello F, Siquini W (eds) Surgery in the Multimodal Management of Gastric Cancer. Springer-Verlag, Milan
20. Liu J, Li JH, Zhai RJ, Wei B et al (2012) Predictive factors improving survival after gastric and hepatic surgical treatment in gastric cancer patients with synchronous liver metastases. Chin Med J (Engl) 125:165-171

21. Ueda K, Iwahashi M, Nakamori M et al (2009) Analysis of the prognostic factors and evaluation of surgical treatment for synchronous liver metastases from gastric cancer. Langenbecks Arch Surg 394:647-653
22. Tiberio GA, Coniglio A, Marchet A et al (2009) Metachronous hepatic metastases from gastric carcinoma: a multicentric survey. Eur J Surg Oncol 35:486-491
23. La Vecchia C, Negri E, Franceschi S (1992) Family history and the risk of stomach and colorectal cancer. Cancer 70:50-55
24. Corso G, Pedrazzani C, Pinheiro H et al (2011) E-cadherin genetic screening and clinico-pathologic characteristics of early onset gastric cancer. Eur J Cancer 47:631-639
25. Lynch HT, Smyrk TC, Watson P (1993) Genetics, natural history, tumour spectrum, and pathology of hereditary nonpolyposis colorectal cancer: an update review. Gastroenterology 104:1535-1549
26. Kinzler KW, Volgestein B (1996) Lessons from hereditary colorectal cancer. Cell 87:159-170
27. Parsonnet J, Friedman GD, Vandersteen DP (1991) Helicobacter Pylori infection and the risk of gastric carcinoma. N Engl J Med 325:1127
28. Yamamoto H, Sawai H, Perucho M (1997) Frameshift somatic mutations in gastrointestinal cancer of the microsatellite mutator phenotype. Cancer Res 57:4420-4426
29. Carr KM, Rosenblatt K, Petricoin EF et al (2003) Genomic and proteomic approaches to study human cancer: prospects for true patient tailored therapy. Ann Rev Genomics Hum Genet 1:134-140
30. Macdonald JS, Smalley SR, Benedetti J et al (2001) Chemoradiotherapy after surgery compared with surgery alone for adenocarcinoma of the stomach or gastroesophageal junction. N Engl J Med 345:725-730

Colon Cancer

3

Francesco Corcione, Pierluigi Angelini and Lucia Miranda

3.1 Epidemiology, Risk and Protective Factors

With ≈1 million of new cases per year separated into 72% for the colon and 28% for the rectum, colorectal cancer (CRC) is the fourth most common cancer in men (after cancer of the lung, prostate and stomach) and the third most common in women (after cancer of the breast and cervix) without significant differences in incidence by sex (male:female ratio of 1.2:1). The areas with the highest incidence rates are Australia and New Zealand, North America, Japan and western Europe [1]. In 2002, it resulted in ≈8% of the 6,724,000 registered deaths for cancer. It is estimated that 83% of cases occur in patients aged >60 years and the average age at diagnosis is 70 years. Unfortunately, the incidence of CRC is escalating in patients younger than 50 years, with an increased rate of 56% for patients aged 40–44 years over the past two decades [2]. Five-year survival is stage-dependent, being 90% in localized disease, 68% for regional disease, and 10% if distant metastases are present. Familial adenomatous polyposis (FAP), hereditary non-polyposis colorectal cancer (HNPCC), personal or in the first- and second-degree relative history of high-risk polyp or colonic cancer and a personal history of inflammatory bowel disease (IBD) are the most important innate risk factors. Race is also important: 20% more African–Americans develop colon cancer than Caucasians. However, geographic factors can modify racial risk: Native Alaskan Americans have an incidence rate of 102.6/100,000 if living in Alaska and 21.0/100,000 if residing in the southwest of the USA. Smoking and diet are the most important variables and acquired risk factors. Diets high in red or

F. Corcione (✉) · P. Angelini · L. Miranda
Department of General Laparoscopic and Robotic Surgery
Ospedale dei Colli-Monaldi-Cotugno-CTO, Naples, Italy
e-mail: francesco.corcione@ospedalideicolli.it

A. Valeri et al. (eds.), *What's New in Surgical Oncology*,
DOI: 10.1007/978-88-470-5310-6_3, © Springer-Verlag Italia 2013

processed meats can increase the risk of developing CRC, especially in smokers (relative risk [RR], 1.5) [3]. A body mass index (BMI) >25 and physical inactivity augment the risk of colon cancer. Smoking and heavy use of alcohol worsen the prognosis of CRC.

Interesting evidence about the protective role of certain drugs is emerging. Taking aspirin or other non-steroidal anti-inflammatory drugs (NSAIDs) such as sulindac and celecoxib is associated with a lower risk of CRC and has been shown to reduce the formation of adenomatous polyps in people with FAP. It also seems that statins and angiotensin-converting enzyme (ACE) inhibitors help lower the risk of polyps and CRC and of relapse. Aspirin can cause stomach ulcers and other side effects, but the association is strong enough that the Aspirin in Dukes C and High-risk Dukes B Colorectal Cancer (ASCOLT) trial was created to study the use of this drug as an adjuvant medication [4].

3.2 New Developments in Genetic-based Treatments

Recent discoveries of inherited genes that increase a person's risk of developing CRC are being used in genetic tests to inform people most at risk. Anti-epidermal growth factor receptor (EGFR) monoclonal antibodies (cetuximab and panitumumab) have been available for some years and have good efficacy for the treatment of metastatic colorectal cancer (mCRC) and in chemotherapy-refractory cases. EGFR regulates cancer-cell proliferation, apoptosis and tumor-induced neo-angiogenesis. Unfortunately, efficacy is limited to a subset of patients: EGFR-independent, constitutive activation of the RAS or RAF kinase pathways impairs the response to anti-EGFR drugs. KRAS links growth-promoting signals from the cell surface to the nucleus. It is a member of the RAS protein group of guanosine triphosphate/ guanosine diphosphate (GTP/GDP) binding proteins, and the wild-type gene works transiently only if growth factor receptors (such as the EGFR) are activated. However, when specific mutations in the KRAS gene occur (usually in codons 12 or 13), the resulting KRAS protein can be constitutively active (it can then function independently of upstream growth factor receptor-driven signals and remain active), thereby verifying the block of anti-EGFR monoclonal antibodies. A different and (not equally clearly defined) mechanism allows a mutation in the gene for B-RAF kinase to permit replication of tumoral cells independently from the EGFR. This is why everyone with advanced colon cancer who is considering an EGFR-targeted therapy such as Erbitux® or Vectibix® should have testing for KRAS and BRAF before treatment starts to spare them (mutation is present in ≈40% of cases) from receiving unnecessary treatments. Data from important and well-powered multicenter studies demonstrated that the KRAS and BRAF mutation was significantly associated with more rapid and aggressive metastatic behavior in CRC, short-interval liver metastases, poor survival after resection of the colon and liver, and a worse prognosis [5]. In a Korean study on patients with metastatic or recurrent CRC, lung metastasis was more frequently the initial metastatic site in patients with KRAS mutations [6]. By better understanding the interactions between KRAS and other genes, we may then take advantage of these synthetic lethal combinations to provide additional options to treat chemotherapy- or cetuximab-refractory CRC patients harboring KRAS mutations. Knowledge of these synthetic lethal interactions may also enable the development of improved targeted therapies that may be more effective without the toxicities of traditional chemotherapy due to off-target killing of normal cells. Continued prospective studies and basic science research is critical in the effort to improve outcomes in CRC patients with this mutation.

3.3 Earlier Detection and Diagnosis

The "adenoma–carcinoma" multistep model of CRC is one of the best known models of carcinogenesis. The aim of a screening program is to detect a polyp before its transformation or a cancer at its earlier stage [7]. The common pattern of tests in program of screening for colon cancer are stool and endoscopic (colonoscopy or sigmoidoscopy) or radiologic (virtual colonscopy and air contrast barium enema) tests. The age to begin screening differs between people with an average risk (start screening at 50 years) or with a family history (start screening at 40 years or 10 years before the age when a relative was diagnosed of with colon cancer). The recent evidence of a younger onset associated with more advanced stage, more aggressive histopathological characteristics, and a worse prognosis when compared with older patients as well as a relative rightward shift over the past three decades of the colonic distribution of cancer are encouraging a preference for colonoscopy over sigmoidoscopy and an ever more early age of screening. Screening colonoscopy also involves risks [8]; perforation and bleeding in the case of polypectomy are estimated to be near 0.1% and 1%, respectively. Chromoendoscopy (which involves the application of stains or pigments) and magnification endoscopy (with or without staining) allows the endoscopist to better visualize mucosal details with up to 100-fold image enhancement. Narrow-band imaging colonoscopy allows better visualization of vascular changes in superficial lesions. The value of these techniques in screening for colon cancer has yet to be established. The effectiveness of colonoscopy is dependent upon the skill and experience of the endoscopist to not only reach the cecum but also to identify small lesions. Despite criticism about the cost and potential morbidity, colonoscopy remains the "gold standard" to evaluate the colonic mucosa. A recent long-term prospective study validated colonoscopic polypectomy, with a 53% reduction in mortality [9]. New imaging and laboratory tests are also being developed. Newer, more accurate ways to look for changes in stools that might indicate CRC have been developed. These include tests that are better able to detect blood in stools and tests that can be used to detect changes in the DNA of cells in the stool ("fecal immunochemical tests").

3.3.1 Double-contrast Barium Enema (DCBE)

Retrospective studies have found that DCBE may miss 15% to 22% of CRCs [10]. Even if abnormalities are found, this test must be followed by colonoscopy for biopsy or excision. The use of DCBE for screening has been declining with the increasing use of endoscopic procedures and computed tomography (CT) colonography (also known as virtual colonoscopy (VC)), but retains its value in areas where colonoscopy resources are limited. It has no role in the surveillance of colon cancer but may be used to evaluate the colon by radiographic means if a stoma reversal is being consiered.

3.3.2 VC

VC is a special type of CT that provides endoluminal visualization of the colon based on two- and three-dimensional imaging that enables the detection of many colorectal polyps and cancers early. To enhance accuracy, patients frequently undergo bowel preparation before the procedure, but recent studies found that it could be helpful in screening even without the patient having to drink large amounts of liquid laxative first. The colon is then insufflated with air or carbon dioxide (or, in some cases, water) to facilitate colonic distention and detection of intraluminal lesions. In addition to its non-invasive nature, VC is associated with enabling the diagnosis of extra-colonic disease and establishing the presence of synchronous lesions in the setting of an obstructive distal cancer that does not permit colonoscopy. Synchronous lesions are thought to occur in 1% to 7% of patients, and a 100% sensitivity rate for the detection of proximal synchronous cancers in the setting stenosing cancers has been observed. Sensitivities and specificities increase according to increasing polyp size (≈80% for polyps of diameter >9 mm and ≈100% for lesions of diameter >15 mm) [11,12].

3.3.3 CT

In newly diagnosed colon cancer, preoperative abdominal and pelvic CT demonstrated variable sensitivity for detecting distant metastasis (75% to 87%), nodal involvement (45% to 73%) or the depth of transmural invasion (≈50%) as well as tumor-related complications such as obstruction, perforation, and fistula formation [13]. CT is not a reliable diagnostic test for low-volume tumors on peritoneal surfaces. The sensitivity for detecting peritoneal implants is <40% neither for large lesions (diameter, 5 mm to 50 mm). The most important feature of preoperative CT is the planning of eventual simultaneous or staged liver metastasectomy or eventual neoadjuvant therapy for high-volume and diffuse, metastatic, non-stenosing and non-bleeding colon cancer. Intraoperative ultrasonography and manual palpation of the liver may provide a better yield than preoperative CT [14], but the latter is precluded in laparoscopic colon resections, and both methods can be hindered by supramesocolic adhesions from previous surgery. A preoperative CT of the chest might be of more value for rectal cancer than for colon cancer depending on the different types of venous drainage.

3.3.4 Magnetic Resonance Imaging (MRI) and Positron Emission Tomography (PET)

Contrast-enhanced MRI and PET or PET/CT have no role in screening or in the routine staging of colon cancer. However, they may have a role in patients thought to be candidates for resection of isolated liver metastases of colon cancer (especially in patients who have not previously undergone therapy), which changes surgical plans in a consistent percentage of patients [15].

Recently, increasing attention has been placed on the application of PET to assist with early detection of disease recurrence, in differentiating it from postoperative scarring, or in the evaluation of patients with unexplained increasing levels of carcinoembryonic antigen (CEA) after initial surgery. In this setting, PET can potentially be used to localize occult disease, permitting the selection of patients who may benefit from exploratory surgery. PET is frequently used in conjunction with CT and demonstrates high sensitivities and specificities (>90%) in association with contrast-enhanced or non-contrast CT [16].

3.4 Preoperative Preparation

Recent demonstration of low septic and anastomotic complications in emergency colectomy without mechanical bowel preparation (MBP) [17], together with the results of prospective studies demonstrating safety in elective surgery of the colon and rectum with avoidance of mechanical bowel cleaning, are changing conceptions about the central role of MBP with or without oral antibiotics in preventing postoperative complications [18,19]. In elderly patients, MBP can produce intravascular depletion and electrolyte abnormalities, thereby increasing surgical risks [20]. A meta-analysis involving seven randomized clinical trials [21], revealed a higher rate of anastomotic dehiscence among patients in the MBP group compared with patients in the non-MBP group (5.6% *vs* 2.8%, respectively, $p = 0.03$) with similar septic peritoneal or wound infections. A review of 26 trials [22] on various intravenous and oral preoperative antibiotic regimens demonstrated that antibiotic prophylaxis decreased the overall infection rate from 36% to 22% and mortality rates from 11.2% to 4.5%, suggesting that antibiotic prophylaxis for colorectal procedures is merited. Some studies based on replacing routine MBP with a single preoperative enema [23] noted significant increases in postoperative morbidity (26 *vs* 9, $p = 0.004$) and wound infection (7 *vs* 1, $p = 0.041$). A well-powered study to assess the relative benefits of no preparation *vs* mechanical preparation alone or in conjunction with antibiotics is required.

3.4.1 Goal-directed Fluid Management

Several recent studies [24, 25] have suggested that a restricted goal-directed fluid regimen that avoids excess fluid administration causing adverse cardiovascular and pulmonary effects and even leading to impairments in wound healing may improve postoperative outcomes in colectomy. A too-restricted fluid regimen can lead to tissue hypoperfusion, anastomotic leaks, and sepsis. Dehydration from preoperative MBP and prolonged perioperative nil-by-mouth regimens can create difficulty in optimizing fluid management that is equally [26] challenging in the operating room. This is because the various medications and anesthetic agents administered can affect urine output and the cardiac parameters commonly used in the assessment of volume status. Given this challenge, several surrogate markers have been used to help guide fluid administration in the perioperative period, including serum lactate levels and mixed venous oxygen saturation. The recent introduction of intraoperative esophageal Doppler to monitor cardiac output by directly measuring flow in the descending aorta seems to be a very good guide for balanced fluid administration [27], mitigating the risk of gut hypoperfusion that can occur. Consequently, application of this method should be considered for patients undergoing colectomy.

3.4.2 Enhanced Recovery After Surgery (ERAS)

Colectomy is a common and major procedure which, unfortunately, is associated with significant morbidity and costs to healthcare systems. Over the past 20 years, there have been two important developments in elective major abdominal surgery—the introduction of laparoscopic surgery and implementation of ERAS programs (also referred to as "fast track" (FT) perioperative care)—with the aims of reducing the length of hospital stay, morbidity and mortality, length of time to return to full function, and to improve patient satisfaction [28,29]. During the mid-1990s, FT perioperative care was pioneered by Henrik Kehlet. FT programs consist of a multidisciplinary approach (dieticians, nurses, surgeons, anesthesiologists) and aim at reducing surgical-stress responses, organ dysfunction, and morbidity, thereby promoting faster recovery after surgery.

FT perioperative care comprises extensive preoperative counselling, no bowel preparation, no sedative premedication, carbohydrate-loaded liquids up to 2 h before surgery, and effective multimodal pain management with short-acting anaesthetics (blocking the neurohormonal response to surgery). The goal is to reduce the risk of organ dysfunction and complications, enable adequate perioperative goal-directed fluid management, use small incisions, and to not use drains and nasogastric tubes. Intraoperative care involves the prevention of hypothermia (because it reduces sympathetic responses), undesirable cardiac events, and wound morbidity [30]. Postoperative care involves early oral feeding, enforced mobilization, early removal of urinary catheters, and standard use of laxatives. NSAID agents and epidural anesthesia/analgesia are used to reduce the perioperative inflammatory responses, leading to a reduction in mediator release and catabolism. Optimal analgesia can permit early ambulation, and diet introduction is probably the most important (and least appreciated) component of an ERAS program [31]. The Laparoscopy and/or FT Multimodal Management Versus Standard Care (LAFA) trial [32] has provided interesting data regarding which of these components is essential to improved outcomes: the focus is on laparoscopy, analgesia, early ambulation, and early resumption of diet. A recent multicentric Dutch trial confronting the four combinations of laparoscopy, open surgery, standard and FT perioperative care showed that the combination of laparoscopic surgery with FT care resulted in a significantly faster recovery after colonic surgery than all other combinations [33]. The challenge of building and enabling the organizational structure around the necessary multidisciplinary group for a successful ERAS program is well documented, but encouraging results are pointing towards such implementation. The multidisciplinary approach of any ERAS program should address the oft-quoted question raised by Henrik Kehlet: "why is the patient in hospital today?"

3.4.3 Stadiation

The American Joint Committee on Cancer (AJCC) has published the seventh edition of its staging manual [34]. Tables 3.1 and 3.2 report the new tumor/node/metastasis (TNM) classification for CRC report, which should be compared with the previous classifications of Dukes and Astler–Coller.

3.4.3.1 Staging Information

The features of the revised staging give more importance to the poor prognostic features of the depth of invasion despite fewer positive nodes.

- T4 is divided between penetration to the surface of the visceral peritoneum and direct gross adherence to adjacent structures;
- T1–2N2 is downstaged from stage IIIC to IIIA or IIIB depending on the number of nodes involved
- Shift T4bN1 from IIIB to IIIC;
- Subdivide T4/N1/N2;
- Resolution of staging for issue of mesenteric deposits where nodal tissue is not identified;
- Revised sub-staging of stage II based on depth of invasion, with addition of stage IIC;

Table 3.1 TNM classification for colon cancer

Primary tumor (T)
TX Primary tumor cannot be assessed
T0 No evidence of primary tumor
T*is* Carcinoma *in situ*: intra-epithelial or invasion of lamina propria
T1 Tumor invades submucosa
T2 Tumor invades muscularis propria
T3 Tumor invades through the muscularis propria into pericolorectal tissues
T4a Tumor penetrates to the surface of the visceral peritoneum
T4b Tumor directly invades or is adherent to other organs or structures
Regional lymph nodes (N)
NX Regional lymph nodes cannot be assessed
N0 No regional lymph node metastasis
N1 Metastasis in 1–3 regional lymph nodes
N1a Metastasis in 1 regional lymph node
N1b Metastasis in 2–3 regional lymph nodes
N1c Tumor deposit(s) in the subserosa, mesentery, or non-peritonealized pericolic or perirectal tissues without regional nodal metastasis
N2 Metastasis in ≥4 lymph nodes
N2a Metastasis in 4–6 regional lymph nodes
N2b Metastasis in ≥7 regional lymph nodes
Distant metastasis (M)
M0 No distant metastasis
M1 Distant metastasis
M1a Metastasis confined to 1 organ or site (e.g., liver, lung, ovary, non-regional node)
M1b Metastases in >1 organ/site or the peritoneum

- Revised sub-staging of stage III based on node number (N1a, 1 node; N1b, 2–3 nodes; N2a, 4–6 nodes; N2b, ≥7 or more nodes);
- Division of metastases to ≥1 sites in recognition of the possibility of a curative approach for aggressive treatment of a single site of metastases.

The seventh edition considers, together with the classic anatomic bases of T, N and M, some other important anatomic and serological prognostic factors validated by clinical studies and which are evidence-based and which assume prognostic value that influences patient care. Among the important anatomical factors are lymphatic vessel invasion (Lx: cannot be assessed; L0: absent; L1: present), venous invasion (V0: absent; V1: microscopic; V2: macroscopic), perineural invasion (PN: 1 present or 0 absent) and the residual tumor (Rx:

Table 3.2 Anatomic stage/prognostic groups

Stage	T	N	M	Dukes	MAC
0	T*is*	N0	M0	--	--
I	T1	N0	M0	A	A
	T2	N0	M0	A	B1
IIA	T3	N0	M0	B	B2
IIB	T4a	N0	M0	B	B2
IIC	T4b	N0	M0	B	B3
IIIA	T1–T2	N1/N1c	M0	C	C1
	T1	N2a	M0	C	C1
IIIB	T3–T4a	N1/N1c	M0	C	C2
	T2–T3	N2a	M0	C	C1/C2
	T1–T2	N2b	M0	C	C1
IIIC	T4a	N2a	M0	C	C2
	T3–T4a	N2b	M0	C	C2
	T4b	N1-N2	M0	C	C3
IVA	Any T	Any N	M1a	--	--
IVB	Any T	Any N	M1b	--	--

T tumor, *N* node, *M* metastasis, *MAC* modified Astler-Coller.

cannot be assessed; R0: no residual; R1: microscopic residual; R2: macroscopic residual). The two principal serological prognostic factors are CEA (Cx: not assessed; C0: <5 ng/mL – normal; C1: >5 ng/ml – elevated) and microsatellite instability (MSI). MSI is a marker of the functionality of the DNA repair enzyme system operating during cellular replication. MSI (higher (H) or lower (L) level) is especially significant in HNPCC and in ≈20% of sporadic cancers.

3.4.4 Sentinel Lymph Node (SLN) Biopsy

Since the 1980s, many studies have been conducted focusing on intraoperative identification of SLNs and/or complete mapping of lymph nodes using different technologies (e.g., vital coloration, intraoperative ultrasound and/or radioimmunoguided nodal mapping) [35,36]. The first aim was to eventually modify the extension of the resection that could be more limited in small lesions (frequently diagnosed in screening programs and eventually removed endoscopically) with negative SLNs, or more extended over the boundaries of classic lymphadenectomy in cases of aberrant lymphatic drainage. Furthermore, microscopic evaluation of node status in colon cancer is based on hematoxylin and eosin (H&E) staining, and has a non-negligible percentage of false-negative values (especially if we consider micrometastases), and cell clusters of diameter <0.2 mm are also associated with relevant recurrence of disease and lower 5-year survival rates. Correct identification of this false stage-II population can be achieved by a more sensible (but more expensive) immunohistochemical (IHC) test. The individualization of a SLN could help to reach this aim.

3.5 Treatment According to Stage of Colon Cancer

3.5.1 Stages

Stage 0: These cancers are in the inner lining of the colon; polypectomy or local excision through a colonoscope is often all that is needed. Colectomy may occasionally be needed if a tumor is too big to be removed by local excision.

Stage I: Several layers of the colon are penetrated from the cancer without spread outside the colon wall (or into nearby lymph nodes). Partial colectomy (i.e., surgery to remove the section of colon that has cancer and nearby lymph nodes) is the standard treatment without the need for additional therapy.

Stage II: Many of these cancers have grown through the wall of the colon and may extend into nearby tissue. They have not yet spread to the lymph nodes. Colectomy is usually the only treatment needed. However, adjuvant chemotherapy may be recommended if the cancer has a higher risk of returning because of certain factors: it looks very abnormal (is high grade) or has a dangerous histotype; shows MSI; has grown into nearby organs; the surgeon did not remove all the cancer and ≥12 lymph nodes; the cancer obstructs the colon or causes a perforation in the colon wall. Many research teams have studied the way to identify stage II because the risk of recurrence is greater. Petersen et al. [37] proposed a sub-classification of the prognostic index (PI) based on four elements subsequently considered by many other authors. Three of them have a score of 1: peritoneal involvement with or without ulceration; extramural or submucosal venous spread; or a involved or inflamed margin. The last element, perforation through the tumor, has a score of 2. Patients in stage II with a PI of ≥2 are to be considered at high risk and could be candidates for adjuvant therapy (see below). Even the pathological aspects of tumor necrosis as well as host systemic and local inflammatory responses are taken into account. Different criteria have been used to measure these variables, such as the Glasgow Prognostic Score [38] for systemic inflammatory responses, the Klintrup–Makinen criteria [39] for local inflammatory infiltrates and for the assessment of tumor necrosis. Richards et al. [40] confirmed by statistical means that tumor necrosis is a marker of a poor prognosis, independent of pathological stage, and that it is associated directly with an increase in the systemic inflammatory response and a decrease in local inflammatory cell infiltrates. This finding suggests that the impact of tumor necrosis on survival from CRC may be explained by close relationships with host inflammatory responses. Patients in stage II with extensive tumor necrosis are to be considered at high risk and could be candidates for adjuvant therapy.

Stage III: There is a spread to nearby lymph nodes, but cancer has not yet spread to other parts of the body. Partial colectomy followed by adjuvant chemotherapy is the standard treatment for this stage.

Stage IV: Distant organs and tissues such as the liver, lungs, peritoneum or ovaries can be affectted by colon cancer. If only a few small metastases are present in the liver or lungs and can be completely removed along with the colon cancer, surgery may prolong life and sometimes may even cure. Chemotherapy is typically given before and/or after surgery. Other options to destroy tumors in the liver include hepatic artery infusion, cryosurgery, radiofrequency ablation, or other non-surgical methods. If the cancer is too widespread to try to cure with surgery, colectomy or diverting colostomy may be needed in cases of bleeding or occlusion. Sometimes, such surgery can be avoided by inserting a stent into the colon during colonoscopy to keep the lumen patent. Most patients with stage-IV cancer will receive chemotherapy and/or targeted therapies to control the cancer.

3.5.2 Recurrent Colon Cancer

Recurrent cancer means that the cancer has returned after treatment. If the cancer comes back locally, surgery (often with previous and/or after chemotherapy) can stop recurrence, prolong life, and eventually cure the patient. If the cancer comes back at a distant site (liver, lung, others), surgery may be an option in some cases. If needed, chemotherapy can be tried first to shrink the tumor(s), and may be followed by surgery. If the cancer is too widespread for a surgical approach, chemotherapy and/or targeted therapies may be used depending on which (if any) drugs were received before the cancer returned and how long ago the patient received them, as well as general health status. Radiotherapy may be an option to relieve symptoms in some cases.

3.6 Adjuvant Therapy

In previous years, the standard of care for stage-III and -IV disease (and even some high-risk stage-II disease) was treatment with 5-fluorouracil (5FU) and leucovorin (LV) for six cycles with surgery or these agents alone in cases without a surgical indication. From 2004, with the results of the Multicenter International Study of Oxaliplatin/5-fluorouracil (FU)/leucovorin (LV) in the

Adjuvant Treatment of Colon Cancer (MOSAIC) trial [41], oxaliplatin became part of the chemotherapy regimen. Also, irinotecan was demonstrated to improve the effectiveness of 5FU and LV. Hence, the principal protocol of adjuvant therapy was FOLFOX (5FU, LV, and oxaliplatin) or FOLFIRI (5FU, LV, and irinotecan). In addition to this regimen, especially in stage-IV disease or stage III refractory to chemotherapy, targeted therapies (see above) [42] have become the first-line therapy in recent years. They demonstrate a good decrease in median progression-free survival and better quality of life in the absence of mutations of KRAS or BRAF.

3.7 Surgical Treatment

3.7.1 Laparoscopic Colectomy (LC)

Laparoscopic surgery for CRC has undergone slow (but tremendous overall) advancement since 1991, when first laparoscopic colonic resection for cancer was described. LC can today be considered the gold standard surgical treatment for colon cancer when indicated appropriately. Randomized clinical trials have shown that this method is safe and effective for malignant disease with oncologic outcomes equivalent to open surgery [43–45]. LC results in a shorter hospital stay as well as less morbidity and postoperative pain than open colorectal surgery.

Nevertheless significant socioeconomic disparities in the use of minimally invasive surgery (MIS) for colorectal disease remain. A recent revision of 211,862 colorectal resections carried out at high-volume hospitals in 2008 in the USA [46] demonstrated that only 16,637 (7.3%) colorectal resections were done using MIS. It was found that racial and socioeconomic factors influenced appreciably the access to MIS for CRC treatment. Laparoscopic surgery for colon cancer is the cornerstone of enhanced recovery programs thanks to its lower level of injury to potentially complex, immune-challenged hosts. The underlying philosophy of FT programs is to capitalize upon small differences to effectuate more important global benefits in overall patient recovery in the hope that the short-term advantages of enhanced-recovery colonic surgery may have important cumulative long-term benefits. Clearly, further investigation is warranted. Under the impact of an ever advancing technology, enhancing the ergonomics and extending the boundaries of MIS, the next few years are expected to be very promising for laparoscopic surgery of colon cancer with prospective randomized studies reaching full maturity and having the possibility to extend the follow-up to a more significant period of 10 years. The integration of enhanced-recovery regimens with laparoscopic methods should also provide greater uniformity of clinical outcomes throughout the world. Furthermore, the previously arduous learning curve will predominantly be addressed in the postgraduate training period. The comparisons of experiences will probably lead, in this decade, to an evermore important technical standardization of colectomies.

3.7.2 Single-incision Laparoscopic Colectomy (SILC)

Single-incision laparoscopic surgery (SILS) represents the latest development in laparoscopic surgery and has been promoted to improve the cosmetic effect and incisional and/or parietal pain as well as to reduce port site-related complications. The initial increases in surgical costs associated with purchasing new equipment do not seem to be mitigated by a significant reduction in morbidity and duration of hospital stay [47]. SILS has several disadvantages compared with multiport laparoscopic surgery with regard to surgical instruments and methods. One of the biggest challenges associated with SILS is the optimal positioning of instruments. Therefore, SILS requires an experienced surgeon to overcome the difficulties of triangulation, pneumoperitoneum leaks, and instrument crowding. In fact, many cases require conversion to open or multiport laparoscopic procedures to get better retraction or aid in colonic mobilization. Some investigators recommend utilizing articulating instruments or variable-length tools, including a bariatric-length bowel grasper or an extra-long laparoscope to minimize external clashing. Most of the experiences in SILC have been in the setting of right hemicolectomy [48] (Fig. 3.1). This is because this procedure was proposed as an intracorporeal ileocolic anastomosis using an Endo stapler and closure of the orifice left from the stapler by the endostitch that requires limited wrist movements to avoid interference with the endoscope. It was also to avoid mesenteric traction occurring with extracorporeal sutures, which often involve enlarging the incision of the multiport device [49]. Further advantages can be gained from the use of particular access ports to allow the introduction of several trocars multiple times, for example using Gelport™ , in which trocars can be kept apart for as long as possible to maintain instrument triangulation and to prevent clashing outside the abdomen. It has recently been suggested [50] that the implementation of robotic technology to SILC could help overcome some of the difficulties associated with conventional SILS.

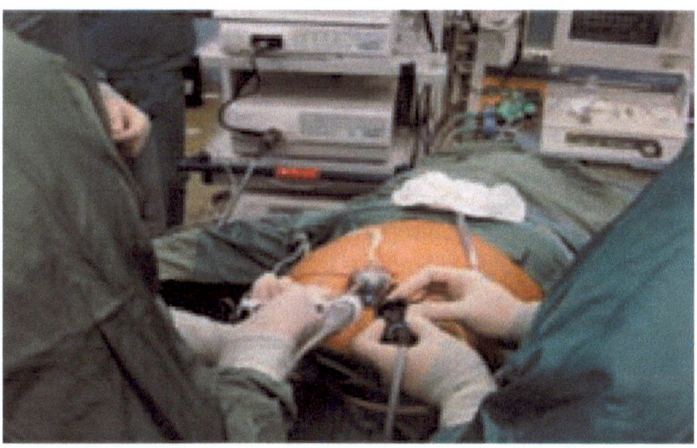

Fig. 3.1 Position of monotrocar in SILS right colectomy

3.7.3 Natural Orifice Transluminal Endoscopic Surgery (NOTES)

In specialist centers around the world efforts are being made to assess various possibilities to transform the new concept of NOTES from the experimental setting into clinical practice. The common focus of these concepts is to minimize trauma to the abdominal wall while gaining access to the peritoneal cavity and/or extracting the surgical specimen through a natural orifice such as the mouth, anus or vagina as well as reducing the incisional complications of pain, infections and hernia. Endoscopic technology is not available to carry out NOTES exclusively for complex procedures such as a colon resection, so a hybrid solution has emerged.

In this setting, there has been renewed interest in a classically described method of natural orifice specimen extraction (NOSE), which was originally proposed by Franklin. This hybrid method uses a natural orifice for instruments and tasks that need a larger diameter of access (>5 mm) to the abdominal cavity. NOSE also allows for laparoscopic assistance *via* small-size trocars to reduce the trauma of access and morbidity. An interesting combination of laparo-endoscopic single-site (LESS) and NOSE was also developed and experimented in sigmoidectomy to push the technical limits of MIS of the colon [52]. A recent review of transvaginal specimen extraction in colorectal surgery [53] reported on 130 patients of which 67 had colonic cancer. Two significant complications, pelvic seroma and rectovaginal fistula, were likely to have been related to transvaginal extraction. The duration of follow-up was specified in only one study. Harvested nodes and negative margins were adequate and reported in 70% of oncological cases. There is relative skepticism about the possibility of propagation of these procedures considering the high costs in terms of instrumentation and prolonged operating time due to the technical difficulties of these procedures.

3.7.4 Robotic Colon Surgery

Theoretically, the demerits of laparoscopic methods such as unstable camera platforms, limited degrees of freedom, two-dimensional imaging, and ergonomic constraints could be overcome by robotic surgery. Its implementation has gained acceptance in rectal surgery, appearing able to ensure a more refined total mesorectal excision accurate with nerve sparing. However, it remains unclear if robot-assisted colectomy (RAC) has significant clinical advantages over laparoscopically assisted colectomy (LAC) in treating colonic cancer. The use of robotic technology for colon resections has been reported in several small series in the past years. In 2004, D'Annibale and colleagues [54] reported on 53 patients undergoing robotic colorectal surgery in which 22 patients underwent surgery for malignant disease. In this series, no significant difference in total operating time was noted between laparoscopic and robotic groups (although a longer time was required to prepare the operating room in the robotic group). Specimen length, number of lymph nodes harvested, intraoperative blood loss, and duration of hospital stay were comparable between the groups. In 2011, Luca and colleagues [55] published the results of a case-matched series in which the outcomes of patients undergoing right hemicolectomy for cancer were compared with patients undergoing open resections. Although the operating time was longer in the robotic cohort, patients in this group demonstrated reduced intraoperative blood loss and a shorter duration of hospital stay than patients in the open surgery cohort. Consistent with the report by D'Annibale and colleagues, patients in both groups had similar specimen lengths and number of lymph nodes harvested.

Despite these promising reports, several challenges must be addressed before robotic technology can be adopted for colon surgery. Robotic surgery is associated with substantive costs, which may prohibit the widespread implementation of this method. Limited robotic instrumentation for intra-abdominal surgery is available, highlighting the importance of continued development of devices. The required machinery is bulky, resulting in difficulties with maneuvering and the need for substantial space in the operating room. As with all new technologies, specialized training and proficiency is required before implementation. With increased experience and familiarity with the procedure, the longer operating times associated with robotic colon resections have been shown to decrease. The feasibility and safety of RAC have been confirmed but prolonged operating time and elevated costs without actual significant benefit to justify the greater cost were reported recently from Shin et al. [56]. Continued advances are undoubtedly expected, although the ultimate utility of this method for routine colon resections remains to be seen.

3.8 Conclusions

Colon cancer remains a major therapeutic challenge. In many ways, the encouraging results achieved from the improvement and dissemination of screening, the good outcomes of MIS and ERAS programs, as well as the deepening of genetic knowledge with the introduction of targeted therapies, has allowed significant progress in the battle against colon cancer. There is no consensus on the role of robotic SILS and NOTES colectomy in the treatment of this serious disease. Technological progress and the results of the first multicenter studies in progress may clarify the true costs and benefits of these treatments.

References

1. Cancer Facts Figures 2011 Available at: http://www.cancer.org/Cancer/ColonandRectumCancer/index.
2. Davis DM, Marcet JE, Frattini JC, Prather AD, Mateka JJ, Nfonsam VN.(2011) Is it time to lower the recommended screening age for colorectal cancer? J Am Coll Surg.: 213(3):352-61.
3. Chao A, Thun MJ, Connell CJ, McCullough ML, Jacobs EJ, Flanders et al. (2005) Meat consumption and risk of colorectal cancer. JAMA.: 12;293(2):172-82.
4. Ali R, Toh HC, Chia WK; ASCOLT Trial Investigators (2011). The utility of Aspirin in Dukes C and High Risk Dukes B Colorectal cancer--the ASCOLT study: study protocol for a randomized controlled trial. Trials. 14;12:261.

5. Andreyev H.J., Norman A.R., Cunningham D., Oates J.R., Clarke P.A.(1998) Kirsten ras mutations in patients with colorectal cancer: The multicenter "RASCAL" study. J. Natl. Cancer Inst.: 90:675–684.
6. Kim M.J., Lee H.S., Kim J.H., Kim Y.J., Kwon J.H., Lee J.O., Bang S.M., Park K.U., Kim D.W., Kang S.B., et al. (2012) Different metastatic pattern according to the KRAS mutational status and site-specific discordance of KRAS status in patients with colorectal cancer. BMC Cancer.: 12:347.
7. Klabunde CN, Lanier D, Breslau ES, Zapka JG, Fletcher RH, Ransohoff DF, Winawer SJ. (2007) Improving colorectal cancer screening in primary care practice: innovative strategies and future directions. J Gen Intern Med.:22(8):1195-205. Review.
8. Gatto NM, Frucht H, Sundararajan V, Jacobson JS, Grann VR, Neugut AI.v (2003) Risk of perforation after colonoscopy and sigmoidoscopy: a population-based study. J Natl Cancer Inst.: 5;95(3):230-6.
9. Zauber AG, Winawer SJ, O'Brien MJ, Lansdorp-Vogelaar I, van Ballegooijen M, Hankey BF et al. (2012) Colonoscopic polypectomy and long-term prevention of colorectal-cancer deaths.N Engl J Med.: 23;366(8):687-96. doi: 10.1056/NEJMoa1100370.
10. Toma J, Paszat LF, Gunraj N, Rabeneck L. (2008) Rates of new or missed colorectal cancer after barium enema and their risk factors: a population-based study. Am J Gastroenterol.: 103(12):3142-8. doi: 10.1111/j.1572-0241.2008.02199.x.
11. Chaparro M, Gisbert JP, Del Campo L, Cantero J, Maté J. (2009) Accuracy of computed tomographic colonography for the detection of polyps and colorectal tumors: a systematic review and meta-analysis. Digestion.:80(1):1-17. doi: 10.1159/000215387. Review.
12. Park SH, Lee JH, Lee SS, Kim JC, Yu CS, Kim HC, Ye BD, Kim MJ, Kim AY, Ha HK. (2012) CT colonography for detection and characterisation of synchronous proximal colonic lesions in patients with stenosing colorectal cancer. Gut.:61(12):1716-22. doi: 10.1136/gutjnl-2011-301135.
13. McAndrew MR, Saba AK. (1999) Efficacy of routine preoperative computed tomography scans in colon cancer. Am Surg.:65(3):205-8.
14. Milsom JW, Jerby BL, Kessler H, Hale JC, Herts BR, O'Malley CM. (2000) Prospective, blinded comparison of laparoscopic ultrasonography vs. contrast-enhanced computerized tomography for liver assessment in patients undergoing colorectal carcinoma surgery.Dis Colon Rectum.:43(1):44-9.
15. Niekel MC, Bipat S, Stoker J. (2010) Diagnostic imaging of colorectal liver metastases with CT, MR imaging, FDG PET, and/or FDG PET/CT: a meta-analysis of prospective studies including patients who have not previously undergone treatment.Radiology.:257(3):674-84. doi: 0.1148/radiol.10100729.
16. Kitajima K, Murakami K, Yamasaki E, Domeki Y, Tsubaki M, Sunagawa M, et al. (2009) Performance of integrated FDG PET/contrast-enhanced CT in the diagnosis of recurrent colorectal cancer: Comparison with integrated FDG PET/non-contrast-enhanced CT and enhanced CT.Eur J Nucl Med Mol Imaging.:36(9):1388-96. doi: 10.1007/s00259-009-1081-5.
17. De U, Ghosh S. (2003) Single stage primary anastomosis without colonic lavage for left-sided colonic obstruction due to acute sigmoid volvulus: a prospective study of one hundred and ninety-seven cases. ANZ J Surg.:73(6):390-2.
18. Bucher P, Gervaz P, Soravia C, Mermillod B, Erne M, Morel P. (2005) Randomized clinical trial of mechanical bowel preparation versus no preparation before elective left-sided colorectal surgery. Br J Surg.:92(4):409-14.
19. Zmora O, Mahajna A, Bar-Zakai B, Hershko D, Shabtai M, Krausz MM, Ayalon A. (2006) Is mechanical bowel preparation mandatory for left-sided colonic anastomosis? Results of a prospective randomized trial. Tech Coloproctol.:10(2):131-5
20. Oliveira L, Wexner SD, Daniel N, DeMarta D, Weiss EG, Nogueras JJ, et al. (1997) Mechanical bowel preparation for elective colorectal surgery. A prospective, randomized, surgeon-blinded trial comparing sodium phosphate and polyethylene glycol-based oral lavage solutions.Dis.Colon Rectum.:40(5):585-91.
21. Bucher P, Mermillod B, Gervaz P, Morel P. (2004) Mechanical bowel preparation for elective colorectal surgery: a meta-analysis. Arch Surg.:139(12):1359-64; discussion 1365.

22. Baum ML, Anish DS, Chalmers TC, Sacks HS, Smith H Jr, Fagerstrom RM. (1981) A survey of clinical trials of antibiotic prophylaxis in colon surgery: evidence against further use of no-treatment controls. N Engl J Med. 1;305(14):795-9.
23. Veenhof AA, Sietses C, Giannakopoulos GF, van der Peet DL, Cuesta MA. (2007) Preoperative polyethylene glycol versus a single enema in elective bowel surgery. Dig Surg.:24(1):54-7; discussion 57-8.
24. Senagore AJ, Emery T, Luchtefeld M, Kim D, Dujovny N, Hoedema R. (2009) Fluid management for laparoscopic colectomy: a prospective, randomized assessment of goal-directed administration of balanced salt solution or hetastarch coupled with an enhanced recovery program. Dis Colon Rectum.: 52(12):1935-40. doi: 10.1007/DCR.0b013e3181b4c35e.
25. Rahbari NN, Zimmermann JB, Schmidt T, Koch M, Weigand MA, Weitz J. (2009) Meta-analysis of standard, restrictive and supplemental fluid administration in colorectal surgery. Br J Surg.: 96(4):331-41. doi: 10.1002/bjs.6552. Review.
26. Chappell D, Jacob M, Hofmann-Kiefer K, Conzen P, Rehm M. (2008) A rational approach to perioperative fluid management.Anesthesiology.:109(4):723-40. doi: 10.1097/ALN.0b013e3181863117. Review.
27. Abbas SM, Hill AG. (2008) Systematic review of the literature for the use of oesophageal Doppler monitor for fluid replacement in major abdominal surgery. Anaesthesia.: 63(1):44-51. Review.
28. Kehlet H, Harling H. (2012) Length of stay after laparoscopic colonic surgery - an 11-year nationwide Danish survey. Colorectal Dis.:14(9):1118-20. doi: 10.1111/j.1463-1318.2011.02922.x.
29. Abraham N, Albayati S. (2011) Enhanced recovery after surgery programs hasten recovery after colorectal resections.World J Gastrointest Surg.: 27;3(1):1-6. doi: 10.4240/wjgs.v3.i1.1.
30. Wong PF, Kumar S, Bohra A, Whetter D, Leaper DJ. (2007) Randomized clinical trial of perioperative systemic warming in major elective abdominal surgery. Br J Surg.:94(4):421-6.
31. White PF, Kehlet H, Neal JM, Schricker T, Carr DB, Carli F; Fast-Track Surgery Study Group. (2007) The role of the anesthesiologist in fast-track surgery: from multimodal analgesia to perioperative medical care. Anesth Analg.: 104(6):1380-96, table of contents. Review.
32. Wind J, Hofland J, Preckel B, Hollmann MW, Bossuyt PM, Gouma DJ, et al. (2006) Perioperative strategy in colonic surgery; LAparoscopy and/or FAst track multimodal management versus standard care (LAFA trial). BMC Surg.: 29;6:16.
33. Vlug MS, Wind J, Hollmann MW, Ubbink DT, Cense HA, Engel AF, et al.; LAFA study group. (2011) Laparoscopy in combination with fast track multimodal management is the best perioperative strategy in patients undergoing colonic surgery: a randomized clinical trial (LAFA-study). Ann Surg.: 254(6):868-75.
34. Edge SB, Compton CC.2010 The American Joint Committee on Cancer: the 7th edition of the AJCC cancer staging manual and the future of TNM.Ann Surg Oncol.:17(6):1471-4. doi: 10.1245/s10434-010-0985-4.
35. Tiernan JP, Ansari I, Hirst NA, Millner PA, Hughes TA, Jayne DG. (2012) Intra-operative tumour detection and staging in colorectal cancer surgery. Colorectal Dis.:14(9):e510-20. doi: 10.1111/j.1463-1318.2012.03078.x.
36. Bianchi P, Andreoni B, Rottoli M, Celotti S, Chiappa A, Montorsi M. (2007) Technique of sentinel lymph node biopsy and lymphatic mapping during laparoscopic colon resection for cancer. Ecancermedicalscience.:1:60. Epub 2007 Nov 15.
37. Petersen VC, Baxter KJ, Love SB, Shepherd NA. (2002) Identification of objective pathological prognostic determinants and models of prognosis in Dukes' B colon cancer. Gut.: 51(1):65-9.
38. Powell AG, Wallace R, McKee RF, Anderson JH, Going JJ, Edwards J, Horgan PG. (2012) The relationship between tumour site, clinicopathological characteristics and cancer-specific survival in patients undergoing surgery for colorectal cancer. Colorectal Dis.:14(12):1493-9. doi: 10.1111/j.1463-1318.2012.03048.x.
39. Klintrup K, Mäkinen JM, Kauppila S, Väre PO, Melkko J, Tuominen H, et al. (2005) Inflammation and prognosis in colorectal cancer. Eur J Cancer.:41(17):2645-54. Epub 2005 Oct 18.

40. Richards CH, Roxburgh CS, Anderson JH, McKee RF, Foulis AK, Horgan PG, McMillan DC. (2012) Prognostic value of tumour necrosis and host inflammatory responses in colorectal cancer. Br J Surg.:99(2):287-94. doi: 10.1002/bjs.7755. Epub 2011 Nov 16.
41. André T, Boni C, Mounedji-Boudiaf L, Navarro M, Tabernero J, Hickish T,et al; Multicenter International Study of Oxaliplatin/5-Fluorouracil/Leucovorin in the Adjuvant Treatment of Colon Cancer (MOSAIC) Investigators. (2004) Oxaliplatin, fluorouracil, and leucovorin as adjuvant treatment for colon cancer. N Engl J Med.: 3;350(23):2343-51.
42. Tol J, Koopman M, Cats A, Rodenburg CJ, Creemers GJ, Schrama JG, et al. (2009) Chemotherapy, bevacizumab, and cetuximab in metastatic colorectal cancer. N Engl J Med.: 5;360(6):563-72. doi: 10.1056/NEJMoa0808268.
43. Guillou PJ, Quirke P, Thorpe H, et al. MRC CLASICC trial group (2005) Short-term endpoints of conventional versus laparoscopic-assisted surgery in patients with colorectal cancer (MRC CLASICC trial): multicentre, randomised controlled trial. Lancet.: 14–20;365(9472):1718–26.
44. Veldkamp R, Kuhry E, Hop WC, et al. COlon cancer Laparoscopic or Open Resection study group (COLOR) (2005) Laparoscopic surgery versus open surgery for colon cancer: short-term outcomes of a randomised trial. Lancet Oncol:6(7):477–84.
45. Bilimoria KY, Bentrem DJ, Merkow RP, et al. (2008) Laparoscopic-assisted vs open colectomy for cancer: comparison of short-term outcomes from 121 hospitals. J Gastrointest Surg.:12(11):2001–9.
46. Robinson CN, Balentine CJ, Sansgiry S, Berger DH. (2012) Disparities in the use of minimally invasive surgery for colorectal disease. J Gastrointest Surg.:16(5):897-903; discussion 903-4. doi: 10.1007/s11605-012-1844-3.
47. Egi H, Hattori M, Hinoi T, Takakura Y, Kawaguchi Y, Shimomura M,et al. (2012) Single-port laparoscopic colectomy versus conventional laparoscopic colectomy for colon cancer: a comparison of surgical results.World J Surg Oncol.: 24;10:61.
48. Waters JA, Rapp BM, Guzman MJ, Jester AL, Selzer DJ, Robb BW,et al. (2012) Single-port laparoscopic right hemicolectomy: the first 100 resections. Dis Colon Rectum.: 55(2):134-9.
49. Morales-Conde S, Barranco A, Socas M, Méndez C, Alarcón I, Cañete J, Padillo FJ. (2012) Improving the advantages of single port in right hemicolectomy: analysis of the results of pure transumbilical approach with intracorporeal anastomosis. Minim Invasive Surg. 2012:874172. Epub 2012 Apr 10.
50. Corcione F. (2011) Minimally invasive surgery: mini or mono? This is the problem!Cir Esp.: 89(8):485-6. doi: 10.1016/j.ciresp.2011.03.001. Epub 2011 Apr 19.
51. Mohiuddin SS, Gonzalez JJ, Glass J, Portillo G, Franklin ME Jr. (2009) Laparoscopic-assisted endoluminal hybrid surgery: a stepping stone to NOTES. Surg Laparosc Endosc Percutan Tech.: 19(6):474-8. doi: 10.1097/SLE.0b013e3181bd9087.
52. Leroy J, Diana M, Wall J, Costantino F, D'Agostino J, Marescaux J. (2011) Laparo-endoscopic single-site (LESS) with transanal natural orifice specimen extraction (NOSE) sigmoidectomy: a new step before pure colorectal natural orifices transluminal endoscopic surgery (NOTES®). J Gastrointest Surg.: 15(8):1488-92. doi: 10.1007/s11605-011-1557-z. Epub 2011 May 17.
53. Diana M, Perretta S, Wall J, Costantino FA, Leroy J, Demartines N, Marescaux J. (2011) Transvaginal specimen extraction in colorectal surgery: current state of the art. Colorectal Dis.: 13(6):e104-11. doi: 10.1111/j.1463-1318.2011.02599.x.
54. D'Annibale A, Morpurgo E, Fiscon V, Trevisan P, Sovernigo G, Orsini C, Guidolin D. (2004) Robotic and laparoscopic surgery for treatment of colorectal diseases. Dis Colon Rectum.: 47(12):2162-8.
55. Luca F, Ghezzi TL, Valvo M, Cenciarelli S, Pozzi S, Radice D, Crosta C, Biffi R. (2011) Surgical and pathological outcomes after right hemicolectomy: case-matched study comparing robotic and open surgery.Int J Med Robot.: 11. doi: 10.1002/rcs.398.
56. Shin JY. (2012) Comparison of Short-term Surgical Outcomes between a Robotic Colectomy and a Laparoscopic Colectomy during Early Experience. J Korean Soc Coloproctol.: 28(1):19-26. doi: 10.3393/jksc.2012.28.1.19.

Carcinomas of the Rectum and Anus

4

Paolo De Paolis, Alberto Bona, Andrea Borasi,
Giuseppe Spinoglio, Ferruccio Ravazzoni, Boris Franzato
and Carlo Augusto Sartori

4.1 Introduction

In recent years, improvements in preoperative staging, surgical methods and histological assessment have helped to ameliorate the long-term outcome of patients undergoing surgery for carcinoma of the rectum and anus. In this chapter, we analyze some features concerning prognostic factors and minimally invasive applications in rectal cancer and anal carcinoma.

4.2 Carcinoma of the Rectum

4.2.1 What are the Oncologic Outcomes for the Different Surgical Options?

The propagation of total mesorectal excision (TME) has significantly improved locoregional control in rectal cancer. Local recurrence rates of ≈10% after quality TME without neoadjuvant treatment have been described in randomized trials [1]. TME is recommended as the standard of care for rec-

P. De Paolis (✉) · A. Bona · A. Borasi
Surgery, Presidio Sanitario Gradenigo, Turin, Italy
e-mail: paolo.depaolis@gradenigo.it

G. Spinoglio · Ferruccio Ravazzoni
Oncologic Surgery, Presidio Ospedaliero SS Antonio e Biagio, Alessandria, Italy

B. Franzato
General Surgery, Presidio Ospedaliero di Castefranco Veneto, Italy

C.A. Sartori
U.O. Chirurgia Generale
General Surgery, Ospedale Sacro Cuore Don Calabria, Negrar (Verona), Italy

A. Valeri et al. (eds.), *What's New in Surgical Oncology*,
DOI: 10.1007/978-88-470-5310-6_4, © Springer-Verlag Italia 2013

tal cancers localized in the middle and lower third of the rectum. Partial mesorectal excision is adequate for rectal cancer localized in the upper third of the rectum (>10–15 cm from anal verge) because it is associated with reduced morbidity [2].

The oncologic value of TME is not in doubt, but there is concern about its significant postoperative complications and long-term side effects. The 'anterior resection syndrome', including functional disorders such as incontinence, urgency, and incomplete rectal evacuation, is considered to be a consequence of TME and low rectal anastomoses.

A recent multicentric trial [3] reported morbidity and mortality rates of about 30% and 5%, respectively. For instance, poor bowel function was noted in 30–60% and genito-urinary disorders were seen in 30% of subjects.

Population-based registries have shown that improvements in oncologic outcome after TME occur mainly in younger patients. Furthermore, 6-month postoperative mortality is significantly increased in elderly patients (≥75 years of age) compared with younger patients (<75 years of age). For elderly patients with diminished physiological reserves and comorbidity, alternative treatments to TME that keep surgical trauma to a minimum and optimize radiotherapy (RT) might be more suitable [2].

However, TME does not seem to be effective in reducing local recurrence rates for low rectal cancers undergoing abdomino-perineal resection (APR). A review pooling >3,600 patients [4] found a 5-year local recurrence rate of 19.7% after APR compared with 11% for anterior resection (AR). Patients managed with APR had an 11% reduction of cancer-specific survival compared with those managed with AR. This is probably not due to the tumor biology but to an increased risk of positive circumferential resection margins (CRMs) and of iatrogenic perforations during APR.

Most of the studies in the last 30 years have confirmed that a positive CRM increases the likelihood of local recurrence by approximately fourfold, and that an inadvertent perforation of the bowel indicates a threefold risk of recurrence [5].

According to den Dulk et al., [4] the rate of CRM involved is 10,6% for APR compared with 5% for AR. The occurrence of a rectal-wall perforation (in the proximity or within the tumor itself) is 13.7% for APR compared with 2.5% for AR. If effective radical surgery is done (without positive CRM or perforation), APR patients share the same prognosis as AR patients [6].

Local excision (LE) of rectal cancer is associated with excellent surgical results and no risk of functional problems, but unfortunately lymph-node staging is not possible. This strategy can be discussed as an alternative to "standard" TME only in case of very early T1 tumors with favorable pathologic features (low grade, absence of blood or lymphatic vessels, superficial invasion of submucosae). In a study by Peng et al., [7], this "low risk" subgroup had a 5-year pelvic recurrence rate after local resection of 1.2% (not so different compared with the 0.4% relapses observed after TME surgery [1] for the same group of tumors) whereas "high risk" lesions with adverse pathological aspects had a local failure rate of 21% (similar to T2 cancers).

Transanal endoscopic microsurgery (TEM) is a technically reliable option to carry out LE. This method allows removal of the full thickness of the rectal wall with a high quality of surgical excision (R0 resection) as well as in cases of mid and upper lesions. According to a study from Moore et al., [8] the R1 resection rate was lower with TEM than with conventional transanal surgery (6% *vs* 31%) whereas morbidity and mortality rates did not differ.

After LE, the specimen must be analyzed carefully to evaluate its integrity, the depth of invasion in the bowel wall, absence of margin infiltration (laterally and deeply), and unfavourable histopathological criteria. In such cases, further radical surgery is required and is usually carried out within 1 month after LE of the tumor [9]. This "delayed" rectal resection does not compromise oncologic outcome compared with primary radical surgery [9] but is associated with a higher rate of surgical-related complications (48% according to a recent study) [10].

Otherwise 'salvage' surgery (resection only if relapse is clinically evident) is associated with very poor outcomes. Three-year cancer-related survival of 50% in patients undergoing salvage APR for local failure after LE of a T1 rectal tumor have been described [11].

Key Concepts

- Good-quality TME for resection for cancer of the middle and low rectum is associated with a local failure rate of ≈10% and is considered to be the "gold standard" for the treatment of these lesions;
- Also with TME, conventional APR is an independent predictor of higher local recurrence and worse cancer-specific survival as compared with AR, with a difference of 10% at 5-years follow-up;
- LE (preferably with a TEM procedure) is an alternative to TME resection in case of T1 tumors with favorable pathological features. If adverse criteria are present on local rectal specimen, further radical surgery is required.

4.2.2 What are the Current Indications for Multimodal Approach to Locally Advanced (T3–4 and/or N+) Rectal Cancer?

The benefit of TME on local control can be increased with preoperative short course RT. This was shown by a large multicentric randomized trial from the Dutch Colorectal Cancer Group [1]. This study found better rates for local failure for stage-II and stage-III disease after preoperative RT followed by TME rather than after surgery alone. In the recently published 12-year follow-up update, the 10-year cumulative local recurrence rate was 5% for integrated treatment compared with 11% for surgery alone [6].

However, preoperative RT does not compensate for positive CRM such as postoperative treatment. In a trial conducted by Sebag-Montefiore et al., [12] patients with CRM involvement on the surgical specimen were managed with postoperative RT, but the 3-year local recurrence was 20,7%.

The optimal sequence of surgery and RT was addressed by the CAO/ARO/AIO-04 trial [13]. This study showed less toxicity and local failure (but no survival benefits) with preoperative therapy compared with postoperative therapy.

Based on these data, nowadays most patients receive preoperative RT followed by TME for locally advanced presentations (e.g., T3–4 and/or N+).

Two neoadjuvant regimens are currently used: "short course" RT and "long course" concomitant chemoradiotherapy (CRT). Phase-III trials have failed to suggest the preferred approach. In a Polish trial [14] comparing preoperative CRT and RT, no difference in survival and local control was found at a median follow-up of 4 years, but the CRT arm had a significantly lower rate of CRM involvement after surgery than the RT arm (4% *vs* 13%) as a consequence of more tumor regression.

Phased array magnetic resonance imaging (MRI) is highly accurate method for the prediction of CRM positivity [15]. MRI can help to define if a lesion is as close as 1 mm or directly involves the mesorectal fascia. In these cases, it has been suggested that a preoperative CRT regimen can manage threatened or involved CRMs better than RT.

Local control is clearly improved by radiotherapy, but there are no definitive data about the efficacy of RT on overall survival. Five meta-analyses have reported conflicting results [2]. The analysis by Camma et al. and the Collaborative Colorectal Cancer Group reported a survival advantage with RT, whereas studies by Munro and Bentley and Fiorica and Cartei did not. The Swedish Council of Technology Assessment in Health Care undertook a systematic review of RT trials and reported that survival is improved by ≈10% using preoperative RT. Probably the reduction in local failure rates in most intermediate cancers after TME standardization is too small to translate into an overall survival benefit irrespective of which RT modality is used.

However, radiotherapy is not free from long-term sequelae. According to a trial from the Dutch Cancer Group [16], the combined RT and surgery arm reported increased rates of long-term fecal incontinence after TME resections compared with surgery alone, (62% *vs* 38%, respectively) and, at 12-year follow-up, there were more deaths for further (not rectal-related) malignancy within the irradiated patients group [6].

Hence, management of rectal cancers demands a tailored approach taking into account an accurate balance of the risk and benefits of RT and surgery.

According to guidelines set by the European Society of Medical Oncology (ESMO), [17] RT or CRT followed by TME is the standard treatment for locally advanced cancers of the middle and low rectum, with the exception of middle rectum T3a/b N0 lesions. This specific subset of tumors without invasion of the mesorectal fascia may be managed in two ways: with short-course RT (minor toxicity compared with CRT [14]) or with surgery alone (because the benefits in local control with radiation may not be worth the risks of the side effects).

Lesions in the upper third of the rectum (>10 cm from the anal verge) are usually managed like colosigmoid cancer without radio(chemo)therapy. Only patients with bulky tumors involving adjacent structures or peritoneal reflection show disease-free benefit with preoperative CRT [12].

Key Concepts

- Preoperative RT is effective in improving local control for locally advanced middle and low rectum tumors and can be discussed for T4 high-rectum lesions;
- Reports suggest that a favorable subgroup of T3N0 middle rectum tumors with low rates of local failure can be managed with surgery alone;
- The preferred neoadjuvant regimen (RT or CRT) remains undetermined. Long-course CRT enhances tumor downstaging. Toxicity-associated rates are probably lower with short-course RT;
- Positive CRM on the surgical specimen is a strong predictor of local recurrence and cannot be compensated by preoperative or postoperative RT. However, the rate of CRM involvement can be reduced by tumor regression after neoadjuvant treatment;
- Use of MRI parameters can help to tailor neoadjuvant regimens.

4.2.3 Pathological Complete Response (pCR) after Neoadjuvant Treatment: a New Prognostic Factor?

Several studies underline the ability of CRT to downstage the tumor and the associated lymph nodes, with complete disappearance of all neoplastic cells in ≤20% of cases [18]. This occurrence is called a pCR and is defined on the surgical specimen using strict histological criteria [2].

Although level-I evidence is lacking, the concept that pCR is a new prognostic factor associated with very good oncologic outcome is supported by data from two recent meta-analyses [18, 19]. The authors analyzed primarily retrospective studies and found that, after TME resection, complete responders showed local recurrence rates (0.7%), 5-year overall survival (90.2%) and disease-free survival (83.3–87.0%) that were comparable with those after R0 proctectomy for stage-I rectal cancer. Notably, the effect of pCR on long-term outcome was independent according to initial clinical T and N category.

Many important questions regarding post-RT downstaging and pCR have not been answered.

The first problem concerns the rate of distant disease despite the apparent disappearance of the primary tumor. Although local recurrence appears to be almost completely eradicated, distant failure is not: ≈9% of pCR tumors developed metastatic disease at 5 years [18, 19]. This finding may be an indication that adjuvant chemotherapy is warranted in these patients. According to Maas et al., [19] ≈39% of complete responders underwent adjuvant chemotherapy after surgery. However, a recent European Consensus Conference failed to reach agreement about the benefit of postoperative chemotherapy after CRT [2].

A second problem is regards predicting the pCR before the onset of RT. Potential predictors of response under investigation are pretreatment tumor volume and certain biological factors (e.g., p53, epidermal growth factor receptor (EGFR), Ki-67, P21, and Bax/bcl-2).

Other foci of research are strategies to maximize pCR rates. Several recent randomized trials have assessed the use of bevacizumab, oxaliplatin and capecitabine as radiosensitizing agents alone or in association with 5-fluorouracil (5FU). The use of these new chemotherapics does not seem to increase the pCR rate. Only the German study CAO/ARO/AIO-04 [13] found a modest augmentation (4.5%) of the pCR with oxaliplatin. Conversely, toxicity rates were higher compared with conventional regimens.

Another simple option for increasing pCR rates is to lengthen the interval between CRT completion and surgery. The Lyon R90-01 trial is the only prospective trial in which patients with locally advanced rectal cancer were assigned randomly to have surgery at two time intervals after CRT. This study found that a 6–8-week interval resulted in a higher response rate compared with a 2-week interval [20].

In two studies, [21, 22] an 8-week interval between CRT and rectal resection was significantly associated with a pCR rate of 32–35% *vs* 16–17% compared with a shorter interval. According to Kalady et al., [22] other benefits were not observed with a resting period >12 weeks.

Key Concepts

- pCR practically eradicates the risk of local recurrence after TME resections (0.7% after 55.5 months);
- However, if local control appears to be almost complete, distant disease is not (8.7% of patients after 5-year follow-up). The indications for adjuvant therapy in this setting are a matter of research;
- Although there are only initial reports, a long resting interval after CRT seems to increase pCR rates;
- Using a combination of new CRT agents increase toxicity without allowing a higher pCR rate.

4.2.4 Can a Tailored Approach be Possible after Major CRT Response?

Keeping in mind the possible complications and side effects of TME, there is a strong suspicion that TME could be an overtreatment of major tumor regression. Some surgeons argue that more conservative strategies are preferable.

4.2.5 Rectum-conserving Strategies

4.2.5.1 Role of LE after CRT

According to a recent review, [23] there are 16 reports on transanal excision of downsized tumors after CRT (especially using TEM). Interpretation of data from these series is difficult due to the different selection criteria and because many studies involved patients who are elderly or unsuitable for surgery, and who are effectively being treated palliatively.

Only two studies involved a large proportion of patients with node-positive tumors, and had contrasting results. Callender et al. [24] found that the local recurrence rate was about fourfold higher for pre-CRT node-positive tumors than for node-negative tumors (23% *vs* 6%). Nair et al. [25] did not find that nodal positivity before irradiation was associated with increased rates of local recurrence.

Nodal positivity is an accepted adverse prognostic factor after CRT, so most studies have assessed the value of TEM after CRT only in patients who were node-negative before treatment on the assumption that they would remain so after CRT.

In a prospective trial [26] on T2 node-negative tumors, 70 patients were randomized to undergo CRT followed by laparoscopic TME resection or transanal excision. At 5 years, there was no difference in disease-free or overall survival between the two groups.

According to the European Society of Medical Oncology/European Society for Radiotherapy and Oncology/European Cancer Organisation (ESMO/ESTRO/ECCO) consensus conference, [2] LE associated with preoperative CRT is an appropriate procedure for T2 tumors only if major surgery is contraindicated or refused.

4.2.5.2 Role of an Observational Strategy

A series of retrospective studies by Habr-Gama and co-workers suggested that simple observation of patients achieving a clinical complete response (cCR) could yield survival rates similar to those of patients who undergo radical surgery with confirmation of a pCR [27].

However, most studies addressing a non-surgical approach are mainly from a research team in Brazil and their results are unique. They have not been replicated in any other center with the exception of a small series (21 patients) from Maas et al. [28] using very strict selection criteria (after CRT, only 11% of patients were considered to be complete responders).

The major challenge with the "wait and see" approach is the clinical definition of response before surgery. No imaging techniques allow an accurate differentiation between residual tumor cells and radiation-induced fibrosis. Some authors recommend execution of a full-thickness biopsy or a TEM to confirm clinical and imaging data. Habr-Gama et al. claim that TEM after CRT results in significant morbidity, wound dehiscence and a readmission rate of 30% [29]. The ongoing Transanal Endoscopic Microsurgery (TEM) After

Radiochemotherapy for Rectal Cancer (CARTS) trial [30] will analyze these aspects.

Staging tools lack sufficient accuracy also for the assessment of lymph nodes. As a consequence, despite an apparent complete luminal and mural tumor response, 2–5% of patients may still have positive nodes [23]. In a recent series from Habr-Gama et al., [31] 1/5 conservatively managed patients had disease recurrence within the first year after an apparent cCR. Notably all these recurrences were endoluminal and amenable to surgical salvage without significant differences in overall or disease-free survival from patients who underwent radical surgery in the first instance. However, other authors suggested that ≤25% of relapses could not be salvaged by surgery because of pelvic recurrence [32]. These conflicting results can be partially explained by different selection of patients and different follow-up programs.

Firstly, Habr-Gama et al. claimed that an observational approach is best for very low, early-stage rectal cancers that are likely to be initially node-negative whereas medium-stage and late-stage large rectal cancers (i.e., pre-CRT T3 or T4) may be best treated with an anterior resection. In their series, only 22% of tumors were node-positive and the average tumor size was only 3,7 cm. In other studies, tumors did not appear to be selected on the basis of site or size. In the only European study for which outcomes are similar to those from the Brazilian group, [28] T3 and T4 lesions were considered eligible, but >1 out of 4 tumors were T1 or T2 cancers.

Secondly, Habr-Gama et al. stated that an exceptionally rigorous follow-up program (monthly clinical assessments, proctoscopy, serial measurement of carcinoembryonic antigen (CEA) and CT) is needed. The lack of international consensus on the type or frequency of follow-up meant that other authors did not appear to have such a meticulous follow-up, so recurrence may have been detected late.

Key Concepts

- Organ preservation represents one of the ongoing topics of surgical research on rectal cancers: there must be clear differentiation between LE of downstaged tumors and simple surveillance after a major response;
- Outcomes of LE are clearly documented for initial N0 tumors whereas studies on N+ tumors are rare because of the concern about the persistence of metastases in locoregional lymph nodes after downstaging;
- In a small (70 patients) prospective trial on T2 N0 tumors which responded to preoperative treatment, LE showed a similar 5-year disease-free and overall survival after LE as conventional TME;
- The "wait-and-watch" philosophy has been adopted in patients where an APR has been the alternative by one research team with impressive results, similar to those seen after RT for anal carcinoma. This treatment policy is an investigational approach and the standard of care remains surgery.

4.2.6 Does Tumor Downsizing Induced by Neoadjuvant Radiotherapy Increase the Likelihood of a Sphincter-saving Procedure?

The extent of resection is usually planned before the onset of RT without reconsidering the surgical strategy after its completion regardless of tumor response. RT can change this philosophy because same surgeons from specialist centers claim that the indication for AR can be reconsidered after tumor downsizing for patients initially earmarked for APR [33]. The *rationale* of this approach is that there is no clear demonstration that a more distal resection margin is required after preoperative treatment. The usual rule of 1–2 cm of a lower margin established for patients managed with primary surgery is probably also valid after RT [34]. Hence, if the distance between the lower pole of the tumor to the anal verge is increased after neoadjuvant RT, a definitive stoma can be avoided. In this setting, CRT should be used due to greater tumor regression rates then short-course RT.

However the evidence from randomized trials supporting the beneficial effect of CRT on avoiding a definitive stoma is still weak. In only three randomized trials on RT the subgroup of patients initially scheduled for APR was clearly defined before the onset of preoperative RT, but results from the three studies [13, 14, 20] were conflicting. In the CAO/ARO/AIO-04 trial, [13] the effect of CRT on sphincter-preservation rates was evident: 39% of candidates for APR could benefit from AR after preoperative irradiation. These findings, however, were not confirmed by a similar analysis of the Lyon R90-01 trial [20] and by a Polish trial [14]. In the latter study, despite significant tumor downsizing with long-course preoperative CRT, (pCR 16% *vs* 1% with short-course RT) no increase in AR was observed. The authors noted that, in some situations, AR was not done even in cases of cCR. Surgeons' willingness to adapt the procedure to tumor shrinkage is of crucial importance; if the final decision on sphincter preservation is based on tumor status at the beginning of treatment and not at the time of surgery, the interpretation of the results becomes impossible.

However sphincter-preserving surgery is related not only to preoperative treatment but also to the technical skill of the surgical team. A clear demonstration of this fact was given in the recent Sphincter-preserving Surgery after Preoperative Treatment for Ultra-low Rectal Carcinoma (GRECCAR I) trial [35]: 85% of cancers at <1 cm from the levator ani could have been treated with AR after CRT. This result was due to tumor downsizing and to the extensive use of intersphinteric resection (3/4) by the authors.

Key Concepts

- According to some surgeons, the decision to carry ou AR or APR should be discussed after neoadjuvant CRT and not before because of the possibility of tumor downstaging induced by irradiation;

- The literature is inconclusive in evaluation of the role of preoperative CRT in promoting sphincter-saving surgery for low-lying tumors (although a subgroup analysis of one randomized trial supports this idea;
- The number of patients with preserved sphincters has increased from 25% up to 50–75% in the last 30 years. The change in attitude to surgery may be at least as important as the effects of preceding CRT in explaining this increase.

4.2.7 Is Extralevator Abdomino-perineal Resection a New Surgical Standard?

The increased number of positive CRMs and iatrogenic perforations with conventional APR (both of which are avoidable) led to a more extensive procedure called "cylindrical" or "extralevator abdomino-perineal amputation". This procedure has the purpose of increasing the size of the specimen at the levator plane. The perineal incision in the anterior direction follows the same plane as the current method whereas, in the posterolateral direction, it is larger than usual, and may also include the coccyx, which will be disarticulated [36]. The dissection proceeds as far as the muscular plane, which is cut very close to the obturator muscle.

During the perineal stage, the patient should be put in the prone position as in the original description of his method by Miles. The prone "jackknife" position allows the rectum to be prolapsed after opening the pelvis, giving excellent visualization of the plane between the rectum and prostate/vagina.

Though extended and conventional APR have never been compared in a randomized trial, according to a recent review, [5] the extralevator method demonstrated local recurrence rate of 6.6% compared with 11.9% for the conventional method as a result of a lower prevalence of a positive lateral margin (9.6% *vs* 15.4%) and of intraoperative visceral perforation (4.1% *vs* 10.4%).

In a recent study on 655 consecutive patients undegoing radical resection for rectal cancer [37], stage-specific local recurrence was not significantly different between cylindrical APR and AR (local recurrence was 6% *vs* 3.1% and 3% *vs* 6%, respectively, for APR and AR in stage I–II and in stage-III rectal cancer). Interestingly, neoadjuvant CRT was not used in this study. Nevertheless, extralevator surgery often requires gluteal flaps or biological meshes for the reconstruction of the perineal region and is associated with increased perineal wound complications (from 20% to 38% according to West et al.), [38] which are usually the main reason of prolonged hospital stay for these patients.

Key Concepts

- According to a recent review focusing on retrospective studies, extralevator APR is associated with a local recurrence rate of 6.6%, which is comparable with AR;

- This method is associated with perineal wound complication in 20% to 30% of cases;
- It seems reasonable to reserve conventional APR for patients who do not have invasion of the external sphincter but ineligible for ultra-low AR because of pre-existing incontinence and to carry out an extralevator APR for more advanced tumors.

4.2.8 Role of Minimally Invasive Surgery

The laparoscopic and, more recently, the robotic approach, in rectal surgery have been increasingly adopted [39–43]. The efficacy and safety of mininvasive rectal resection has been demonstrated in randomized controlled studies, with better short-terms results than open procedures, and with the same long-term oncological outcomes [39–43].

Robotic technology was developed in an attempt to reduce the limitations of laparoscopic pelvic surgery, which requires a considerable learning curve. The robotic system has many advantages: three-dimensional vision; stable camera; multi-articulated instruments; and elimination of tremor and subsequent improved dexterity (especially in the narrow, deep pelvis, which permits a more accurate nerve-sparing TME) [42–43]. The da Vinci Surgical System Si HD© with four arms allows a single-docking, full robotic procedure, as described initially by Kim et al. [44].

In rectal surgery, innovative imaging with indocyanine green near infrared (ICG-NIR) fluorescence is a new and wide field of research using a dedicated platform. The components of this system are: a surgical endoscope capable of white-light and NIR imaging; a three-dimensional, high-definition stereoscopic camera head that is coupled to the endoscope; and an endoscopic illuminator that provides visible light and NIR illumination through the surgical endoscope *via* a flexible light guide. By intravenous injection of dye it is possible to visualize, in real time, the vascular anatomy to evaluate perfusion in the large bowel stump before stapling. Also, by injecting the dye in a peritumoral, subserosal or submucosal manner, it is possible to obtain lymphatic mapping and "rectal tumor tattooing" [45–46].

Key Concepts

- Minimally invasive surgery for rectal cancer is safe and effective, with better short-term results than open procedures and identical long-term oncological outcomes;
- Robotic technology was developed to reduce the limitations of laparoscopic pelvic surgery;
- Imaging with ICG-NIR fluorescence allows visualization, in real time, the vascular anatomy and permits lymphatic mapping.

4.3 Carcinoma of the Anus

Despite its short length, the anal canal can produce various tumors. These tumor types can be categorized as: squamous cell tumors, adenocarcinoma, neuroendocrine neoplasms, malignant melanoma, mesenchymal tumors and malignant lymphoma.

Anal squamous cell carcinomas account for ≈70% of all anal cancers in the USA [47]. Various etiologies have been implicated in their development, the most significant being human papillomavirus (HPV) infection [48]. Adenocarcinoma of the anal canal accounts for ≈10% (range, 5–19%) of all anal canal cancers [49]. Crohn's disease or other inflammatory conditions that result in chronic anal fistulas may predispose to the development of fistula-associated adenocarcinomas [50].

Anal melanomas account for ≈4% of anal canal tumors and <1% of all melanomas [51].

Although various mesenchymal tumors may occur in the anal canal, the most common ones are smooth muscle tumors and gastrointestinal stromal tumors (GISTs).

4.3.1 Treatment

Most anal canal carcinomas are managed using CRT [52]. For all stages of localized squamous cell cancers of the anal canal, concurrent chemotherapy and RT is recommended over RT alone to improve local control and decrease colostomy rates. The optimal drug combination for squamous cell cancer of the anal canal is 5FU plus mitomycin C (MMC), concurrently with RT [53].

Randomized controlled trials have shown a significantly lower local failure rate with CRT compared with RT alone with a significantly higher disease-free and colostomy-free survival with the addition of MMC [54]. Combined chemotherapeutic regimens have been advocated in the treatment of metastatic disease but these treatments have not been standardized [55]. There are no data on the efficacy of biological agents combined with CRT (though several trials are in progress) [56]. Initial cCR rates were reported in 7 of 9 patients (78%). There are ongoing trials such as ECOG E3205, AMC045 trials, and the FNLCC trial (which has been modified after early toxicity was reported).

4.3.1.1 External Beam Radiation Therapy

Martenson and colleagues from the Mayo Clinic [57] published a retrospective study of 18 patients treated with external beam radiation only for stage-T1 and -T2 tumors. They showed a high tumor control rate with 100% freedom from local recurrence, and a 5-year survival rate of 94%. The radiation doses used in this study were higher than those used previously, reaching 67 Gy in total. Researchers from the Memorial Sloan Kettering Cancer Center suggested that a select group of patients with small lesions were candidates for initial excisional biopsy followed by postoperative radiation with a limited dose of 30 Gy, this being adequate for disease control [58]. There is evidence of a radiation dose response; little more than 30 Gy may be needed to control areas in which there is only a risk of microscopic tumor burden. Gross tumor may require doses >55 Gy to give optimal probability of disease eradication. As in many other curative treatment situations, continuous-course irradiation apparently confers an advantage over split-course radiation [52]. Surveillance regimens after CRT are not standardized, and controversies exist regarding evaluation for recurrent disease [55]. It is well known that anal cancers continue to regress well after treatment, but the exact timing of maximal tumor regression is not clear [55]. Routine biopsy is controversial for monitoring the response to CRT, with some clinicians advocating multiple random biopsies every 3 months, whereas others target only clinically suspicious lesions [55]. After CRT, 10–15% of subjects will have persistent disease and around 10–30% of patients can be expected to have subsequent recurrence. The standard treatment for persistent and recurrent disease is APR [59].

Assessment of clinical response usually takes place 6–8 weeks after completion of treatment, with 60–85% of patients expecting to achieve a cCR [60]. Residual or recurrent tumors must be confirmed histologically before considering radical surgery [52]. Haboubi et al. [61] showed that, in salvage surgery, the prognosis is worse for certain categories: non-responders more than those with recurrence; initial tumor size of ≥5 cm; depth of invasion into and beyond the levator ani; patient age ≥55 years; and lymph-node involvement. Recent guidelines from ESMO [52] suggest that LE can be considered only for small well-differentiated carcinomas of the anal margin (T1 N0), i.e., <2 cm in diameter, without evidence of nodal spread. Several studies in rectal cancer specimens have demonstrated that histological quantification of tumor regression is useful for determining tumor response to CRT, and showed prognostic significance with regard to local recurrence and disease-free survival [62]. The three-category system described by Ryan et al. in 2005 is recommended because it provides good interobserver reproducibility and prognostic information [63]:

- Grade 0: no viable cancer cells (complete response);
- Grade 1: single cells or small groups of cancer cells (moderate response);
- Grade 2: residual cancer outgrown by fibrosis (minimal response);
- Grade 3: extensive residual cancer (poor response).

For Grade 0, a complete pathological response is combined with grade 1 in the classification described by Ryan et al.

Key Concepts

- The paradigm of external beam radiation therapy with concurrent 5FU and MMC developed over 30 years ago remains first-line treatment;
- Surgery is reserved for small N0 anal cancers, and for persistent or

Table 4.1 Ongoing trials for anal cancer. Reproduced with permission from [64]

Phase II trials	N.	Design	RT dose	CR	Median F/U	3 yr DFS	3 yr CFS	OS
RTOG-0529 phase II completed accrual March 2008	63	5FU 1000 mg/m2 days 1-4 and 29-33 2 doses of MMC 10 mg/m2 days 1, 29 Total dose = 20 mg/m2	IMRT dose acc to T stage 50,4 Gy/28# T2NO 54 Gy/30# for T3/T4NO 54 Gy/30# for T3/T4NO	34/61 67% at 8 weeks	No data	No data	No data	No data
ECOG E320510	62	NACT cisplat/5FUx2 induction, then 5FU/ cisplat/cetuximab during RT in immunocompetent	54 Gy/30# for T3/T4NO	Study suspended 11/3/2008	No data	No data	No data	No data
AMC045 NCT0032444	47 15	5FU 1000 mg/m2 days 1-4, cisplatin day 1, 29 cetuximab during RT in HIV+	54 Gy/30# for T3/T4NO	Study ongoing	No data	No data	No data	No data
FNCLCC NCT009551	77 40	Cisplatin and 5FU with cetuximab	65 Gy	Study ongoing	No data	No data	No data	No data
Total	245							

N number, *RT* radiotherapy, *CR* complete clinical response, *DFS* disease free survival, *CFS* colostomy free survival, *OS* overall survival, *IMRT* intensity modulated radiotherapy, *5FU* 5-fluorouracil, cisplat cisplatinum, *MMC* mitomycin C, *F/U* follow-up, *NACT* neoadjuvant chemotherapy, *HIV* human immunodeficiency virus.

recurrent disease. National and international trials in this disease site [64] to evaluate new treatment modalities are ongoing throughout Europe (Table 4.1);

- New experimental regimens may achieve better results in advanced stage anal cancer than those achieved so far.

References

1. Peeters KC, Marijnen CA, Nagtegaal ID et al (2007) Dutch Colorectal Cancer Group the TME trial after a median follow-up of 6 years: increased local control but no survival benefit in irradiated patients with resectable rectal carcinoma. Ann Surg 246:693-701
2. Valentini V, Aristei C, Glimelius B et al (2009) Multidisciplinary Rectal Cancer Management: 2nd European Rectal Cancer Consensus Conference (EURECA-CC2). Radiother Oncol 92:148-163
3. Fazio VW, Zutshi M, Remzi FH et al (2007) A randomized multicentric trial to compare long-term functional outcome, quality of life, and complications of surgical procedures for low rectal cancers. Ann Surg 246:481-488
4. den Dulk M, Putter H, Collette L et al (2009) The abdominoperineal resection itself is associated with an adverse outcome: the European experience based on a pooled analysis of five European randomised clinical trials on rectal cancer. Eur J Cancer 45:1175-1183

5. Stelzner S, Koehler C, Stelzer J et al (2011) Extended abdominoperineal excision vs. standard abdominoperineal excision in rectal cancer-a systematic overview. Int J Colorectal Dis 26:1227-1240
6. van Gijn W, Marijnen CA, Nagtegaal ID et al (2011) Preoperative radiotherapy combined with total mesorectal excision for resectable rectal cancer: 12-year follow-up of the multicentre, randomised controlled TME trial. Lancet Oncol 12:575-582
7. Peng J, Chen W, Sheng W et al (2011) Oncological outcome of T1 rectal cancer undergoing standard resection and local excision. Colorectal Dis 13:14-19
8. Moore JS, Cataldo PA, Osler T et al (2008) Transanal endoscopic microsurgery is more effective than traditional transanal excision for resection of rectal masses. Dis Colon Rectum 51:1026-1030
9. Hahnloser D, Wolff BG, Larson DW et al (2005) Immediate radical resection after local excision of rectal cancer: an oncologic compromise? Dis Colon Rectum 48:429-437
10. Piessen G, Gabral C, Benoist S et al (2012) Previous transanal full-thickness excision increases the morbidity of radical resection for rectal cancer. Colorectal Dis 14:445-452
11. Doornebosh PG, Ferenschild FT, de Wilt JH et al (2010) Treatment of recurrence after transanal endoscopic microsurgery (TEM) for T1 rectal cancer. Dis Colon Rectum 53:1234-1239
12. Sebag-Montefiore D, Stephens RJ, Steele R et al (2009) Preoperative radiotherapy versus selective postoperative chemoradiotherapy in patients with rectal cancer (MRC CR07 and NCIC-CTG C016): a multicentre, randomised trial. Lancet 373:811-820
13. Roedel C, Becker H, Fietkau R et al (2011) Preoperative chemoradiotherapy and postoperative chemotherapy with 5-fluorouracil and oxaliplatin versus 5-fluorouracil alone in locally advanced rectal cancer: First results of the German CAO/ARO/AIO-04 randomized phase III trial. J Clin Oncol 29(suppl): abs 3505
14. Bujko K, Nowacki MP, Nasierowska-Guttmejer A et al (2006) Long-term results of a randomized trial comparing preoperative short-course radiotherapy with preoperative conventionally fractionated chemoradiation for rectal cancer. Br J Surg 93:1215-1223
15. MERCURY study group (2007) Extramural depth of tumor invasion at thin-section MR in patients with rectal cancer: results of the MERCURY study. Radiology 243:132-139
16. Peeters KC, van den Velde CJ, Leer JW et al (2005) Late side effects of short-course preoperative radiotherapy combined with total mesorectal excision for rectal cancer: increased bowel dysfunction in irradiated patients-a Dutch colorectal cancer group study. J Clin Oncol 23:6199-6206
17. Schmoll HJ, Van Cutsem E, Stein A et al (2012) ESMO Consensus Guidelines for management of patients with colon and rectal cancer. A personalized approach to clinical decision making. Ann Oncol 23:2479-2516
18. Martin ST, Heneghan HM, Winter DC (2012) Systematic review and meta-analysis of outcomes following pathological complete response to neoadjuvant chemoradiotherapy for rectal cancer. Br J Surg 99:918-928
19. Maas M, Nelemans PJ, Valentini V et al (2010) Long-term outcome in patients with a pathological complete response after chemoradiation for rectal cancer: a pooled analysis of individual patient data. Lancet Oncol 11:835-844
20. Francois Y, Nemoz CJ, Bauliex J et al (1999) Influence of the interval between preoperative radiation therapy and surgery on downstaging and on the rate of sphincter-sparing surgery for rectal cancer: the Lyon R90-01 randomized trial. J Clin Oncol 17:2396-2402
21. Tulchinsky H, Shmueli E, Figer A et al (2008) An interval >7 weeks between neoadjuvant therapy and surgery improves pathologic complete response and disease-free survival in patients with locally advanced rectal cancer. Ann Surg Oncol 15:2661-2667
22. Kalady MF, de Campos-Lobato LF, Stocchi L et al (2009) Predictive factors of pathologic complete response after neoadjuvant chemoradiation for rectal cancer. Ann Surg 250:582-589
23. Smith FM, Waldron D, Winter DC (2010) Rectum-conserving surgery in the era of chemoradiotherapy. Br J Surg 97:1752-1764
24. Callender GG, Das P, Rodriguez-Bigas MA et al (2010) Local excision after preoperative

chemoradiation results in an equivalent outcome to total mesorectal excision in selected patients with T3 rectal cancer. Ann Surg Oncol 17:441-447
25. Nair RM, Siegel EM, Chen DT et al (2008) Long-term results of transanal excision afterneoadjuvant chemoradiation for T2 and T3 adenocarcinomas of the rectum. J Gastrointest Surg 12:1797-1805
26. Lezoche G, Baldarelli M, Guerrieri M et al (2008) A prospective randomized study with a 5-year minimum follow-up evaluation of transanal endoscopic microsurgery versus laparoscopic total mesorectal excision after neoadjuvant therapy. Surg Endosc 22:352-358
27. Habr-Gama A, Perez RO, Nadalin W et al (2004). Operative versus nonoperative treatment for stage 0 distal rectal cancer following chemoradiation therapy: long term results. Ann Surg 240:711-717
28. Maas M, Beets-Tan RG, Lambregts DM et al (2011) Wait-and-see policy for clinical complete responders after chemoradiation for rectal cancer. J Clin Oncol 29:4633-4640
29. Perez RO, Habr-Gama A, Sao Juliao GP et al (2011) Transanal endoscopic microsurgery for residual rectal cancer after neoadjuvant chemoradiation therapy is associated with significant immediate pain and hospital readmission rates. Dis Colon Rectum 54:545–551.
30. Bökkerink GM, de Graaf EJ, Punt CJ et al (2011) The CARTS study: Chemoradiation therapy for rectal cancer in the distal rectum followed by organ-sparing transanal endoscopic microsurgery. BMC Surg 11:34
31. Habr-Gama A, Perez RO, Proscurshim I et al (2006) Patterns of failure and survival for nonoperative treatment of stage c0 distal rectal cancer following neoadjuvant chemoradiation therapy. J Gastrointest Surg 10:1319-1328
32. Glynne-Jones R, Hughes R (2012) Critical appraisal of the 'wait and see' approach in rectal cancer for clinical complete responders after chemoradiation. Br J Surg 99: 897-909
33. Rouanet P (2009) Impact des traitements néo-aduvants sur la conservation sphinctérienne des cancers du bas rectum. In Cancer du rectum. Faucheron JL, Rullier E (eds) Arnette, Paris pp 80-87
34. Slim K et al (2009) Cancérologie digestive: pratiques chirurgicales. Raccomandations de la Sociétè de Chirurgie Digestive (SFCD) et de l'Association de Chirurgie Hépatobilaire et de la Transplantation Hépatique (ACHBT). J Chir 146(suppl2):S54
35. Rouanet P, Rivoire M, Lelong B (2006) Sphincter preserving surgery after preoperative treatment for ultra-low rectal carcinoma. A French multicenter prospective trial: GRECCAR 1. J Clin Oncol 24: abs 3527
36. Holm T, Ljung A, Häggmark T et al (2007) Extended abdominoperineal resection with gluteus maximus flap reconstruction of the pelvic floor for rectal cancer. Br J Surg 94:232-238
37. Mathis KL, Larson DW, Dozois EJ et al (2012) Outcomes following surgery without radiotherapy for rectal cancer. Br J Surg 99:137-143
38. West NP, Finan PJ, Anderin C et al (2008) Evidence of the oncologic superiority of cylindrical abdominoperineal excision for low rectal cancer. J Clin Oncol 26:3517-3522
39. Jayne DG, Thorpe HC, Copeland J et al (2010) Five-year follow up of the medical Research Council CLASSIC Trial of laparoscopically assisted versus open surgery for colorectal cancer. Br J Surg 97:1638-1645
40. Quarati R, Summa M, Priora F et al (2011) Single centre retrospective evaluation of laparoscopic rectal resection with TME for rectal cancer: 5-Year cancer-specific survival. Int J Surg Oncol. 2011:473614
41. Kang SB, Park JW, Jeong SY et al (2010) Open versus laparoscopic surgery for mid or low rectal cancer after neoadjuvant chemoradiotherapy (COREAN trial): short-term outcomes of an open-label randomised controlled trial. Lancet Oncol 11: 637-645
42. Bianchi PP, Ceriani C, Locatelli A et al (2010) Robotic versus laparoscopic total mesorectal excision for rectal cancer: a comparative analysis of oncological safety and short-term outcomes. Surg Endosc 24:2888-2894
43. Kang J, Yoon KJ, Min BS et al (2012) The impact of robotic surgery for mid and low rectal cancer: a case-matched analysis of 3-arm comparison — open, laparoscopic, and robotic surgery. Ann Surg. 2012 Oct 10 Epub ahead of print
44. Koh DC, Tsang CB, Kim SH (2011). A new application of the four-arm standard da Vinci®

surgical system: totally robotic-assisted left-sided colon or rectal resection. Surg Endosc 25:1945-1952
45. Kudszus S, Roesel C, Schachtrupp A et al (2010) Intraoperative laser fluorescence angiography in colorectal surgery: a noninvasive analysis to reduce the rate of anastomotic leakage. Langenbecks Arch Surg 395:1025-1030
46. Hutteman M, Choi HS, Mieog JS et al (2011) Clinical translation of ex vivo sentinel lymph node mapping for colorectal cancer using invisible near-infrared fluorescence light. Ann Surg Oncol 18:1006-1014
47. Frisch M, Melbye M (2006) Cancer Epidemiology and Prevention. 3rd ed. NewYork, NY: Oxford University Press
48. De Vuyst H, Clifford GM, Nascimento MC et al (2009) Prevalence and type distribution of human papillomavirus in carcinoma and intraepithelial neoplasia of the vulva, vagina and anus: a meta-analysis. Int J Cancer 124:1626-1636
49. Beal KP, Wong D, Guillem JG et al (2003) Primary adenocarcinoma of the anus treated with combined modality therapy. Dis Colon Rectum 46:1320-1324
50. Belkacemi Y, Berger C, Poortmans P et al (2003) Management of primary anal canal adenocarcinoma: a large retrospective study from the Rare Cancer Network. Int J Radiat Oncol Biol Phys 56:1274-1283
51. Chang AE, Karnell LH, Menck HR (1998) The National Cancer Data Base report on cutaneous and noncutaneous melanoma: a summary of 84,836 cases from the past decade: the American College of Surgeons Commission on Cancer and the American Cancer Society. Cancer 83:1664-1678
52. Glynne-Jones R, Northover JM & Cervantes A on behalf of the ESMO Guidelines Working Group (2010) Anal cancer: ESMO Clinical Practice Guidelines for diagnosis, treatment and follow-up. Annals of Oncology 21 (Supplement 5): v87-v92
53. Spithoff K, Cummings B, Jonker D et al (2009) Gastrointestinal Cancer Disease Site Group. Management of squamous cell cancer of the anal canal. Toronto (ON): Cancer Care Ontario; 2009 Mar 31. Program in Evidence-based Care Evidence-Based Series No.: 2-8
54. (1996) UKCCCR Anal Cancer Working Party. Epidermoid Anal Cancer: results from the UKCCCR randomised trial of radiotherapy alone versus radiotherapy, 5-fluorouracil and Mitomycin. Lancet 348:1049-1054
55. Fleshner PR, Chalasani S, Chang GJ et al (2008) Practice parameters for anal squamous neoplasms. Dis Colon Rectum 51:2-9
56. Olivatto LO, Meton F, Bezerra M et al (2008) Phase I study of cetuximab (CET) in combination with 5-flurouracil (5FU), cisplatin (CP) and radiotherapy (RT) in patients with locally advanced squamous cell anal carcinoma (LAAC). J Clin Oncol 26(15S):240 [abstract 4609]
57. Martenson Jr JA, Gunderson LL (1993) External radiation therapy without chemotherapy in the management of anal cancer. Cancer 71:1736-1740
58. Hu K, Minsky BD, Cohen AM et al (1999) 30 Gy may be an adequate dose in patients with anal cancer treated with excisional biopsy followed by combined-modality therapy. J Surg Oncol 70:71-77
59. Cummings BJ, Keane TJ, O'Sullivan B et al (1991) Epidermoid anal cancer: treatment by radiation alone or by radiation and 5-fluorouracil with and without mitomycin C. Int J Radiat Oncol Biol Phys 21:1115-1125
60. Engstrom PF, Arnoletti JP, Benson AB et al (2010) NCCN clinical practice guidelines in oncology. Anal carcinoma. J Natl Compr Canc Netw 8:106-120
61. Haboubi NY, Edilbe MW, Hill J (2007) Justification for staging of epidermoid anal carcinoma after salvage surgery: a pathological guideline. Colorectal Dis 9:238-244
62. Rodel C, Martus P, Papadoupolos T et al (2005) Prognostic significance of tumor regression after preoperative chemoradiotherapy for rectal cancer. J Clin Oncol 23): 8688-8696
63. Ryan R, Gibbons D, Hyland JM et al (2005) Pathological response following long-course neoadjuvant chemoradiotherapy for locally advanced rectal cancer. Histopathology 47:141-146
64. Lim F, Glynne-Jones R (2011) Chemotherapy/chemoradiation in anal cancer: a systematic review. Cancer Treat Rev 37:520-532

Hepatobiliary Cancer

5

Lorenzo Capussotti, Luca Viganò and Nadia Russolillo

5.1 Introduction

Hepatobiliary surgery has had an extraordinary evolution in recent decades. In the 1970s, it was a high-risk procedure undertaken by few surgeons treating advanced diseases having a poor prognosis. To date, hepatobiliary surgery is a standardized procedure, carried out routinely, reaching near-zero mortality rates and offering a chance of cure to many cancer patients. Furthermore, the surgeon is no more the only "actor" in patient treatment. He/she has been inserted into a multidisciplinary setting in which his/her expertise is combined with that of oncologists, gastroenterologists, radiologists and radiotherapists to optimize management of patients. Hepatobiliary surgery is now considered a separate specialty undertaken by dedicated surgeons. Even if the centralization of hepato-biliary oncology and surgery has not yet been standardized, many data are in favor of this direction, and referral centers can be easily identified. We will try to depict the most important ad innovative data during recent years in hepatic and biliary surgical oncology. Solid evidences and new perspectives will be analyzed. Due to the unfeasibility of analyzing every issue, the most significant ones will be considered briefly.

5.2 Hepatocellular Carcinoma (HCC)

In the past, liver surgery for HCC was associated with high rates of mortality and liver failure due to the underlying cirrhosis and poor functional reserve of the liver. Today, the fragility of these patients remains and should not be for-

L. Capussotti (✉) · L. Viganò · N. Russolillo
HPB and Digestive surgery, Ospedale Mauriziano Umberto I, Turin, Italy
e-mail: lcapussotti@mauriziano.it

A. Valeri et al. (eds.), *What's New in Surgical Oncology*,
DOI: 10.1007/978-88-470-5310-6_5,

gotten, but simple selection criteria help in the identification of good candidates for surgery. Together with the traditional Child–Pugh score (only class-A patients are amenable to surgery), the indocyanine green retention test can be adopted as well as the Model for End-Stage Liver Disease (MELD) score in combination with plasma sodium values to refine patient selection. Mortality rates lower than 5% are the present standard, reaching 0% in some series. These advances have allowed the extension of indications to more complex procedures.

5.2.1 Indications

In 2000, the Barcelona Clinic Liver Cancer (BCLC) Consensus Conference and the subsequent guidelines from the European Association for the Study of the Liver (EASL) and the American Association for the Study of Liver Diseases (AASLD) defined, as a candidate for surgery, the Child–Pugh class A patient with a single tumor of diameter <5 cm without macrovascular invasion or portal hypertension [1]. In these patients, surgery achieves excellent survival results over 60% at 5 years. Unfortunately, the same guidelines contraindicated resection in patients affected by advanced HCC, that are the majority of cases. For such patients, only palliative treatments were proposed. In practice, liver surgeons regularly break guidelines and schedule surgery for patients with large and oligonodular HCC, with a tumor thrombus in branches of the portal vein or hepatic veins and with mild portal hypertension. Many authors have reported favorable outcomes. The most important series involved 2,046 patients from 10 large centers worldwide [2]. Half of the patients were affected by advanced HCC. Ninety-day mortality was less than 3% and overall survival at 5 years was 56% (60% for BCLC class 0-A and B patients, 38% for class-C patients). These results largely exceed the survival expectancy after palliative treatments, and strongly suggest the need for an update of the guidelines.

5.2.2 Anatomic vs. Non-anatomic Resection

HCC has a typical pattern of spread along the portal branches. Satellite nodules may be found into the same liver segment even distant from the primary lesion. Hence, theoretically anatomic segmental resection should be the standard treatment to prevent local recurrence. For many years, the superiority of anatomic over non-anatomic resection has been debated and no clear benefits of survival after anatomic resection have been demonstrated. In 2008, a Japanese survey collected more than 5,500 patients undergoing liver resection for single HCC [3]. The authors demonstrated a prognostic superiority of anatomic resection only for HCC ranging from 2 cm to 5 cm. In HCC of diameter <2 cm, atypical resection was adequate, whereas in large HCC other prognostic determinants needed to be considered.

5.2.3 Surgery vs. Radiofrequency Ablation (RFA)

Three potentially curative treatments of HCC are available: liver resection, liver transplantation, and RFA. Their respective indications are difficult to define because the optimal candidates for each procedure are almost identical. Considering RFA, patients with HCC >3 cm are usually excluded because of the high risk of treatment failure. A debate is ongoing for lesions up to 3 cm. The largest study is from Japan. It involved 7,135 patients with 1–3 HCCs up to 3 cm and compared the outcomes of surgery and RFA [4]. Overall survival was similar (at 2 years 93% in the RFA group *vs* 94.5% in the resection group), but the risk of recurrence was significantly lower in resected patients (2-year time-to-recurrence rate was 55.4% vs. 35.5%, $p<0.0001$). Conversely, Livraghi et al. reported a series of 218 HCCs up to 2 cm treated by RFA having a 97% sustained local complete response. It corresponded to a 5-year survival of 68.5%, reproducing the outcome of liver resection [5]. A recent meta-analysis involving one randomized trial and nine controlled studies demonstrated the superiority of resection over RFA, but differences between the two options disappeared for HCC <3 cm [6]. At present, as also suggested by Japanese guidelines, RFA is an alternative to surgery only for HCC up to 2 cm in diameter. A gray area of competence between RFA and surgery remains for lesions between 2 cm and 3 cm.

5.2.4 Surgery and Liver Transplantation: Alternative or Complementary?

The respective roles of liver resection and liver transplantation are not clear and strongly debated. Within the Milan criteria (single HCC <5 cm or 2–3 HCCs <3 cm) liver transplantation achieves excellent outcomes (up to 70% survival at 5 years) but in the same subset of patients similar results have been reported recently even after resection [7]. Furthermore, in the case of recurrence, transplantation was still possible in most cases. Conversely, many authors have attempted to extend the indications for transplantation out of the Milan criteria to offer this ideal treatment (cure of HCC and underlying cirrhosis) to as many patients as possible. The debate is ongoing and far from solution. In a "what's new" perspective, the authors want to state that liver resection and liver transplantation are evolving towards cooperation rather than opposition. At least three possible "combinations" are possible, even if no rules can be recommended: liver surgery as first-line treatment, considering transplantation as a "salvage" option in case of recurrence or liver failure; liver resection as a "bridge" treatment before liver transplantation while on the waiting list; liver resection as initial therapy to select (on the basis of pathology examination) high-risk patients who may benefit from early "*de principe*" liver transplantation.

5.2.5 Chemotherapy and Target Therapies (Sorafenib)

Chemotherapy has failed to achieve survival benefit in patients with HCC in comparison with best supporting care. Some promising data derive from target therapies. There are 56 molecular therapies under evaluation in HCC treatment, but sorafenib is the only approved one.

Sorafenib is a multikinase inhibitor that blocks Raf signaling, vascular endothelial growth factor (VEGF), platelet-derived growth factor (PDGF), and c-Kit. As demonstrated by the Sorafenib HCC Assessment Randomized Protocol (SHARP) trial, it improves overall survival of Child–Pugh class-A patients with untreatable HCC (10.7 *vs* 7.9 months) [8]. These results have been confirmed by the Asian Pacific trial (overall survival 6.5 *vs* 4.2 months). Its role in Child–Pugh class-B patients is under evaluation. Further indications have to be explored, such as sorafenib as adjuvant treatment after resection/ablation or transarterial chemoembolisation (TACE). Preliminary data showed a high response rate (52%) after the combination of TACE and sorafenib, which was superior to that seen with TACE alone.

5.2.6 Selective Internal Radiation Treatment (SIRT)

SIRT is a promising option for HCC patients. It is a form of brachytherapy with intra-arterial injection of ^{90}Y-loaded microspheres (Fig. 5.1). Side effects are minimal. A recent review reported response rates of 25–50% and stable disease in 77–90% of patients after a mean interval of 6.6 months [9]. Only retrospective series or non-controlled prospective studies are available, but they have collected about 700 cases. The candidates for SIRT are patients with advanced HCC progressing after TACE or sorafenib as well as those excluded from TACE because of portal-vein thrombosis or multiple bilobar lesions. In selected cases, even downstaging to surgery has been reported.

5.3 Colorectal Liver Metastases (CRLMs)

CRLMs are the most common indication for liver surgery. Since the 1980s, the beneficial impact of resection on prognosis has been clearly demonstrated. Surgery is the established "gold standard" treatment with excellent short- and long-term results (mortality lower than 2%, survival up to 50–60% at 5 years in selected cases) [10, 11], mainly in high-volume centers [12]. Even a curative role of surgery has been recently demonstrated by reports of 10-year actual survivors in 15–20% of cases.

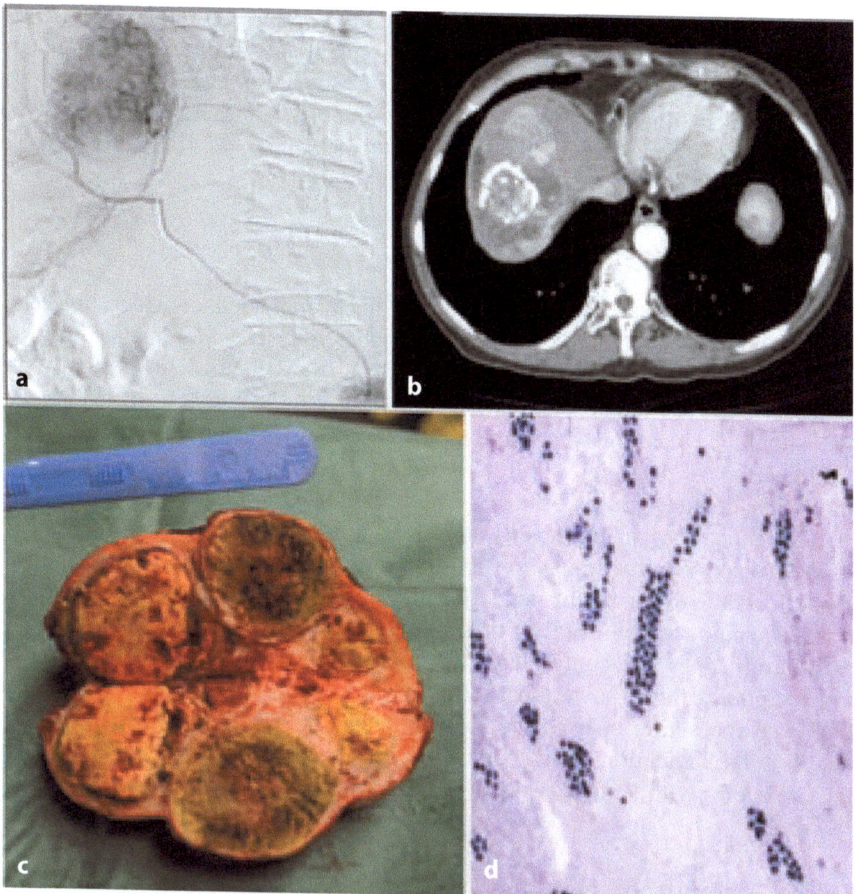

Fig. 5.1 A large HCC in a 75-year-old HCV-positive patient treated by selective internal radiation treatment (SIRT). (**a**) Angiographic image during SIRT. (**b**) CT after SIRT. (**c**) The specimen after a right trisectionectomy. (**d**) At final pathology, 90% necrosis was evident; resin microspheres were visible in the vessels

5.3.1 Staging

Together with computed tomography (CT), a significant contribution to staging has been offered by magnetic resonance imaging (MRI) of the liver. It has achieved extremely high sensitivity and specificity for the detection and characterization of hepatic lesions, especially thanks to contrast agents and diffusion-weighted images [13].

The role of positron emission tomography-computed tomography (PET-CT) is controversial. Even if it offers additional data, the high rate of false-positive (inflammation) and false-negative (especially after chemotherapy) images limit its impact [13]. It has a role in doubtful cases or in patients with advanced disease to disclose extrahepatic deposits.

5.3.2 Indications

The surgical indications for CRLM have been expanded considerably. The number and diameter of lesions, extra-hepatic disease, and synchronicity of metastases are no longer a contraindication [10]. Patients with lymph-node metastases beyond the hepatic pedicle do not show a clear benefit from surgery and should be cautiously scheduled for resection. The only absolute contraindication is the impossibility of achieving complete surgery. A debate about the adequate width of the surgical margin is ongoing. Evidence suggests that a negative margin is probably sufficient, but de Haas et al. recently reported even a non-negative impact of a 0-mm margin (R1 surgery) [14]. It probably reflects the extension of indications to more complex cases in which large margins cannot be achieved. In these patients, the impossibility to avoid a 0-mm margin does not contraindicate surgery. Nevertheless, it should not be considered a pathway toward palliative surgery.

Recurrences after liver resection often occur (≤60% of cases). Re-resection has the same indications as the first liver resection (surgery whenever technically feasible) with similar survival outcome.

5.3.3 Chemotherapy

In the last 15 years, effective chemotherapy drugs have been introduced, such as oxaliplatin and irinotecan. Median survival in unresectable patients (80–90% of cases) passed the threshold of 20 months. In some cases (≈10–15%), chemotherapy obtains a significant tumor shrinkage that even enables the patient to undergo resection. In 1996, Bismuth et al. were the first to report resection after "conversion chemotherapy". Several series have reported encouraging long-term results (5-year survival, ≈30%), even if high recurrence rates have been observed [15]. The effectiveness of chemotherapy in unresectable patients let some authors consider its application in "borderline-resectable" cases. The aim was to obtain tumor shrinkage, to enable easier and more conservative resections, and to select good candidates for surgery. Neoadjuvant chemotherapy is now commonly adopted even if supported by little evidence. The next step has been the proposal of systematic chemotherapy in all resectable patients. The European Organisation for Research and Treatment of Cancer (EORTC) randomized trial 40983 published in 2008 (surgery alone *vs* surgery + perioperative oxaliplatin-based chemotherapy) tried to validate this policy. Even though the primary endpoint (higher disease-free survival at 3 years in the chemotherapy group) was achieved, the difference was limited (+8%) and no differences in overall survival were observed [16]. Further trials are ongoing to clarify this issue.

5.3.3.1 Response to Chemotherapy

The response to chemotherapy has been demonstrated to have a prognostic impact. Radiological disease progression at restaging has even been considered to be a contraindication to surgery because of extremely poor outcome (8% at 5 years). More recent studies better reclassified it as a relative contraindication to surgery: in selected patients (up to 3 metastases, <50 mm, CEA <200 ng/mL), resection can be undertaken with good outcome despite disease progression [17]. On the basis of pathological examination, Rubbia-Brandt et al. proposed a tumor regression grade to assess metastatic responses to chemotherapy [18]. It has a strong prognostic impact, clearly more precise than that seen for radiological data.

5.3.3.2 Disadvantages of Chemotherapy

Firstly, chemotherapy-related liver injuries have been depicted, for example, sinusoidal injuries and nodular regenerative hyperplasia after oxaliplatin-based treatments and steatohepatitis after irinotecan-based therapies. These lesions increase postoperative morbidity and, in case of steatohepatitis, even surgical mortality due to liver failure [19]. Chemotherapy-related liver injuries increase together with the number of chemotherapy cycles, whereas their clinical impact decreases upon prolonging the interval between chemotherapy and surgery. A short duration of chemotherapy and an adequate interval between chemotherapy and surgery are the rules to respect to limit these problems.

A further disadvantage of chemotherapy is the disappearance of metastases, especially small ones. Unfortunately, this finding does not correspond to the true sterilization of neoplastic foci. In 2006, Benoist et al. showed that 80% of disappeared lesions either was still present at surgery or recurred at follow-up [20]. More favorable data have been reported by recent studies (residual disease in only 30%), especially if intra-arterial chemotherapy was administered. In any case, surgeons should look at the radiological disappearance of CRLMs with suspicion.

5.3.4 Targeted Therapies

In association with chemotherapy, targeted therapies show a significant contribution to disease control and tumor shrinkage. The most common targeted therapies are bevacizumab (anti-epidermal growth factor receptor (EGFR) antibody) and cetuximab (anti-VEGF-A antibody). Their association with chemotherapy increases the response rate by up to 78%. Even a benefit in terms of overall and progression-free survival has been reported [21, 22]. With regard to cetuximab, a molecular predictor of effectiveness has been identified: the k-Ras gene. Only patients with a wild-type k-Ras gene may benefit from this treatment. A prognostic impact of k-Ras mutations has been also suggested.

5.3.5 Surgical Strategies

Due to the excellent outcome of surgery, surgeons have implemented strategies to increase resectability to offer a chance of cure to as many patients as possible. In those with multiple bilobar lesions, the need for complete surgery has to be integrated with the need for an adequate future liver remnant (FLR). In 2000, Adam et al. proposed a two-stage hepatectomy to solve this problem. They scheduled two subsequent liver resections to achieve R0 surgery to allow liver hypertrophy between the two procedures. This procedure was better codified by Jaeck et al. in 2004: (i) extirpation of lesions in the planned FLR, usually the left lobe, during the first operation; (ii) portalve in occlusion, usually the right one (intraoperative ligation or postoperative embolization); (iii) major hepatectomy (usually a right hepatectomy or right trisectionectomy) 4 weeks later provided adequate FLR hypertrophy [23]. About 75–80% of patients will complete the treatment and achieve excellent long-term results (5-year survival of 30–50%), similar to those observed after one-stage resections. Recently, a new proposal has been advanced: the association of liver partition to portalvein ligation at the time of the first resection to achieve an extremely rapid volume increase (within 1 week). This strategy, called "associating liver partition and portal vein ligation for staged hepatectomy" (ALPPS), allows completion of the second procedure within the same hospitalization (7–10 days after the first procedure) and avoids the drop-out risk between the first and second stage [24]. Only few preliminary reports are available on ALPPS.

Another important issue is the management of patients with synchronous metastases. The debate between simultaneous and delayed resection is ongoing, but an interesting new proposal has been advanced: the "reverse strategy". Mentha et al. reported it first in 2006. The authors proposed to treat first the liver metastases and then the primary tumor in two separate procedures. This strategy allows prioritizing hepatic deposits, which are the true determinants of the prognosis. In 2012, the Mentha research team compared this strategy with the classic approach (colorectal resection followed by liver surgery): the reverse approach guaranteed the same outcome as the standard one [25]. In the authors' opinion, the reverse strategy is of interest, especially for patients with locally advanced rectal tumors in whom chemoradiotherapy before rectal surgery should be scheduled. Theoretically, reverse strategy allows carrying out chemoradiotherapy after having completed liver surgery before rectal resection. *Ad hoc* trials are needed to clarify this issue.

Finally, it is important to underline the evolution of surgery in CRLM treatment towards a parenchymal-sparing policy. Major liver resections are carried

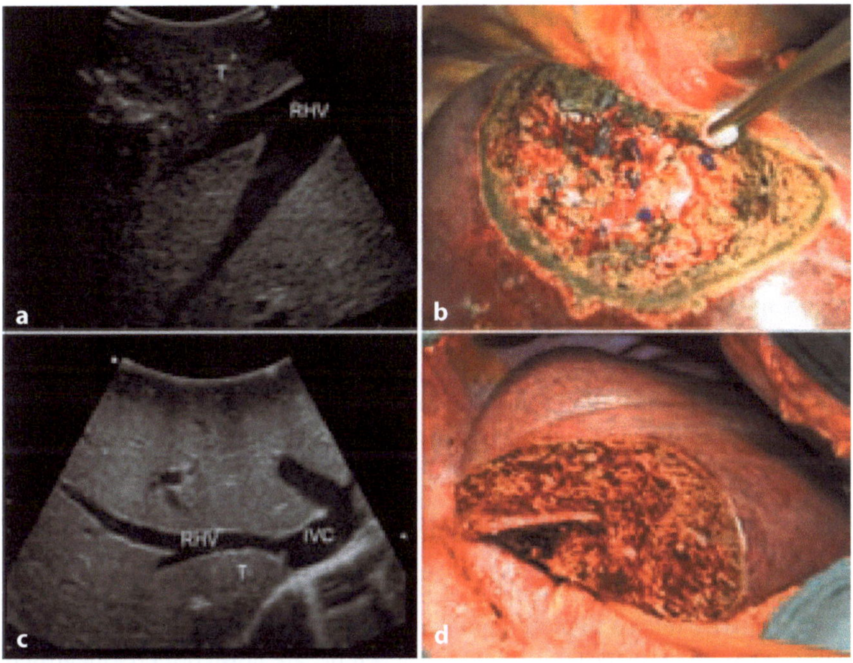

Fig. 5.2 Parenchymal-sparing strategy in resection of colorectal liver metastases. (**a**) Intraoperative ultrasonography shows a metastasis in contact with the right hepatic vein without infiltration. (**b**) Wedge resection of segments 7 and 8 sparing the right hepatic vein that has been exposed on the raw cut surface. (**c**) Intraoperative ultrasonography shows a metastasis compressing (but not infiltrating) the right hepatic vein. (**d**) Resection of Sg7 with exposure of the right hepatic vein on the raw cut surface

out less often to reduce the risk of liver dysfunction and to increase the opportunities of re-resection. Wedge resections and segmentectomies guarantee adequate ongological treatment if planned appropriately. Intraoperative ultrasonography is an essential tool to safely undertake these resections (Fig. 5.2).

5.3.6 Interstitial Treatments

After their successful application in HCC, interstitial treatments have been proposed for CRLMs. Their appeal relies on easy application, brief hospitalization, and excellent short-term outcome. Anyway, strong evidence is against their application to resectable CRLMs [26]. In comparison with surgery, RFA is associated with higher local recurrence rates and lower overall and disease-free survival. The same poor results have been observed even for small lesions (<3 cm). RFA is not an alternative to surgery. It can be combined with surgery to achieve complete treatment by ablating deeply located lesions that were otherwise unresectable. Even for these patients, outcome is lower in comparison with those receiving surgery alone.

5.4 Biliary Tumors

In comparison with CRLMs, biliary tumors have had a more limited evolution in recent years. This is due to their rarity, the need for large and high-risk surgical procedures (mortality rates, 5–10%) and the lack of effective medical treatments.

It is possible to distinguish intrahepatic cholangiocarcinoma, hilar cholangiocarcinoma (Klatskin tumor), distal bile duct cancer, and gallbladder cancer. Tumors of the middle bile duct are no longer considered because, according to the level of tumor, hepatic or pancreatic surgery is needed.

5.4.1 Peripheral Cholangiocarcinomas (CCCs)

CCCs have had a marked increase of incidence in recent years. This finding could be partly related to their improved diagnosis: hepatic lesions previously classified as "liver metastases of unknown origin" are now correctly identified as CCC.

With respect to surgical treatment, few series are available. Some recent multicenter studies tried to codify indications and outcome [27, 28]. Surgical mortality was ≈5%, but excellent survival results have been reported (≈40% at 5 years). Resection is indicated if complete surgery can be done, but radical resection is finally achieved in only 75–85% of patients. Lymph-node dissection is essential in all patients because of the high percentage of N+ patients (more than one-third of cases). Metastatic lymph nodes are not an absolute contraindication to surgery but are associated with poor outcome. Together with R1 resection, N status is the strongest prognostic determinant.

5.4.2 Hilar Cholangiocarcinomas

The treatment of hilar cholangiocarcinomas has had several modifications in recent years [29]. Preoperative staging can be complete without invasive examination: CT and magnetic resonance cholangiopancreatography (MRCP) clearly show the biliary and radial extension of the tumor. The surgical procedure is now standardized. Isolated bile duct resection has been abandoned in almost all patients. The mucosal and submucosal spread of cancer requires wide margins. The combination of biliary and liver surgery increases the completeness of resection and prolongs survival. Similarly, segment 1 must be removed systematically because it can be a site of direct infiltration by the tumor or perineural/biliary neoplastic diffusion. Lymph-node dissection should be systematic because of the high risk of metastatic deposits (30% to 60%), but positive lymph nodes at the hepatic pedicle do not contraindicate resection.

Liver resection for hilar cholangiocarcinomas has been traditionally associated with high mortality rates (up to 10–15%). A combination of biliary drainage and portal-vein embolization in patients with inadequate FLR has improved the safety of these procedures, even reaching 0% mortality in some series. Nevertheless, the indications for preoperative biliary drainage are controversial because not all patients need it (low bilirubin values, left-sided resections) and because severe sepsis due to bile-duct contamination may occur. Biliary drainage is essential whenever portal-vein embolization is required, and should drain only the FLR.

Improving surgical outcomes have enabled surgeons to treat even advanced diseases aggressively. Type-IV hilar cholangiocarcinomas (bilateral involvement of second biliary divisions) are no longer absolute contraindications. Patients can be scheduled for right or left trisectionectomies with complex biliary reconstructions (Fig. 5.3). Resections and reconstructions of vascular structures can also be associated. Survival benefits have been clearly demonstrated for portal-vein resections whereas, in the case of resection and reconstruction of the hepatic artery, outcomes are controversial [30].

Surgical margins are key factors in the treatment of hilar cholangiocarcinomas. Firstly, a negative biliary margin is essential. Even if the first resection margin is involved by the tumor, a re-resection achieving negative margins improves outcome [31]. Furthermore, the radial margin must be considered. The neoplasm diffuses early into surrounding soft tissue, reaching the portal vein and hepatic artery. Dissection of the bile duct from these vessels could expose the tumor or even make surgery incomplete. At the end of the 1990s, a new proposal was advanced by Neuhaus et al., the "no-touch technique" for right-sided hilar cholangiocarcinomas. The authors proposed to systematically

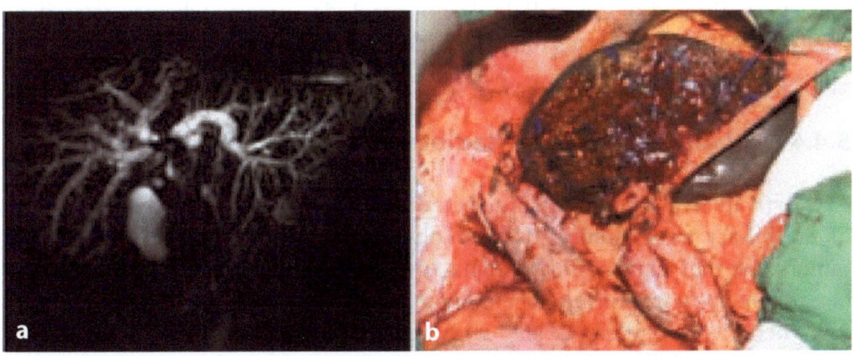

Fig. 5.3 Surgery for hilar cholangiocarcinoma. (**a**) Preoperative MRCP shows a type-IIIa hilar cholangiocarcinoma. (**b**) A right trisectionectomy extended to Sg1 with the bile duct confluence resection was carried out

carry out a right hepatectomy/right trisectionectomy associated with resection and reconstruction of a bifurcation in the portal vein to avoid tumor dissection. Mortality rates was high (10%), but survival outcome was excellent (58% at 5 years) [32].

Finally, the indications for liver transplantation for hilar cholangiocarcinoma have been re-discussed. Preliminary studies reported unsatisfactory results with high recurrence rates. In 2005, the Mayo Clinic Group published the outcome of a protocol including chemotherapy and radiotherapy followed by transplantation: the 5-year survival rate was 82% [33]. As suggested for the no-touch technique, these data could open new opportunities, but further validations are needed.

5.4.3 Gallbladder Cancer

The treatment and outcome of gallbladder cancer is strictly dependent upon tumor stage. In the early stages, the role of surgery is well codified: cholecystectomy is adequate for T1a tumors, whereas liver resection (bisegmentectomy Sg4b-5/gallbladder bed resection) and lymph-node dissection are needed for T1b and T2 tumors. This is due to the high rate of lymph-node metastases (10–15% for T1b and 40–50% for T2) and to the risk of direct, perineural and lymphatic diffusion of the tumor to the liver parenchyma. Even if the diagnosis is after a simple cholecystectomy, prompt and adequate radicalization is needed to offer a chance of cure for these patients (overall survival at 5 years, 60–100%). A debate persists about more advanced stages (T3 or T4). Evidence-based treatment is lacking, but some suggestions can be offered. The involvement of the common bile duct is no longer a contraindication to surgery [34], whereas the need for a duodenopancreatectomy should be evaluated cautiously. Even if some authors have reported good outcomes, in the authors' experience (11 patients) no clear survival benefits were achieved (0% survival at 2 years). As reported for hilar cholangiocarcinomas, lymph-node metastases limited to the pedicle do not preclude surgery, whereas retro-pancreatic or celiac metastases must be evaluated on a case-by-case basis.

5.4.4 Chemotherapy and Radiotherapy

Few data are available regarding chemotherapy in patients affected by tumors of the biliary tract. Studies have involved few patients with mixed types of tumors. Further cholangiocarcinomas and gallbladder cancers have shown a heterogeneity in response to chemotherapy. In 2010, Valle et al. showed a survival benefit for patients treated with gemcitabin and cisplatin in comparison with those receiving cisplatin alone [35]. The impact of targeted therapies, especially anti-EGFR, is under investigation, but promising results have been anticipated. More robust data are needed. Similarly, few data have been reported for external radiotherapy or endoluminal brachytherapy. Some studies have reported tumor shrinkage in inoperable patients, but no recommendations can be formulated.

5.5 Surgical Technique and Prognosis

The technique of hepato-biliary surgery has evolved rapidly in recent years. Technical issues have been analyzed to verify their impact on the prognosis. Even if little evidence is available, some interesting topics can be considered.

5.5.1 Laparoscopic and Robotic Surgery of the Liver

The minimally invasive approach to hepatic and biliary surgery was first reported at the beginning of the 1990s. The initial evolution and propagation have been extremely slow, but the situation has changed in the last decade: laparoscopic hepatobiliary surgery has been applied and developed widely to reach >3,000 published procedures. Numbers are smaller for robotic surgery due to its limited availability, but are increasing. The beneficial impact of a laparoscopic approach on short-term outcomes has, by and large, been proved, whereas its oncological safety is under evaluation. The strongest evidence concerns HCC: the margin width and the survival outcomes are similar to those seen for open surgery [36]. Data about colorectal metastases are weaker, but evolving into the same direction. Biliary tumors have rarely been treated with a laparoscopic approach due to the complexity of the procedures required. For good candidates (lesions <5 cm into the anterolateral segments of the liver away from vascular structures), laparoscopic and robotic surgery can be considered a safe alternative. Further technical evolutions will probably allow extending the indications to more advanced hepatic diseases and biliary tumors.

5.5.2 Anterior Approach

Liver resection in patients with large tumors of the right lobe can be problematic: bleeding may occur during liver mobilization, especially in the presence of adhesions with the diaphragm; the right hepatic vein and the inferior vena cava are difficult to isolate and control; the tumor is manipulated, increasing the risk of dissemination or even rupture of neoplastic cells. In 1996, Lai et al. proposed to treat these patients by an "anterior approach", i.e., carrying out the parenchymal transection before mobilization of the right liver. In 2001, Belghiti et al. refined this method by introducing the "hanging maneuver" (a retrohepatic loop that allows "hanging" the liver during transection) to protect the vena cava at the end of the resection. In 2006, the Hong Kong Group published the results of a randomized controlled trial about this issue (anterior *vs* classic approach) which involved 120 HCC patients (60 per arm) [37]. The anterior approach was associated with a lower transfusion rate, lower rate of massive bleeding, and higher overall survival rates. These data have been confirmed recently by a Chinese study. Few data are available for tumors other than HCC, but similar benefits can be expected. Should the anterior approach be adopted systematically during a right hepatectomy, even for small tumors? The authors recently published a randomized trial about this issue, and did not show any difference between the two approaches [38]. The anterior approach should be the standard only in patients with large right-sided tumors.

5.5.3 Pedicle Clamping

Since its introduction in 1908, pedicle clamping has enabled safer and easier liver resections. Randomized trials demonstrated its positive impact on blood losses and transfusions. This dogma has been placed in doubt recently: thanks to improvements in surgical and anesthesiological technique, liver resection can be carried out safely without pedicle clamping. At the same time, experimental studies demonstrated that the inflow occlusion might negatively impact the prognosis: ischemia/reperfusion damage stimulated the outgrowth of pre-established micrometastases and consequently increased the recurrence risk. To date, these data have not been confirmed in the clinical setting [39, 40]. While waiting for further studies every surgeon should adopt his/her preferred clamping policy by considering the type of resection to be undertaken and the characteristics of the parenchyma to be resected.

References

1. Llovet JM, Ducreux M, Lencioni R et al (2012) EASL-EORTC clinical practice guidelines: management of hepatocellular carcinoma. J Hepatol 56:908-943
2. Torzilli G, Belghiti J, Kokudo N et al (2012) A snapshot of the effective indications and results of surgery for hepatocellular carcinoma in tertiary referral centres: is it adherent to the EASL/AASLD recommendations? An observational study of the HCC east-west study group. Ann Surg, in press
3. Eguchi S, Kanematsu T, Arii S et al (2008) Comparison of the outcomes between an anatomical subsegmentectomy and a non-anatomical minor hepatectomy for single hepatocellular carcinomas based on a Japanese nationwide survey. Surgery 143:469-475
4. Hasegawa K, Makuuchi M, Takayama T et al (2008) Surgical resection vs. percutaneous ablation for hepatocellular carcinoma: a preliminary report of the Japanese nationwide survey. J Hepatol 49: 589-594
5. Livraghi T, Meloni F, Di Stasi M et al (2008) Sustained complete response and complications rates after radiofrequency ablation of very early hepatocellular carcinoma in cirrhosis: Is resection still the treatment of choice? Hepatology 47:82-89
6. Zhou Y, Zhao Y, Li B, et al (2010) Meta-analysis of radiofrequency ablation versus hepatic resection for small hepatocellular carcinoma. BMC Gastroenterol 10:78
7. Cherqui D, Laurent A, Mocellin N et al (2009) Liver resection for transplantable hepatocellular carcinoma: long-term survival and role of secondary liver transplantation. Ann Surg 250(5):738-746

8. Llovet JM, Ricci S, Mazzaferro V et al (2008) Sorafenib in advanced hepatocellular carcinoma. N Engl J Med 359:378-390
9. Sangro B, Iñarrairaegui M, Bilbao JI (2012) Radioembolization for hepatocellular carcinoma. J Hepatol.;56:464-473
10. Adam R, De Gramont A, Figueras J et al (2012) The oncosurgery approach to managing liver metastases from colorectal cancer: a multidisciplinary international consensus. Oncologist 17:1225-1239
11. Viganò L, Russolillo N, Ferrero A, et al (2012) Evolution of long-term outcome of liver resection for colorectal metastases: analysis of actual 5-year survival rates over two decades.Ann Surg Oncol 19:2035-2044
12. Viganò L, Langella S, Ferrero A et al (2012) Colorectal cancer with synchronous resectable liver metastases: monocentric management in a hepatobiliary referral center improves survival outcomes. Ann Surg Oncol, in press
13. Floriani I, Torri V, Rulli E et al (2010). Performance of Imaging Modalities in Diagnosis of Liver Metastases From Colorectal Cancer: A Systematic Review and Meta-analysis J Magn Reson Imaging 31:19–31
14. de Haas RJ, Wicherts DA, Flores E, et al (2008) R1 resection by necessity for colorectal liver metastases: is it still a contraindication to surgery? Ann Surg 248:626-637
15. Capussotti L, Muratore A, Mulas MM et al (2006). Neoadjuvant chemotherapy and resection for initially irresectable colorectal liver metastases. Br J Surg 93(8):1001-6
16. Nordlinger B, Sorbye H, Glimelius B, et al (2008) Perioperative chemotherapy with FOLFOX4 and surgery versus surgery alone for resectable liver metastases from colorectal cancer (EORTC Intergroup trial 40983): a randomised controlled trial. Lancet 371:1007-1016
17. Viganò L, Capussotti L, Barroso E, et al (2012) Progression while receiving preoperative chemotherapy should not be an absolute contraindication to liver resection for colorectal metastases. Ann Surg Oncol 19:2786-2796
18. Rubbia-Brandt L, Giostra E, Brezault C et al (2007) Importance of histological tumor response assessment in predicting the outcome in patients with colorectal liver metastases treated with neo-adjuvant chemotherapy followed by liver surgery. Ann Oncol 18(2):299-304
19. Vauthey JN, Pawlik TM, Ribero D et al (2006) Chemotherapy regimen predicts steatohepatitis and an increase in 90-day mortality after surgery for hepatic colorectal metastases. J Clin Oncol 24:2065–2072
20. Benoist S, Brouquet A, Penna C et al (2006) Complete response of colorectal liver metastases after chemotherapy: does it mean cure? J Clin Oncol 24:3939–3945
21. Hurwitz H, Fehrenbacher L, Novotny W et al (2004) Bevacizumab plus irinotecan, fluorouracil, and leucovorin for metastatic colorectal cancer. N Engl J Med 350(23):2335-42
22. Loupakis F, Cremolini C, Salvatore L et al (2012) Clinical impact of anti-epidermal growth factor receptor monoclonal antibodies in first-line treatment of metastatic colorectal cancer: meta-analytical estimation and implications for therapeutic strategies. Cancer 118(6):1523-32
23. Jaeck D, Oussoultzoglou E, Rosso E et al (2004) A two-stage hepatectomy procedure combined with portal vein embolization to achieve curative resection for initially unresectable multiple and bilobar colorectal liver metastases. Ann Surg 240(6):1037-49
24. Schnitzbauer AA, Lang SA, Goessmann H et al (2012) Right portal vein ligation combined with in situ splitting induces rapid left lateral liver lobe hypertrophy enabling 2-staged extended right hepatic resection in small-for-size settings. Ann Surg 255(3):405-14
25. Andres A, Toso C, Adam R et al. A Survival Analysis of the Liver-First Reversed Management of Advanced Simultaneous Colorectal Liver Metastases: A LiverMetSurvey-Based Study. Ann Surg 256(5):772-779
26. Cirocchi R, Trastulli S, Boselli C, Montedori et al (2012) Radiofrequency ablation in the treatment of liver metastases from colorectal cancer. Cochrane Database Syst Rev 13;6:CD006317
27. Ribero D, Pinna AD, Guglielmi A et al (2012). Surgical Approach for Long-term Survival of Patients With Intrahepatic Cholangiocarcinoma: A Multi-Institutional Analysis of 434 Patients. Arch Surg 20:1-7

28. Farges O, Fuks D, Boleslawski E et al (2011). Influence of surgical margins on outcome in patients with intrahepatic cholangiocarcinoma: a multicenter study by the AFC-IHCC-2009 study group. Ann Surg 254(5):824-29
29. Nagino M, Ebata T, Yokoyama Y et al (2012) Evolution of Surgical Treatment for Perihilar Cholangiocarcinoma: A Single-Center 34-Year Review of 574 Consecutive Resections. Ann Surg, in press
30. de Jong MC, Marques H, Clary BM et al (2012) The impact of portal vein resection on outcomes for hilar cholangiocarcinoma: a multi-institutional analysis of 305 cases. Cancer 118(19):4737-47
31. Ribero D, Amisano M, Lo Tesoriere R et al (2011) Additional resection of an intraoperative margin-positive proximal bile duct improves survival in patients with hilar cholangiocarcinoma. Ann Surg 254(5):776-81
32. Neuhaus P, Thelen A, Jonas S et al (2012) Oncological superiority of hilar en bloc resection for the treatment of hilar cholangiocarcinoma. Ann Surg Oncol 19(5):1602-8
33. Rea DJ, Heimbach JK, Rosen CB et al (2005) Liver transplantation with neoadjuvant chemoradiation is more effective than resection for hilar cholangiocarcinoma. Ann Surg 242(3):451-8
34. Nishio H, Ebata T, Yokoyama Y et al (2011) Gallbladder cancer involving the extrahepatic bile duct is worthy of resection. Ann Surg 253(5):953-60
35. Valle J, Wasan H, Palmer DH et al (2010) Cisplatin plus gemcitabine versus gemcitabine for biliary tract cancer. N Engl J Med 362(14):1273-81
36. Mirnezami R, Mirnezami AH, Chandrakumaran K et al (2011) Short- and long-term outcomes after laparoscopic and open hepatic resection: systematic review and meta-analysis. HPB 13(5):295-308
37. Liu CL, Fan ST, Cheung ST et al (2006) Anterior approach versus conventional approach right hepatic resection for large hepatocellular carcinoma: a prospective randomized controlled study. Ann Surg 244:194-203
38. Capussotti L, Ferrero A, Russolillo N et al (2012) Routine anterior approach during right hepatectomy: results of a prospective randomised controlled trial. J Gastrointest Surg 16(7):1324-1332
39. Giuliante F, Ardito F, Pulitanò C et al (2010) Does hepatic pedicle clamping affect disease-free survival following liver resection for colorectal metastases? Ann Surg 252(6):1020-1026
40. Ferrero A, Russolillo N, Viganò L et al (2010) Does Pringle maneuver affect survival in patients with colorectal liver metastases? World J Surg 34(10):2418-2425

Pancreatic Adenocarcinoma

6

Marco Filauro, Gian Andrea Rollandi, Filippo Grillo Ruggieri, Gianni Coccia, Lorenzo Bacigalupo, Alberto Gozza and Andrea Barberis

6.1 Radiological Work-up for Correct Indications for Surgery

Pancreatic cancer represents a challenge for the imaging modalities that are most commonly used: ultrasound, computed tomography (CT), magnetic resonance imaging (MRI), and positron emission tomography-computed tomography (PET-CT). Imaging is used to identify the pancreatic lesion and help in the diagnosis of the different forms of pancreatic cancer in different clinical settings.

To establish the correct indication for surgery, imaging procedures have to be used in a diagnostic algorithm that allows local and distant staging. The goal of imaging procedures is to obtain, in a non-invasive manner, the information for which laparoscopy is considered the "gold standard" (although it has some limitations). The main information that is needed is: primary tumor (T), peri-pancreatic vascular alterations and anatomic anomalies, regional lymph nodes (N), and liver as well as peritoneal metastases (M). To obtain these data, in recent years, new methods have been developed and older methods improved upon.

M. Filauro (✉) · A. Barberis
General, Hepatobiliary and Pancreatic Surgery, Ospedali Galliera, Genoa, Italy
e-mail: marco.filauro@galliera.it

G.A. Rollandi · L. Bacigalupo
Radiodiagnostics, Ospedali Galliera, Genoa, Italy

F. Grillo Ruggieri
Radiotherapy, Ospedali Galliera, Genoa, Italy

G. Coccia
Gastroenterology, Ospedali Galliera, Genoa, Italy

A. Gozza
Oncology, Ospedali Galliera, Genoa, Italy

A. Valeri et al. (eds.), *What's New in Surgical Oncology*,
DOI: 10.1007/978-88-470-5310-6_6, © Springer-Verlag Italia 2013

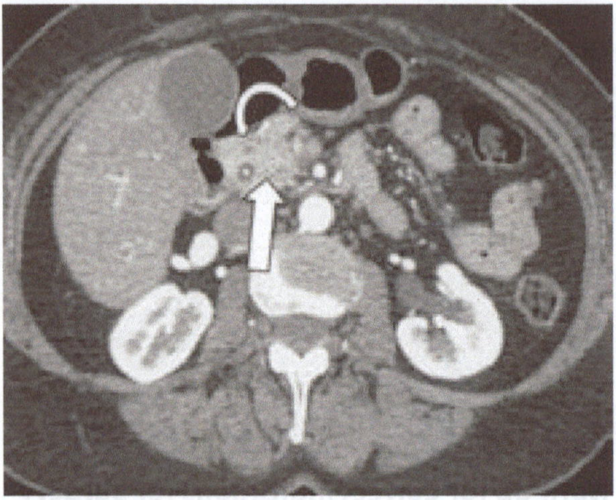

Fig. 6.1 Axial contrast-enhanced arterial phase MDCT demonstrates dilatation of the distal common bile duct (*) due to isoattenuating adenocarcinoma (*arrow*) of the pancreatic head. The main pancreatic duct of body and tail is not dilated (not shown) due to a compensating Santorini duct (*curved arrow*)

Ultrasound devices have recently being upgraded with software and probes that allow the evaluation of the viscoelastic properties of tissues. Some of these methods, such as acoustic radiation force impulse (ARFI), allow qualitative and quantitative assessment. According to some authors, ARFI could be used to aid in the evaluation of pancreatic cystic lesions [1]. Complete evaluation of the pancreas with ultrasound is usually limited, so CT and MRI are needed for unambiguous and complete assessment of the pancreas. In some cases, second-look ultrasound after CT and/or MRI may allow real-time assessment of the relationships of the tumor with adjacent vessels and structures.

With the high spatial resolution obtained by multidetector computed tomography (MDCT), it is possible to assess (in extreme detail) patients with pancreatic cancer, in particular minimal alterations of the peri-pancreatic vessels.

CT protocols for pancreatic cancer usually involve at least three vascular phases: arterial, portal and venous/late phase. According to some authors, the pancreatic phase (obtained at 35 s from the arterial peak of enhancement in the aorta) maximizes the difference in density between the normal pancreas and pancreatic adenocarcinoma. Isoattenuating pancreatic cancer at MDCT is not uncommon (5.4% according to some authors). In these cases (Fig. 6.1), it is very important to assess alterations in the pancreatic ductal system and eventual anomalies (e.g., a compensating Santorini duct) that can explain the absence of ductal dilatation in the pancreatic body in patients with a lesion of the pancreatic head and dilatation of the common bile duct [2]. Isoattenuating pancreatic cancer appears to have a better prognosis than other forms of pancreatic cancer [2].

MDCT can help in the assessment of the “T parameter”. In particular, infiltration of retroportal fat tissue can be assessed by MDCT with 80% sensitivity and 84% specificity according to some authors.

Vascular assessment is very important to define the surgical strategy and define "borderline resectable pancreatic tumors" (BRPTS). In BRPTS, current protocols advise neoadjuvant chemo(radio)therapy. MDCT allows assessment of the vessels, and extensive analyses of the MDCT findings may help to define "true" BRPTs.

One interesting study found that preoperative assessment of body-fat distribution by MDCT, as a surrogate for fatty pancreas infiltration, can help to predict clinically significant pancreatic fistulas after pancreaticoduodenectomy [3].

Many cases of suspected or established pancreatic cancer undergo MRI assessment for further evaluation after MDCT. MRI protocols for the assessment of the pancreas have been expanded with the inclusion of different sequences. The sequence that has been investigated and used most widely in recent years in oncologic imaging is diffusion-weighted imaging (DWI). DWI-MRI permits measurement of the diffusion of water in tissues and quantification of this parameter as apparent diffusion coefficient (ADC). The images that can be obtained with DWI MRI are similar to those of PET-CT and, in fact, in many clinical settings, DWI-MRI is challenging PET-CT in oncologic imaging.

Cystic pancreatic lesions are readily detected at imaging and their assessment has been focused on differentiating malignant from benign lesions, DWI-MRI can aid in the assessment of these types of lesions. Boraschi et al. found that the mean ADC values of different types of pancreatic lesions (intraductal papillary mucinous tumor (IPMT), mucinous cystoadenoma, serous cystoadenoma, pseudocyst) were significantly different ($P<0.05$). Therefore, the authors concluded that DWI-MRI may be helpful in the differential diagnosis of cystic pancreatic lesions [4]. In the work of Sandrasegaran et al., ADC values were found to be helpful in deciding the malignant potential of IPMT. However, ADC values were not useful for differentiating malignant from benign lesions, or for characterizing cystic pancreatic lesions [5].

In pancreatic adenocarcinoma, DWI-MRI can be added to standard MRI protocols and, although the lesion may not be clearly delineated in ≤47% of cases, signal alteration in the pancreas distal to the malignant lesion may provide an adjunct sign for the classic radiological findings in pancreatic adenocarcinoma. Other authors have also found limited improvement with DWI-MRI compared with MDCT in the detection of pancreatic cancer in a high-risk population with main pancreatic duct (MPD) dilatation. Instead, DWI and T2-weighted images used together may help in the depiction of pancreatic neuroendocrine tumors that, in some cases, may be difficult to identify with standard MRI sequences.

In our experience, DWI may help in the diagnosis of intrapancreatic spleen, which can be readily confused with a neuroendocrine lesion of the pancreatic tail. In these cases, the ADC of the intrapancreatic spleen is the same as that of the spleen.

An interesting use of DWI is in the assessment of pancreatitis caused by pancreatic cancer (Fig. 6.2), DWI can, in some cases, be used to detect a

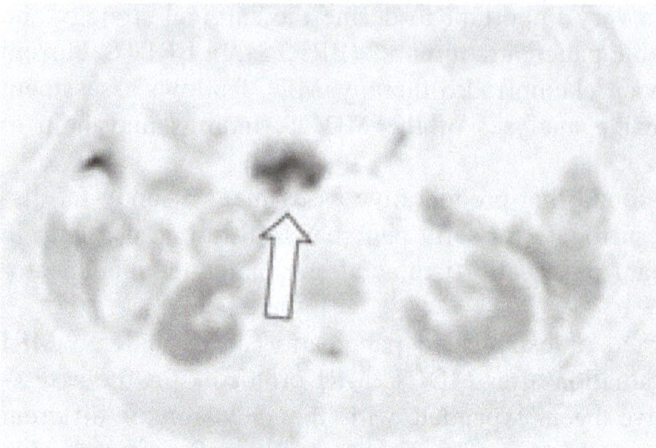

Fig. 6.2 Axial DWI MRI shows a high signal in the pancreatic head that had a low ADC (not shown). This finding is compatible with a diagnosis of pancreatitis due to cancer (*arrow*) of the pancreas head

malign pancreatic lesion with restricted water diffusion within the edematous pancreatic parenchyma with the increased water diffusion (due to increased water content) related to pancreatitis.

ADC measurements can also be helpful for differentiating between normal pancreatic tissue and mass-forming focal pancreatitis. However, the overlap in ADC values of pancreatic cancer and mass-forming focal pancreatitis does not allow their correct distinction in real-world practice [6].

DWI may also aid in the identification of lymph nodes but not in the definition of a "true" metastatic lymph node. Furthermore, often metastatic lymph nodes are of very small diameter (3 mm) and are therefore difficult to detect.

In a pilot study, DWI performed significantly better than contrast-enhanced 64-slices MDCT in the detection of liver metastases in patients with pancreatic tumors. Therefore, DWI may help to optimize therapeutic management in such patients in the future (Fig. 6.3) [7]. In the assessment of hepatic metastases, hepatobiliary contrast agents may be helpful (Fig. 6.4), These contrast media are widely used because they cannot be taken up correctly in the delayed hepatobiliary phase by pancreatic metastases (in general, by all liver metastases).

In our experience, DWI can be used to depict the small foci of peritoneal carcinomatosis that may be unrecognized on standard MRI sequences and MDCT.

Unenhanced MRI can be used to evaluate vascular structures with the use of particular sequences. This elicits results that can be compared with those of contrast-enhanced MRI vascular studies. This research field is being developed. In general, state-of-the-art contrast-enhanced MRI and contrast-enhanced MDCT protocols should be substantially equal in the assessment of pancreatic cancer.

PET-CT has had a small impact in the management of pancreatic cancer. According to some authors, the improvement in PET-CT devices (and particularly the use of iodated contrast media) allows better results [8].

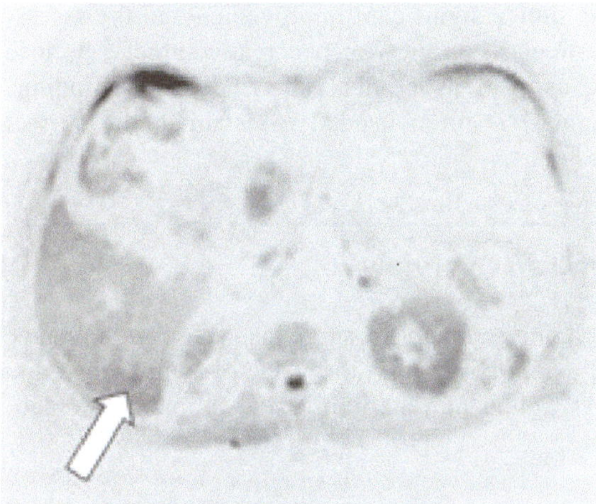

Fig. 6.3 Small metastasis (*arrow*) of pancreatic adenocarcinoma visible only in DWI MRI in hepatic segment VI

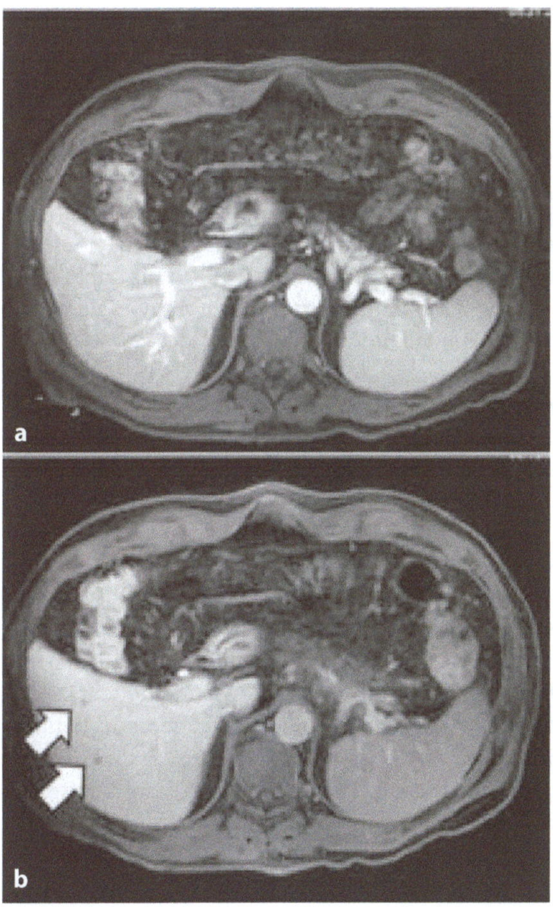

Fig. 6.4 Two small metastases (arrows) of pancreatic adenocarcinoma in segments V and VI. They are hard to identify on portal phase images (**a**) but readily depicted as hypointense lesions in the hepatobiliary delayed (80 min) image after intravenous injection of contrast media (**b**) (gadobenate dimeglumine)

In conclusion, imaging has shown significant improvements in the assessment of pancreatic cancer, particularly in view of pancreatic surgery. A close correlation between imaging as well as clinical and endoscopic findings (including endoscopic ultrasound) is often needed to establish the correct treatment.

6.2 Surgical Treatment: an Overview

Pancreatic tumors are a challenging problem for surgeons. Many authors have discussed the indications and extent of surgery, the value of lymph-node dissection, vascular resections, As well as minimally invasive approaches to neoplastic diseases of the pancreas.

6.2.1 Surgical Methods

The Whipple–Kausch pancreatoduodenectomy (PD) and pylorus-preserving pancreatoduodenectomy (PP-PD) are the treatments of choice for tumors of the pancreatic head. Both procedures comprise resection of the pancreatic head together with the duodenum, with (PD) or without (PP-PD) distal gastrectomy. The reconstruction of the biliary and alimentary tract is usually undertaken with a gastro-jejunal anastomosis (PD) or a duodeno-jejunal (PP-PD) anastomosis and a biliary anastomosis between the hepatic duct and jejunum. A recent review demonstrated no differences among the two methods with regard to morbidity, mortality and overall survival. PP-PD is superior in terms of intraoperative blood loss and operating time. Most authors carry out duodeno-jejunal anastomosis in the antecolic position [9].

6.2.1.1 Lymphadenectomy

The value of extended lymphadenectomy is controversial. There have been many debates about the results of extended lymphadenectomy for adenocarcinoma of the pancreatic head [10]. The conclusion of these articles is that extended lymphadenectomy does not benefit long-term survival and no further studies are required to assess this issue.

6.2.1.2 Pancreatic Reconstruction

Many authors have discussed the type of anastomosis in the pancreatic and alimentary tracts. Two reconstructions are used: pancreatogastrostomy and pancreaticojejunostomy. The main issue is the prevalence of pancreatic fistulas, the "Achilles' heel of pancreatic surgery". In this regard, many studies have been conducted without evidence of the superiority of one type of anastomosis over another. Berger et al. [11] found a lower rate of fistulas with invagination of the pancreas in the jejunal loop with respect to the duct to the jejunum anastomosis (Fig. 6.5). Peng et al. described promising method called

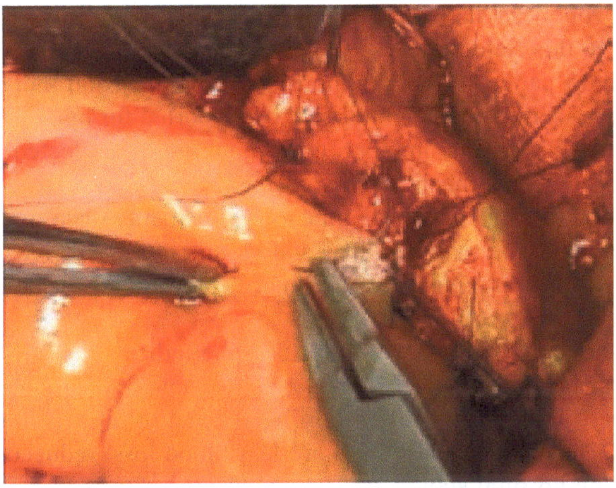

Fig. 6.5 Duct-to-mucosa Wirsung jejunal anastomosis

a "binding pancreaticojejunostomy" [12]: an end-to-end anastomosis with invagination of the pancreas in a jejunal loop in which the mucosa was previously cauterized. Somatostatin seems to have a prophylactic function with respect to postoperative morbidity and fistula formation [13].

With regard to stenting of the MPD, external stents seem to have a better outcome in terms of postoperative complications and pancreatic fistulas compared with internal stents or no stent, but further studies are required [14]. In conclusion, given the relatively high rate of complications in this type of surgery, the choice of pancreatic anastomotic method should be based on individual experience, and the best anastomosis after PD is based upon the preference and experience of the surgeon [15].

6.2.1.3 Vascular Resection

Several studies have been conducted to assess the results of vascular resections to achieve R0 margins during PD for advanced adenocarcinoma with vascular involvement. Even if vascular resection can be achieved safely, the overall 3-year survival in PD with vascular resection shows no differences from PD without vascular resection [16]. In a retrospective analysis of 3,582 patients undergoing PD for malignant disease, Castleberry et al. [17] demonstrated increased 30-day morbidity and mortality in PD associated with vascular resections.

6.2.1.4 Laparoscopic Surgery

Laparoscopic approaches to pancreatic-head tumors are controversial. The criticism originates from the prolonged operating time and the often reduced accuracy in dissection and reconstruction time. Several authors have reported small series of laparoscopic PD, and showing no substantial advantages of minimally invasive surgery (MIS). Looking to the future, widespread and less expensive propagation of robotic-assisted laparoscopic methods could provide a sense of MIS approach in this field.

In a recent study with 15 patients [18], the morbidity, mortality and incidence of pancreatic fistulas seemed to be similar to those reported for open or laparoscopic surgery, as well as the number of lymph nodes collected. Compared with a laparoscopic approach, robotic surgery seems to have a lower conversion rate, blood loss and operating time as well as better oncological results [19]. MIS applied to the treatment of distal tumors of the pancreas (body and tail) has shown encouraging results primarily due to increasing experiences of many researchers worldwide.

In the early days of MIS for distal pancreatic lesions, the indications were limited strictly to benign and borderline diseases (cystic tumors, neuroendocrine tumors). However, authors are now reporting on malignant tumors treated by this approach. The advantages of MIS are less blood loss, reduced postoperative morbidity and hospital stay.

Venkat et al., in their meta-analysis of 1,814 patients, reported similar oncological results and margin-free resections [20]. Moreover, recent retrospective studies from Fox et al. highlight the lower cost (postoperative and total) in the laparoscopic group compared with open pancreatectomy [21].

A matter of concern is the possibility of spleen preservation, which seems to be higher in MIS of the distal pancreas. Two methods can be used to save the spleen. The first involves dissecting out the splenic artery and vein with division between the pancreas and the splenic artery and vein. The second is by resecting the splenic vessels along with the pancreas but with careful preservation of the vascular collaterals in the splenic hilum, which allows the spleen to survive on the short gastric vessels (Warshaw method). Only retrospective studies are available regarding this issue. However, these studies seem to confirm that spleen preservation gives a lower morbidity rate compared with splenectomy associated with this type of pancreatic resection. Distal pancreatectomy plus splenectomy seems to impair postoperative pancreatic leaks, fatigue, cold or flu. Tsiouris et al. noticed more pancreatic leaks in a spleen-preserving group [22]. With regard to the method (splenic vessels resection *vs* vessel preservation), postoperative complications were not different between the two groups; a low occurrence of perigastric varices was detectable in the splenic vessel resection group.

In distal pancreatectomies, robotic-assisted laparoscopic surgery seems to allow promising results in terms of the accuracy of surgical field dissection, harvesting of lymph nodes, blood loss and postoperative recovery due to the well-known advantages of robotic movements. In the next few years we will surely observe propagation of these methods, and obtain results from larger series.

6.2.1.5 Ablative Methods

Some investigators have assessed the feasibility and complications of radiofrequency ablation (RFA) applied to pancreatic tumors that are suitable for complete resection. Complications are related mainly to thermal injuries to the nearest organs, such as the biliary tract, duodenum, portal vein and transverse colon, and the prevalence of such injuries is ≈24%. Promising results have come from the association of RFA with radiochemotherapy or systemic chemotherapy: median survival is 25.6 months with an intra-abdominal morbidity rate of 26.2% [23].

6.3 Preoperative Radiotherapy for Borderline Resectable and Unresectable Disease

A preliminary consideration on the use of preoperative radiotherapy is to discriminate between localized resectable disease and unresectable advanced tumors. This is because treatment goals and consequent treatment approaches will be different between the two groups of tumors with regard to the choice of chemotherapy association (i.e., with 5-Fluorouracil (5FU), capecitabine or gemcitabine) and the treatment dose and volume of radiotherapy

However, there is increasing awareness of a distinct intermediate group of patients who show locally advanced tumors that are borderline resectable. They can be defined according to several parameters:

- tumors confined to the pancreatic bed and nodes without distant metastasis;
- arterial involvement (including encasement of the gastroduodenal artery, short segment encasement or abutment of the hepatic artery (but not the celiac axis), and abutment of the superior mesenteric artery with circumpherential involvement of ≤180°);
- involvement of the superior mesenteric or portal vein, including abutment, lumen constriction and encasement;
- short segment occlusion from thrombosis or constriction is included if vessel length proximal or distal to the occlusion allows vascular reconstruction.

Other parameters combined with local resectability include suspected liver and/or peritoneal metastasis or low performance status.

6.3.1 Rationale and Method

Preoperative radiotherapy, combined with chemotherapy, has a strong *rationale* from oncological and radiobiological viewpoints. Firstly, a rapid start of local and systemic therapy shortly after the diagnosis rather than several weeks after possible surgery is important. Secondly, the untreated tumor is relatively well perfused and so there is less risk of radioresistance from hypoxia. Thirdly, the time interval for neoadjuvant treatment allows assessment for aggressive tumors with rapid onset of metastasis to avoid futile attempts at surgical intervention. Fourthly, disease downstaging can potentially render operable a previous borderline or unresectable tumor.

Patients with locally advanced disease rarely benefit from irradiation of regional lymph nodes that increases gastrointestinal toxicity with ensuing treatment interruptions and decrease in activity. Therefore, the clinical target volume (CTV) is confined to the gross tumor volume (GTV), as delineated by the radiation oncologist with contrast-enhanced CT, MRI and CT-PET integrated with the radiotherapy CT simulation images. These include the infiltrated vascular areas where tumor regression could allow subsequent resection. Before delineating these volumes, discussion with the surgeon, diagnostic radiologist and medical oncologist to decide the aim of therapy can be very helpful.

The CTV is then enlarged selectively (5–10 mm) along the longitudinal, axial and anteroposterior axis to take into account organ motion and uncertainties in patient repositioning for radiotherapy sessions to obtain the planning target volume (PTV) that must receive ≥95% of the prescribed dose. The liver, kidneys, spinal cord, stomach and duodenum are dose-limiting organs. The radiation oncologist must compromise among different dose contributions to the PTV from three-dimensional conformed beams along anteroposterior and laterolateral orientations to keep these organs within acute and late tolerance dose constraints. The linear accelerator X-ray energy must be ≥6 MV (preferably 15 MV or 18 MV). The prescribed dose ranges from 45 Gy to 50.4 Gy in 25–28 daily fractions, whereas shorter regimens of 30 Gy in 10 daily fractions are used in those with poor performance status. Three-dimensional conformal radiotherapy (3DCRT) is the standard and intensity-modulated radiation therapy (IMRT) can be used to increase the dose contribution with simultaneous boost (SIB) to part of the PTV without increasing toxicity.

6.3.2 Results

Despite widespread opinion that neoadjuvant chemoradiotherapy may convert locally advanced pancreatic tumors to resection, preliminary stringent definitions of resectability are necessary to evaluate the true frequency of successful downstaging. In fact, two early series from Memorial Sloan–Kettering Cancer Center (MSKCC) and MD Anderson Cancer Center (MDACC) show that true unresectable patients were converted to resectability in only 1 out of 87 and 6 out of 114 cases, respectively. Other data from MDACC show that, after gemcitabine-based chemoradiotherapy, almost 40% of borderline resectable patients underwent resection, R0 in 94% of cases, with median overall survival of 40 months [24]. Even high-resolution CT restaging after preoperative treatment may underestimate the number of patients suitable for resection because inflammation may obliterate the fat plane between the tumor and the vessel, whereas margin vessel scars may simulate tumors. In the Duke University experience, 11 of 49 patients considered unresectable at restaging CT were resected successfully, and in 6 patients no viable tumor was found. Therefore, other surrogates of response must also be considered, such as pain disappearance, large decrease in cancer antigen (Ca)19.9 values, and overall decrease in tumor size. More recent data from a meta-analysis on 536 patients showed a resectability rate of 65.8% in the initially defined resectable group and 31.6% in the initially borderline resectable group, and median survival was similar in resected patients of both groups [25].

6.4 Medical Oncology with a Focus on Neoadjuvant Therapy

Pancreatic cancer is the seventh most frequent cancer and the fifth most common cause of cancer-related death in Europe. The overall 5-year survival rate is <5%. The only potentially curative treatment is resection, but only 15–20% of patients are resectable at presentation. The high mortality rate is related to late diagnosis, early metastases, and poor response to medical treatments.

Until recently, the approach for patients with metastatic disease was gemcitabine; there have been many phase-III studies looking at gemcitabine-based doublets. However, trends for improvements were observed in the combination arms without statistically significant improvement in overall survival. Only a pooled analysis by Heinemann et al. from five studies of gemcitabine plus a platinum analog showed a statistically significant improvement in overall survival. A recent phase-III trial employing a combination of 5FU, leucovorin, irinotecan and oxaliplatin (FOLFIRINOX) *vs* gemcitabine showed a significant improvement in median survival rates (from 6.8 months with gemcitabine to 11.1 months with FOLFIRINOX), and in progression-free survival (from 3.4 months to 6,4 months). However, the FOLFIRINOX regimen should be chosen only for certain patients (younger men, good performance status, low bilirubin levels) because of the high toxicity profile (grade-3 and -4 myelosuppression and fatigue). Febrile neutropenia occurred in 5% of patients receiving FOLFIRINOX, and ≈42% of patients required granulocyte-colony simulating factor. Thus, modified regimens are likely to be developed to reduce toxicity without affecting efficacy. In this study, tumors arose from the head of the pancreas in <40% of patients, suggesting that only a small percentage of patients had biliary stents *in situ* and consequently a low risk of ascending cholangitis and biliary sepsis. Furthermore, performance status may influence the choice of treatment: only patients with a good Eastern Cooperative Oncology Group (ECOG) performance status should receive combination therapy, whereas monotherapy with gemcitabine should be used in patients with worse performance status. Currently, FOLFIRINOX is tested in locally advanced disease and neoadjuvant settings.

A new drug is nab-paclitaxel, an albumin-stabilized paclitaxel formulation that showed clinical activity when administered in combination with gemcitabine. It may be useful in advanced pancreatic cancer because albumin-binding proteins such as secreted protein acidic and rich in cysteine (SPARC) are overexpressed in some patients. This drug has not been approved for pancreatic cancer. Nevertheless, data from a phase-II trial in terms of response rate and decreases in Ca19.9 levels have led to a promising phase-III study.

Targeted therapeutic agents are disappointing for various clinical and biological reasons. Erlotinib, bevacizumab and cetuximab have been evaluated in this setting, but only erlotinib has shown a very modest improvement in median survival. Thus, there is no evidence supporting the use of biological agents in pancreatic cancer.

Patients with locally advanced pancreatic cancer need to be treated differently from those with metastatic disease. Phase-III studies of gemcitabine-based combinations have included patients with locally advanced and metastatic disease together that indeed should have been distinguished. The use of additional radiotherapy also needs to be taken into consideration. Trials comparing chemoradiotherapy with chemotherapy alone reported contradictory results: whether sequencing of chemoradiotherapy and chemotherapy itself are necessary remains an open question. A systematic review of trials of chemoradiotherapy in patients without progression after 3 months of treatment with gemcitabine demonstrated an improvement of survival with chemoradiotherapy. Depending on the definition of borderline disease, the percentage of patients converted to be able to undergo successful surgery ranges from 1% to 30%. Borderline-resectable disease represents a distinct category defined by radiological findings and is open to interpretation by radiologists and surgeons. Retrospective and phase-II prospective studies presented at the 2012 American Society of Clinical Oncology (ASCO) Annual Meeting showed that neoadjuvant chemoradiotherapy was associated with higher rates of resection of negative margins and better survival. Prospective studies of novel agents or combination regimens are needed in this setting.

In the case of resectable pancreatic disease, an initial approach involving neoadjuvant therapy may provide advantages, such as early delivery of systemic treatment, downstaging of borderline-resectable disease, and exclusion from surgery in patients with early progression during treatment. Evidence to support neoadjuvant chemoradiotherapy was established from phase-II trials that showed trends towards improved resectability and survival. However, randomized trials comparing neoadjuvant therapy followed by resection to upfront resection or a neoadjuvant approach *vs* the adjuvant approach are not available. A large meta-analysis involving 11 studies and 4,394 patients showed that about one-third of patients with unresectable disease at diagnosis may undergo successful resection after neoadjuvant therapy. On the basis of a promising outcome in metastatic cancer, it is likely that neoadjuvant FOLFIRINOX could improve surgical outcome. Combination chemotherapy and multimodal therapy for non-metastatic stages of disease (locally advanced, borderline-resectable and resectable disease) are promising, but the optimal treatment approach needs to be clarified.

6.5 Endoscopic Diagnosis and Stenting for Biliary and Duodenal Obstruction

Since its early days, endoscopic ultrasonography (EUS) proved an accurate imaging modality for the gastrointestinal tract, the pancreas and extrahepatic biliary tree. Introduction of linear-array echoendoscopes and the possibility of carrying out EUS-guided fine-needle biopsies (FNAs), increased the diagnostic yield of EUS and allowed the evolution for interventional methods mainly for diseases of the pancreas and biliary tract.

In patients with solid pancreatic masses, the sensitivity, specificity, positive and negative predictive value of EUS-FNA reaches 95%, 100%, 100% and 85%, respectively. Unfortunately the sensitivity of EUS-FNA is lower for the differential diagnosis of chronic pancreatitis and pancreatic cancer (75%). New methods are developing in this field, particularly contrast-enhanced harmonic endoscopic ultrasound (CE-EUS) and EUS elastography (EUS-EG).

CE-EUS offers information on vascularization and indicates the blood-flow patterns of tissues. The most used agent approved in the European Union is SonoVue® (Bracco, Italy), which contains phospholipid-stabilized microbubbles of sulfur hexafluoride, which are stable and pressure-resistant. CE-EUS has been used for pancreatic cancer. Color and power Doppler CE-EUS demonstrate a relatively hypovascular pattern in pancreatic adenocarcinoma with a sensitivity and specificity comparable with that seen with cytopathology, and an accuracy of 90% in the differential diagnosis of pancreatic cancer and chronic pancreatitis. EUS-EG is a promising modality with high accuracy for the differential diagnosis of solid pancreatic tumors. Introduction of second-generation EUS-EG has allowed the quantitative analysis of tissue stiffness. Malignant lesions are harder, with heterogeneous elastic properties with respect to benign tumors. In a recent study, sensitivity, specificity and overall accuracy were 100%, 85.5%, and 94%, respectively [26].

Many interventional EUS-guided methods have been reported. EUS can guide biliary drainage if endoscopic retrograde cholangiopancreatography (ERCP) is unsuccessful in patients affected by obstructive jaundice. However, this procedure carries a risk of severe morbidity, including bile leakage, bleeding or pneumoperitoneum. EUS-guided oncologic interventions have been described. Injection of various chemotherapeutic agents in advanced pancreatic cancer or EUS-guided brachytherapy may be useful in temporary pain relief with marginal survival benefit. EUS-guided celiac plexus block using ethanol and bupivacaine is a safe procedure with proven efficacy with a complication rate <2% in the treatment of pancreatic cancer pain [27]. Most of these interventional EUS-guided methods are experimental, and more innovations and endoscopic devices are necessary to safely carry out these procedures.

The goal of palliative care is to prevent and relieve suffering and support the best possible quality of life for patients and their families, regardless of the state of the disease. Obstruction is a major complication of gastrointestinal cancers. Obstructive jaundice is a common complication of pancreatic cancer; endoscopic stenting is the standard treatment. Endobiliary stents can be plastic or self-expanding metal stents (SEMS).

Most plastic stents are made of polyethylene; diameters range from 5 F to 11.5 F. The most popular caliber is 10 F with a length of 7–10 mm. SEMS are made of different materials and are all equally effective in palliating biliary

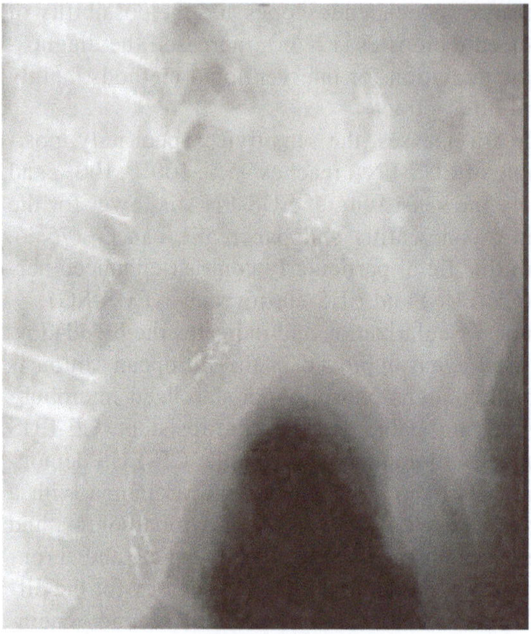

Fig. 6.6 Biliary self-expanding metal stent

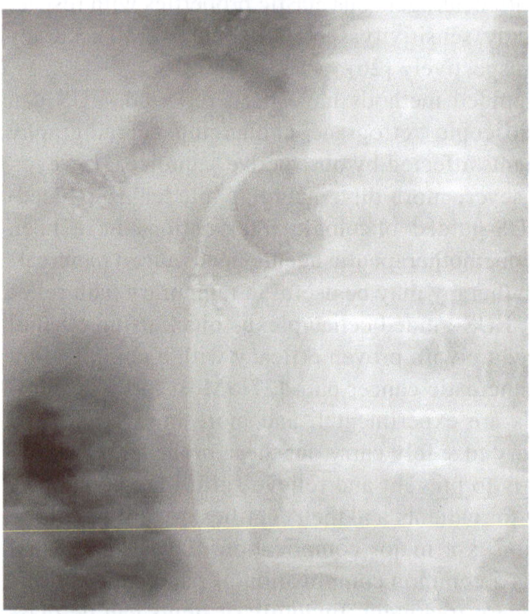

Fig. 6.7 Biliary and duodenal self-expanding metal stent

obstruction (Fig. 6.6). Their larger caliber (10 mm) allows a longer patency and avoids repeated endoscopic sessions for stent exchange. Nevertheless, SEMS are cost-effective in patients with life expectancy >3 months. Partially and totally covered SEMS have been developed to prevent cancer ingrowth. Multiple studies have compared uncovered with partially covered and totally covered SEMS and found no difference in stent patency [28]. In addition, severe adverse events occurred more frequently in partially covered SEMS, mainly due to stent migration. Experimental treatment with drug-eluting metal stents has been proposed to extend the duration of biliary patency. Paclitaxel was mixed with polyurethane and tetrahydrofuran to create a stent membrane that slowly released the drug. The mean patency of these stents was 429 days in 21 patients with unresectable malignant biliary obstruction [29]. Pancreatic cancer is the most common cause of malignant gastroduodenal obstruction and occurs in 11–20% of patients. Endoscopic palliation with duodenal SEMS is the treatment of choice (Fig. 6.7). Duodenal SEMS are similar to biliary, but are longer (6–12 cm), larger (18–23 mm) and uncovered to prevent migration and ampulary occlusion. Technical success is achievable in 92–100% of patients and clinical success in 81–92% [30]. Complications range from 11% to 43%, generally due to the migration or occlusion of stents. Endoscopic enteral stenting appears to be cost-effective compared with surgical bypass with less morbidity and comparable improvement in quality of life.

References

1. D'Onofrio M, Gallotti A, Falconi M et al (2010) Acoustic radiation force impulse ultrasound imaging of pancreatic cystic lesions: preliminary results. Pancreas 39:939-40
2. Kim JH, Park SH, Yu ES, et al (2010) Visually isoattenuating pancreatic adenocarcinoma at dynamic-enhanced CT: frequency, clinical and pathologic characteristics, and diagnosis at imaging examinations. Radiology 257:87-96
3. Tranchart H, Gaujoux S, Rebours V et al (2012) Preoperative CT scan helps to predict the occurrence of severe pancreatic fistula after pancreaticoduodenectomy. Ann Surg 256:139-45
4. Boraschi P, Donati F, Gigoni R et al (2010) Diffusion-weighted MRI in the characterization of cystic pancreatic lesions: usefulness of ADC values. Magn Reson Imaging 28:1447-55
5. Sandrasegaran K, Akisik FM, Patel AA et al (2011) Diffusion-weighted imaging in characterization of cystic pancreatic lesions. Clin Radiol. 2011 Sep 66:808-14
6. Hur BY, Lee JM, Lee JE et al (2012) Magnetic resonance imaging findings of the mass-forming type of autoimmune pancreatitis: comparison with pancreatic adenocarcinoma. J Magn Reson Imaging 36:188-97
7. Holzapfel K, Reiser-Erkan C, Fingerle A et al (2011) Comparison of diffusion-weighted MR imaging and multidetector-row CT in the detection of liver metastases in patients operated for pancreatic cancer. Abdom Imaging 36:179–184
8. Wu LM, Hu JN, Hua J et al (2012) Diagnostic value of diffusion-weighted magnetic resonance imaging compared with fluorodeoxyglucose positron emission tomography/computed tomography for pancreatic malignancy: A meta-analysis using a hierarchical regression model. J Gastroenterol Hepatol. 2012 27:1027-35
9. Diener MK, Fitzmaurice C, Schwarzer G et al (2011) Pylorus-preserving pancreaticoduodenectomy (pp Whipple) versus pancreaticoduodenectomy (classic Whipple) for surgical treatment of periampullary and pancreatic carcinoma. Cochrane Database Syst Rev 11:CD006053
10. Nimura Y, Nagino M, Takao S et al (2012) Standard versus extended lymphadenectomy in radical pancreatoduodenectomy for ductal adenocarcinoma of the head of the pancreas. J Hepatobiliary Pancreat 19:230–241
11. Berger AC, Howard TJ, Kennedy EP et al (2009) Does Type of Pancreaticojejunostomy af-

ter Pancreaticoduodenectomy decrease Rate of Pancreatic Fistula? A Randomized, Prospective, Dual-Institution Trial. J Am Coll Surg 208:738–749

12. Peng SY, Wang JW, Lau WJ et al (2007) Conventional Versus Binding Pancreaticojejunostomy after pancreaticoduodenectomy. Ann Surg 245:692–698
13. Gurusamy KS, Koti R, Fusai G et al (2012) Somatostatin analogues for pancreatic surgery (Review) Cochrane Database Syst Rev. 2012 Jun 13:CD008370
14. Xiong JJ, Altkaf K, Mukherjee R et al (2012) Systematic review and meta-analysis of outcomes after intraoperative pancreatic duct stent placement during pancreaticoduodenectomy. Br J Surg 99:1050-61
15. Tewari a, Hazrah P, Kumar V et al (2010) Options of restorative pancreaticoenteric anastomosis following pancreaticoduodenectomy: A review. Surg Oncol. 19:17-26
16. Carrere N, Sauvanet A, Goere D et al (2006) Pancreaticoduodenectomy with Mesentericoportal Vein Resection for Adenocarcinoma of the Pancreatic Head. World J Surg 30:1526–1535
17. Castleberry AW, White RR, De La Fuente SG et al (2012) The Impact of Vascular Resection on Early Postoperative Outcomes after Pancreaticoduodenectomy: An Analysis of the American College of Surgeons National Surgical Quality Improvement Program Database. Ann Surg Oncol [Epub ahead of print]
18. Zeh EJ, Zureikat AH, Secrest A et al (2012) Outcomes After Robot-Assisted Pancreaticoduodenectomy for Periampullary Lesions. Ann Surg 19:864–870
19. Daouadi M, Zureikat AH, Zenati MS et al (2012) Robot-Assisted Minimally Invasive Distal Pancreatectomy Is Superior to the Laparoscopic Technique. Ann Surg [Epub ahead of print]
20. Venkat R, Barish E, Richard DS et al (2012) Laparoscopic Distal Pancreatectomy Is Associated With Significantly Less Overall Morbidity Compared to the Open Technique. Ann Surg 255:1048–1059
21. Fox AM, Pitzul K, Bhojani F et al (2012) Comparison of outcomes and costs between laparoscopic distal pancreatectomy and open resection at a single center. Surg Endosc 26:1220–1230
22. Tsiouris A, Cogan CM, Velanovich V et al (2011) Distal pancreatectomy with or without splenectomy: comparison of postoperative outcomes and surrogates of splenic function. HPB (Oxford) 13:738-44
23. Cantore M, Girelli R, Mambrini A et al (2012) Combined modality treatment for patients with locally advanced pancreatic adenocarcinoma. Br J Surg 99:1083-8
24. Katz MH, Pisters PW, Evans DB et al (2008) Borderline resectable pancreatic cancer: the importance of this emerging stage of disease. J Am Coll Surg 206:833-46
25. Assifi MM, Lu X, Eibl G, et al (2011) Neoadjuvant therapy in pancreatic adenocarcinoma: a meta-analysis of phase II trials. Surgery 150:466-73
26. Dawwas MF, Taha H, Leeds JS et al (2012) Diagnostic accuracy of quantitative EUS elastography for discriminating malignant from benign solid pancreatic masses: a prospective, single-center study. Gastrointest Endosc 76:953-61
27. Puli SR, Reddy JB, Bechtold ML et al (2012) EUS-guided celiac plexus neurolysis for pain due to chronic pancreatitis or pancreatic cancer pain: a meta-analysis and systematic review. Dig Dis Sci 54:2330-7
28. Yoon WJ, Lee JK, Lee KH et al (2006) A comparison of covered and uncovered Wallstents for the management of distal malignant biliary obstruction. Gastrointest Endosc 63:996-1000
29. Suk KT, Kim JW, Kim HS et al (2007) Human application of a metallic stent covered with a paclitaxel-incorporated membrane for malignant biliary obstruction: multicenter pilot study. Gastrointest Endosc 66:798-803
30. Maetani I, Tada T, Ukita T et al (2004) Comparison of duodenal stent placement with surgical gastrojejunostomy for palliation in patients with duodenal obstructions caused by pancreaticobiliary malignancies. Endoscopy 36:73-8

7 Pancreatic Cystic Tumors

Marco Farsi, Fabio Francesco di Mola and Pierluigi di Sebastiano

7.1 Introduction

Pancreatic cystic tumors represent a diagnostic and therapeutic challenge. These lesions are being discovered incidentally because multidetector computed tomography (MDCT) is being used more often for the diagnosis of abdominal complaints. Over the past decade, there has been a tenfold increased incidence of pancreatic cystic tumors due to increased use of CT and endoscopic ultrasound (EUS) [1]. There is an increased number of resected cystic lesions because more patients with pancreatic cystic lesions are being referred to hepatopancreatobiliary (HPB) surgeons [1, 2].

The vast majority of pancreatic cystic lesions are cystic neoplasms [3] whereas pseudocysts account for ≈30%. Rarely, non-neoplastic cysts are true congenital cysts, polycystic disease, or cystic fibrosis. Cystic pancreatic neoplasms account for 1–20% of all primary pancreatic tumors (1).

The first authors to propose a classification for pancreatic cystic lesions were Compagno and Oertl [4]. The tumors were divided into serous cystic neoplasms (benign) and mucinous cystic neoplasms (MCNs) with overt and latent malignancy. More recently, Basturk and Adsay [2] reported a classification based on pathologic, pathogenetic and biologic features (Table 7.1). They classified cystic lesions of the pancreas on presumed cell origin. In this classification, neoplastic cysts are 60%, and the most frequent are those from a ductal lineage: mucinous type (30%) and serous (clear cell) type (20%). Solid

M. Farsi (✉)
Department of Oncology, Oncologic Surgery Unit, Careggi Hospital, Florence, Italy
e-mail: marcofarsi@tin.it

F. di Mola · P. di Sebastiano
Oncologic Surgery Unit, Policlinico SS. Annunziata
ASL 2 Chieti, Italy

A. Valeri et al. (eds.), *What's New in Surgical Oncology*,
DOI: 10.1007/978-88-470-5310-6_7, © Springer-Verlag Italia 2013

Table 7.1 Types of cystic lesions in the pancreas. Reproduced with permission from [2]

Injury-related and inflammation-related cysts (30%)
• Pseudocyst • Paraduodenal wall cyst • Infection-related cysts
Neoplastic cysts (60%)
Ductal lineage *Mucinous type (30%)* • Intraductal papillary mucinous neoplasm • Mucinous cystic neoplasm • Intraductal oncocytic papillary neoplasm • "Retention cyst", "mucocele" and "mucinous non-neoplastic cyst" • Cystic change in ordinary ductal adenocarcinoma • Other invasive carcinomas *Serous (clear-cell) type (20%)* • Serous cystadenoma • Oligocystic (macrocystic) variant of serous cystadenoma • von Hippel-Lindau syndrome and associated pancreatic cysts • Serous cystadenocarcinoma *Not otherwise specified* • Intraductal tubular carcinoma **Endocrine lineage (< 5%)** • Cystic pancreatic endocrine neoplasm **Acinar lineage (< 1%)** • Acinar cell cystadenoma (cystic acinar transformation) • Acinar cell cystadenocarcinoma • Cystic/intraductal acinar cell carcinoma **Endothelial lineage (< 1%)** • Lymphangioma **Mesenchymal lineage (< 1%)** **Undetermined lineage (5%)** • Solid-pseudopapillary neoplasm **Other** • Mature cystic teratoma
Congenital cysts (< 1%)
• Duplication (enterogenous) cysts • Duodenal diverticula • Others
Miscellaneous cysts (< 5%)
• Lymphoepithelial cyst • Squamoid cyst of pancreatic ducts • Epidermoid cysts within intrapancreatic accessory spleen • Cystic hamartoma • Endometriosic cysts • Secondary tumors

pseudopapillary neoplasms are ≈5% and in the undetermined lineage group. The World Health Organization [5] has classified cystic tumors of the pancreas by considering the most frequent and important ones. Cystic neoplasms are divided into benign (acinar cystadenoma and serous cystoadenoma, SCA), premalignant lesions (neoplasms with low-, intermediate- or high-grade dysplasia) and malignant (cystoadenocarcinoma or invasive associated carcinoma, solid pseudo-papillary neoplasms).

7.2 Serous Cystic Neoplasms

SCAs arise from the centracinar cell/intercalated duct system. They are more frequent in females than males (2:1) and present at a mean age of 75 years. SCAs usually present as large masses measuring up to 25 cm, with 50% located within the head of the pancreas. They are usually single, but multifocal lesions may be associated with von Hippel–Lindau disease [7]. Most patients present with abdominal fullness, vomiting, dyspepsia, weight loss and other vague symptoms [1, 8]; jaundice may be observed; 30% of cases are asymptomatic.

Macroscopically, their surface shows numerous small, thin-walled cysts (spongelike or honeycomb appearance) arranged around a central stellate scar (present in 13–18%) caused by calcification of fibrous stroma (Fig. 7.1). There is no communication with the Wirsung duct. Microscopically, they have a single layer of cuboidal or flattened cells lining small cysts [2]. SCAs express cytokeratins (AE1/AE3, CAM 5.2, CK7, CK8, CK18,CK19) and α-inhibin without immunoreactivity to carcinoembryonic antigen (CEA). The rare oligocystic (macrocystic) variant is composed of larger loculi without a central scar and sometimes making the differential diagnoses with mucinous tumors and pseudocysts is difficult [2].

In 90% of patients, it is possible to make the correct diagnosis with clinical and imaging findings. Ultrasound is usually the first step in diagnostic

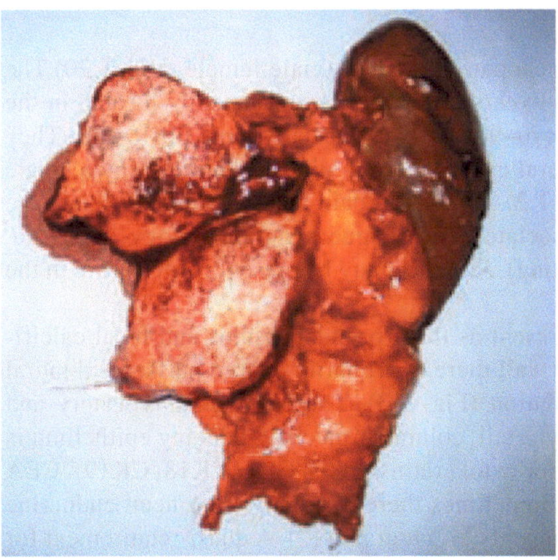

Fig. 7.1 Microcystic serous adenoma in the body of the pancreas. The cut surface shows numerous small, thin-walled cysts arranged around a central stellate scar

imaging for suspect SCAs, but there are two reasons why the microcystic pattern may not be recognized: (i) in spongelike masses, the multiplicity of the small cysts and the fibrous stroma appears as a solid tumor and (ii) in cases of mixed tumors, the macrocystic component conceals the microcystic component, resulting in a macrocystic mass [9].

Unenhanced CT shows from a poorly defined to a thin, well-defined capsule. Contrast-enhanced CT demonstrates enhancement of septa and well-delineated small cysts in honeycomb patterns with central scars and capsulae enhancement [10]. Sometimes, the distal pancreas may be atrophic and the common bile duct dilated. Magnetic resonance imaging (MRI) shows a honeycomb shape with low signal intensity on T1-weighted images and high intensity on T2-weighted images. It is possible to see small cysts and septa as high signal, grape-like clusters on T2-weighted images. Unlike CT, central calcification is rarely visualized with MRI [1]. EUS may help in the diagnosis if the cysts are unilocular and similar to mucinous neoplasms. The analysis of aspirated fluid demonstrates the absence of mucin.

7.2.1 Therapy

The management of asymptomatic pancreatic SCAs is observation with serial follow-up using axial imaging studies. The median growth rate for this neoplasm is 0.6 cm/year, whereas it is significantly greater in large (>4 cm) SCAs, which are more likely to be symptomatic. Therefore, expectant management is reasonable in small asymptomatic tumors. Resection is recommended for large SCAs regardless of the presence or absence of symptoms [11].

7.3 MCNs

MCNs can be present in perimenopausal females (male:female ratio, 1:20) The mean age of presentation is 48 years. They are more frequently located in the body and tail of the pancreas (70–90%) and are usually large (7–10 cm). They are usually composed by several cysts >2 cm in diameter but also by a single macrocystic lesion [12] (Fig. 7.2). Epigastric pain and abdominal fullness are more frequent symptoms associated with vague symptomatology (anorexia, weight loss, nausea and vomiting). Jaundice may be present if MCNs are in the head of the pancreas.

These cystic neoplasms present as thick pseudocapsules and focal calcification at the periphery. In the wall there is primarily a large mass, solid mural nodules, and "velvety" papillation (Fig. 7.3). The cyst contains watery and mucoid fluid. Microscopically, a tall, columnar mucin-producing epithelium is demonstrated that is positive for cytokeratins (CK7, CK8, CK18, CK19), CEA and mucin5AC (MUC5AC). Sometimes there is positivity to neuroendocrine markers such as synaptophysin and chromogranin [2]. A quasi-requirement for

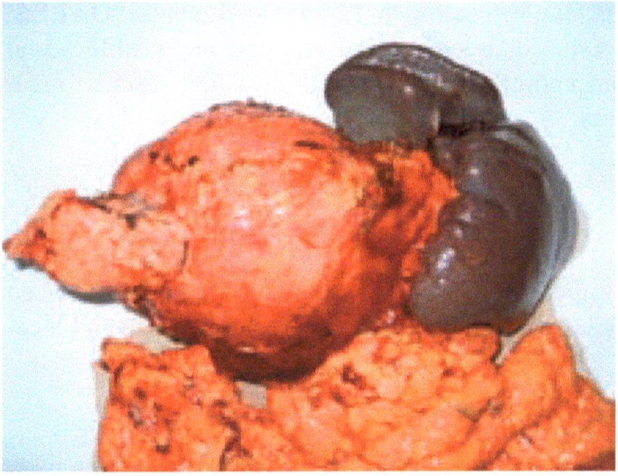

Fig. 7.2 Mucinous cystoadenoma of the pancreas of a 60-year-old female patient. Macroscopic appearance after distal spleno-pancreatectomy

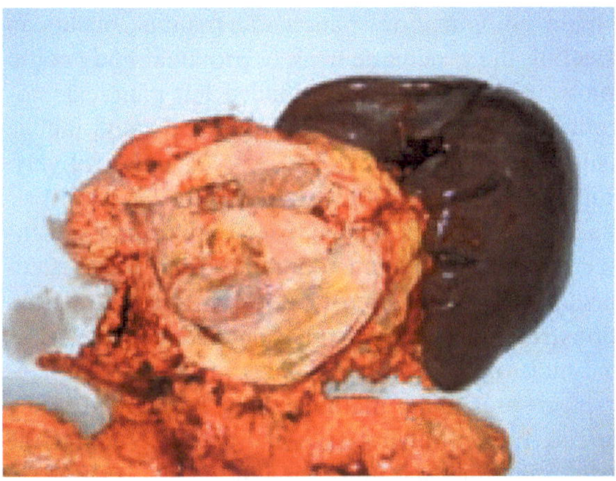

Fig. 7.3 Mucinous cystoadenoma of the pancreas (cut surface). Velvety papillations are present in the cyst wall

the diagnosis is densely packed spindle cells with sparse cytoplasm and uniform, elongated nuclei (ovarian stroma). MCNs regularly express progesterone receptors and, to lesser degree, estrogen receptors. Cells in the stroma stain for α-inhibin an calretinin.

CT shows a large mass with “near water” density, as well as enhancement of septa and the peripheral wall. Typical calcifications (i.e. “eggshell” calcifications) in the peripheral wall and septa may indicate malignancy, in 95% of patients [6]. Also, mural nodules and papillary excrescences are predictive of cystoadenocarcinoma. In these cases, local invasion by obliteration of fat planes and the margins of adjacent organs may be demonstrated [1]. T1-weighted MRI may demonstrate hypodense signal intensity in case of fluid content, whereas protein-based or hemorrhagic liquids appears with hyperdense signal intensity.

Septa and mural nodules may be seen with T2-weighted images. On EUS, mucinous neoplasms are revealed as complex cysts, and are visible septal mural nodules, calcifications and other signs of local invasion, vascular invasion, and lymph-node masses.

7.3.1 Therapy

The therapy of MCNs is surgical excision. This treatment may be influenced by patient age, surgical risk, as well as the histological features, size and location of the tumor.

7.3.1.1 Distal Pancreatic Resection

The localization of mucinous cystic adenomas is often in the pancreatic body or tail, so distal pancreatectomy is the procedure of choice. It is a safe procedure in high-volume centers (morbidity ranges from 5% to 50% and the mortality rate is 0%) and its main complication, pancreatic fistulas, occurs in 15–20% of cases. MCNs affecting the pancreatic neck or proximal body could require an extended right or, more frequently, an extended left pancreatectomy. These extended resections of normal pancreatic tissue may induce endocrine and exocrine insufficiency in 30–35% and 15–20%, respectively, which in a benign or premalignant disease could be important.

Distal pancreatectomy can be undertaken with splenectomy or in a spleen-preserving fashion. Studies comparing patients undergoing distal pancreatectomy with or without splenectomy show no significant differences in relation to perioperative complications, mean operation time, pancreatic fistula rate, duration of hospital stay, and mortality. However, to carry out complete oncological lymphadenectomy, spleen-preserving methods must be avoided in the presence of large tumors or risk factors for invasive malignancy, such as the size of the lesion, eggshell calcifications and mural nodules.

Spleen preservation can be undertaken with or without preservation of the splenic artery and vein [13]. Although the procedure without preservation of the splenic artery and vein appears to be technically less difficult and can be achieved in a shorter operating time, it has been associated with a higher incidence of vascular insufficiency in the spleen.

7.3.1.2 Central Pancreatectomy

MCNs located at the proximal body or neck of the pancreas are suitable for central pancreatectomy. Although the procedure is associated with low mortality, the overall morbidity ranges from 25% to 35%, and the overall prevalence of pancreatic fistulas is 22–45%. This method preserves the spleen and, compared with extended left pancreatectomy or pancreatico-duodenectomy, also preserves endocrine and exocrine functions [14]. Indeed, the prevalence of endocrine and exocrine insufficiency after central pancreatectomy has been reported to be 4–7% and 5–8%, respectively. This surgical method is technically demanding, and associated with a higher prevalence of postoperative complications as well as with the risk of recurrence from potentially residual neoplasms.

7.3.1.3 Tumor Enucleation

Tumor enucleation has been proposed for patients with MCNs <2 cm (which carry a very low probability of malignancy). The benign features and superficial localization of these tumors direct the choice of surgical strategy. Enucleation avoids postoperative pancreatic insufficiency and can be done without the risk of recurrence. However, it has been associated with a higher prevalence of pancreatic fistulas (30–50%) [15].

7.3.1.4 Whipple Procedure

A major oncologic resection such as pancreaticoduodenectomy with or without pylorus-preserving surgery is recommended for MCNs localized in the head of the pancreas. Surgical mortality ranges from 0% to 5%, and is generally related to complications due to the pancreatic anastomosis. However, the most common postoperative complications are delayed gastric emptying and pancreatic fistulas, which occur in 5–10% and 6–20% of cases, respectively. When an enucleation is not possible or contraindicated, MCNs localized in the pancreatic head can be treated by a duodenum-preserving total pancreatic head resection (DPPHR). This procedure shows significant advantages when compared with pancreaticoduodenectomy in relation to postoperative rate of morbidity and mortality, glucose metabolism, hospitalization and cost.

7.3.1.5 Lymphadenectomy

Pancreatectomy with lymph-node dissection must be carried out whenever suspicion of malignancy exists. There is no evidence of invasive mucinous cystic adenocarcinoma with distant lymph-node metastases, so only locoregional lymphadenectomy is justified. In addition, the probability of malignancy is very low in cases of small MCNs without nodules, so lymphadenectomy can be avoided in these cases.

7.3.1.6 Laparoscopy

In patients with benign-appearing and small malignant lesions (<5 cm), a minimally invasive method must be considered. In general, the laparoscopic approach decreases the duration of hospital stay and minimizes the cosmetic impact of the surgical wound. Recent experiences from high-volume centers have demonstrated that laparoscopic left pancreatectomy for MCNs of the body and tail of the pancreas is feasible and safe. The complication rate of laparoscopic left pancreatectomy ranges between 15% and 20% with a mortality rate of 0% whereas, in spleen-preserving laparoscopic pancreatic resection, the overall morbidity ranges from 25% to 40%. The overall prevalence of pancreatic fistulas was 5–8% and 10–15% after laparoscopic spleen-preserving distal pancreatectomy and laparoscopic left pancreatectomy, respectively [16].

7.4 Intraductal Papillary Mucinous Neoplasms (IPMNs)

IPMNs are characterized by the intraductal proliferation of mucinous cells which form papillae and lead to cystic dilation of the pancreatic ducts to form masses [2]. Main-duct intraductal papillary mucinous neoplasms (MD-IPMNs) usually involve dilation of the main pancreatic ducts with or without the associated involvement of the branch ducts ("combined IPMNs"). Mucin production causes ductal ectasia and multiloculated masses (Fig. 7.4). In branch-duct intraductal papillary mucinous neoplasms (BD-IPMN), the side branches of the duct system are involved and the cystic lesions communicate with the non-dilated main pancreatic duct [1, 17].

IPMNs represent ≈1% of all pancreatic neoplasms and 25% of cystic neoplasms. The incidence in pancreatic resection specimens is 5% [2]. IPMNs occur slightly more frequently in men than women, with a mean age at diagnosis of 68 years. In 25% of patients, they are asymptomatic. If symptoms are present, the most frequent are abdominal pain (65%), weight loss (44%), pancreatitis (23%), diabetes mellitus (12%) and jaundice (17%). In 30% of cases, IPMNs can be associated with synchronous or metachronous benign and malignant tumors (digestive tract). This may be explained by the increased medical surveillance of patients with IPMNs and common genetic or extragenomic risk factors for IPMN and other tumors [18]. In some patients, elevated serum CEA (3.8%) and cancer antigen (CA19.9; 13.1%) are possible [19]. A total of 75% of MD-IPMNs are located in the head of the pancreas but tend to spread to the remaining pancreatic duct. BD-IPMNs are more frequent in uncinate processes but may be located in all the other sides of the pancreas. Microscopically, they can be classified into benign (adenoma), borderline (moderate dysplasia) and malignant (*in situ* carcinoma and invasive carcino-

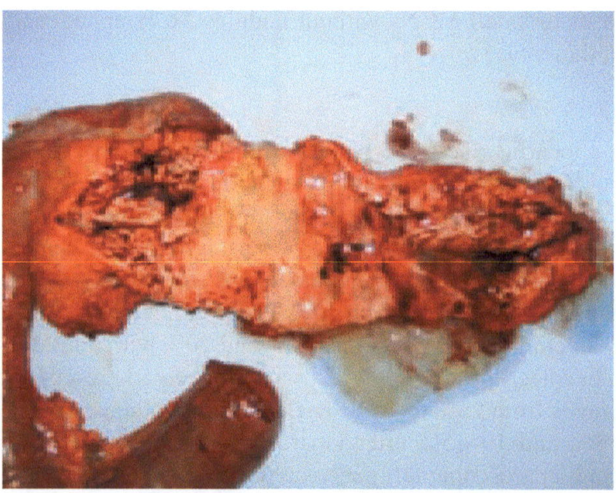

Fig. 7.4 Total pancreatico-duodenectomy for an intraductal papillary mucinous neoplasm. After incision of the pancreas, abundant quantities of mucin and gelatinous material are evident

ma). Very important and complicated is the histological patterns of papillae usually formed by columnar cells with a different spectrum of atypical cytoarchitecture.

Immunohistochemical patterns show four cell types according to MUC and CDX2. The type MUC2+/CDX2+ are intestinal type with a good prognosis, whereas MUC2-/CDX2-/MUC1+ is a pancreatobiliary type with a worse prognosis [18]. The malignancy rate is higher (49–92%) in MD-IPMNs than in BD-IPMNs (6–46%). It may be possible to recognize different grades of dysplasia within the same surgical specimen. Otherwise, the average age of patients with malignant MD- IPMNs is 6.4 years older than patients with adenoma or borderline tumors, which supports the theory of clonal progression to malignancy [18]. Larger size (>3 cm), thick cyst wall, proximal location, mural nodules, and mucin leakage from patulous ampullae are predictors of malignancy for IPMNs (20).

With respect to the genetic role in the pathogenesis of IPMNs, a high rate (65%) of KRAS mutations in these patients has been noted. Otherwise, several other genetic alterations may be present in IPMNs, such as activation of AKT/PKB and HER2/EGFR or mutation of STK11/LKB1. Many of these overexpressed genes are also highly expressed in pancreatic adenocarcinoma. Recently, some authors have suggested a role for the sonic hedgehog (SHH) pathway in IPMN pathogenesis, whereas fascin expression seems to be higher in borderline neoplasms and carcinomas than in adenomas, suggesting overexpression in the progression of IPMN [18].

On CT, it is possible to see the dilated and tortuous main pancreatic duct in MD-IPMNs, whereas BD-IPMNs appear as lobulated cystic lesions with characteristic grape-like clusters (Fig.7.5). MRI imaging (more in T2-weighted) is

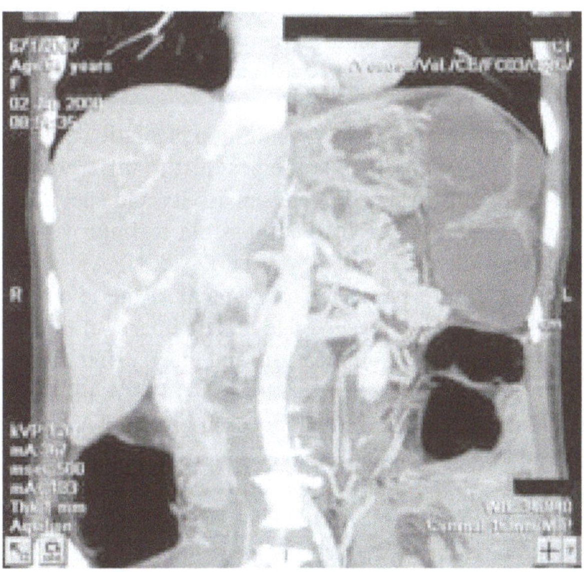

Fig. 7.5 Contrast-enhanced CT in a 64-year-old female patient with a diffuse intraductal papillary mucinous neoplasm

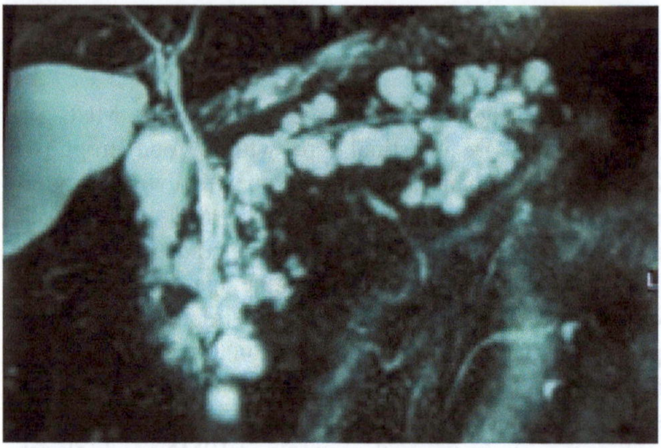

Fig. 7.6 MRI in a 65-year-old female patient with an intraductal papillary mucinous neoplasm of the entire pancreas

useful for demonstrating main-duct dilatation and the characteristics of cystic masses. Magnetic resonance cholangiopancreatography (MRCP) can show not only the main pancreatic duct, but also the cyst and its possible communication with the main duct. With MRCP, it may be possible to undertake a differential diagnosis between MD-IPMNs and BD-IPMNs [1]. Secretin-stimulated MRI (Fig. 7.6) can be used to highlight the ductal anatomy, and it is commonly used in pancreatic centers, but its superiority to non-secretin studies in the evaluation of IPMNs has not been proven [21]. ERCP is helpful if the triad of Ohashi (bulging ampulla of Vater, mucin secretion, dilated pancreatic duct) is present. The injection of contrast may demonstrate intraluminal filling defects representing small papillary projections (1).

EUS is useful for the assessment of the characteristics of cysts, ductal anatomy, pancreatic parenchyma, peripancreatic invasion of tumor, and lymphadenopathy as well as other signs of malignancy. EUS is operator-dependent with low sensitivity (50–60%) [1, 10].

Use of EUS with fine-needle aspiration is increasing in pancreatic centers. The fluid analysis for CEA (< or > 192 ng/mL) is the best test to differentiate a mucinous cyst from a non-mucinous cyst [22]. The sensitivity and specificity for CEA is 73% and 84%, respectively, but it is possible to improve the analysis by combining CEA and molecular analyses (total DNA, KRAS mutation). It is recommended that the fluid be sent for assessment of the levels of CEA, amylase, lipase and/or cytology. Analyses of levels of lipase and amylase can aid determination of ductal communication and may differentiate mucinous neoplasms from IPMNs [21]. High viscosity (>1.6 Pa·s) and CEA >6,000 ng/mL is diagnostic for mucinous cystoadenocarcinoma. CEA levels <6,000 ng/mL and viscosity >1.6 Pa·s are predictive of mucinous cystoadenomas [23]. Recently, some authors stated that the level of CEA in cyst fluid is not predictive of invasive cancer in patients with IPMNs [24]. Table 7.2 shows the most important fluid characteristics of cystic lesions of the pancreas.

Table 7.2 Most important characteristics in the fluid patterns of cystic lesions of the pancreas after endoscopic ultrasound-fine-needle aspiration

Pancreatic cysts	Fluid analyses
Pseudocyst	↑ Amylase ↓ Viscosity
Serous cystic neoplasm	↓ Amylase ↓ CEA ↓ CA19-9 ↓ Viscosity
Mucinous cystic neoplasm	↓ Amylase ↑ CEA ↑ CA 19-9 ↑ Viscosity ↑ Mucin ↑ Mucinous cells
Intraductal papillary mucinous neoplasms	↑ Amylase ↑ CEA ↑ Viscosity ↑ Mucin ↑ Mucinous cells

7.4.1 Therapy

The surgical planning to treat IPMN is often complex. Preoperative studies show a dilated pancreatic duct, but the intraductal mass is often too small to be detected. Indeed, because IPMNs extend along the pancreatic duct, it is important to rule out tumors in the margin. In addition, because of the overproduction of mucus, dilation can occur proximal and distal to the tumor, and neoplasm localization becomes problematic. The therapeutic recommendations for IPMNs are based on a consensus report and on case series from the past decade [20].

7.4.1.1 Non-surgical Approaches

Distinction between IPMNs involving the main duct (MD) or branch duct (BD) plays a central part in therapy. MD-IPMNs constitute an indication for surgery, whereas the treatment of BD-IPMNs is dependent upon clinical, morphological, and imaging criteria. In theory, endosonography with aspiration cytology could be used to determine the malignant potential of BD-IPMNs <3 cm in diameter. However, whether this examination is sufficient is controversial. Asymptomatic BD-IPMNs with a diameter <10 mm should merit annual follow-up, whereas lesions of diameter 10–20 mm should be monitored every 6–12 months. In BD-IPMNs of diameter >20 mm, the indication for surgery should be according to clinical status and discussed with the patient. According to published guidelines, BD-IPMN >3 cm should be resected because of malignant potential. Furthermore, surgery is indicated for symptoms, enlarged lymph nodes, or a distended main duct. However, if no changes have occurred after 2 years of monitoring, the interval of follow-up may be extended.

7.4.1.2 Surgical treatment of IPMNs

Due to the malignant potential of MD-IPMNs, surgery is essential [25]. Conversely, the need for resection for BD-IPMN needs to be defined according to the risk of malignancy. The probability of a malignant BD-IPMN ranges between 30% for symptomatic subjects and <5% in asymptomatic individuals. In case of unclear tumor malignancy, the indication for resection should be defined liberally because only surgical treatment offers an opportunity for cure.

Resections include pylorus-preserving pancreaticoduodenectomy, distal pancreatectomy, and total pancreatectomy in multifocal lesions. Intraoperative histological frozen sections are used to determine the extent of the resection. Tumor-free resection margins are required for all IPMNs. If higher-grade dysplasia is found in the resection margin, then the resection should be continued until a negative margin has been achieved, even at the risk of total pancreatectomy, depending on the age and condition of the patient.

7.5 Solid-pseudopapillary Neoplasms (SPNs)

SPNs are rare (1–2% of exocrine pancreas tumors and 4.6% of cystic neoplasms of the pancreas). Usually, they occur in the third or fourth decade in females (mean age, 28 years; male to female ratio, 1:20). Most SPNs are large (8–9 cm in diameter), often encapsulated, and distributed through the pancreas (Fig. 7.7). The cavities are not true cysts, but instead represent a necrotic/degenerative process [2]. The cut surface shows a variable appearance depending on the degree of hemorrhage and necrosis. This neoplasm is one of very few tumors for which the direction of differentiation of neoplastic cells has yet to be established. No evidence exists for ductal, acinar, or frank endocrine differentiation [26]. Immunohistochemically, the neoplastic cells diffusely and strongly express vimentin, α_1-antitrypsin, β-catenin, CD10, and c-kit (CD117) (Fig.7.8). Cells are less commonly positive for synaptophysin and neuron-specific enolase and negative for chromogranine. The cells express progesterone receptors and only the beta form of estrogen receptors, suggesting a role for hormones in the origin of these neoplasms.

Most patients present with abdominal fullness, vomiting, dyspepsia, weight loss and other vague symptoms, and frequently are asymptomatic; jaundice is rare. The most important symptom is pain, and is mostly due to large masses. Usually, they are benign tumors but in 15% of patients peritoneal and liver matastases are possible (Fig. 7.9).

Ultrasound shows an encapsulated mass with hyper-isoechoic areas for solid patterns (usually peripheric) and hypo-anechoic areas in the cystic part of the tumor (more frequently in the tumor center). Unenhanced CT shows hypodensity in cystic lesions and hyperdensity in solid forms, whereas contrast-enhanced CT demonstrates enhancement of capsulae and calcifications in 30% of cases. MRI shows low signal intensity on T1-weighted images and moderate/high intensity on T2-weighted images. On T1- and T2-weighted

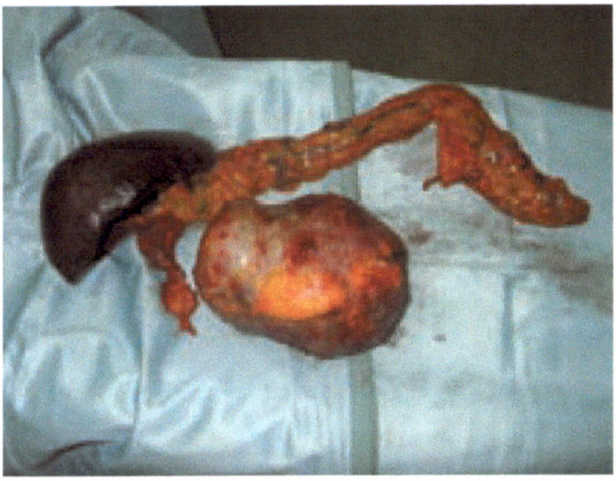

Fig. 7.7 Solid pseudopapillary carcinoma of the pancreas in a 26-year-old female patient. Macroscopic features after distal spleno-pancreatectomy

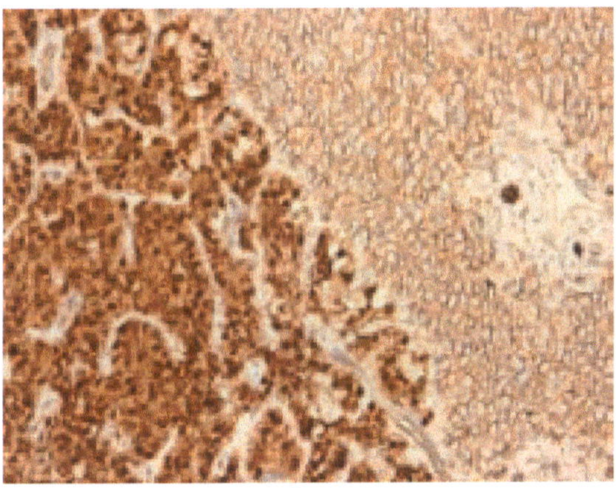

Fig. 7.8 Histologic pattern in hepatic metastasis of solid pseudopapillary carcinoma. Cytoplasmic and nuclear β-catenin immunostaining (*left*) of metastatic tissue are evident in comparison with normal hepatic microscopic morphology

images, hemorrhagic areas demonstrate high intensity while capsulae showing low-intensity signals [27]. EUS- and CT-guided FNA may help in the diagnosis with demonstration of papillary structures by showing cells with cytoplasmic vacuoles and round/oval and uniform nuclei with finely stippled chromatin [28]. CT, MRI and positron emission tomography (PET) help in the diagnosis and localization of metastasis (Fig.7.10).

7.5.1 Therapy

Resection is the main therapeutic approach for SPNs [29]. Intraoperative pathological frozen slices, tumor localization, and range of invasion are important for the choice the optimal surgical strategy. They may be characterized by a non-aggressive behavior, an excellent prognosis, and may present a dense capsule: hence a favourable curative effect could be achieved by minimized resection [30].

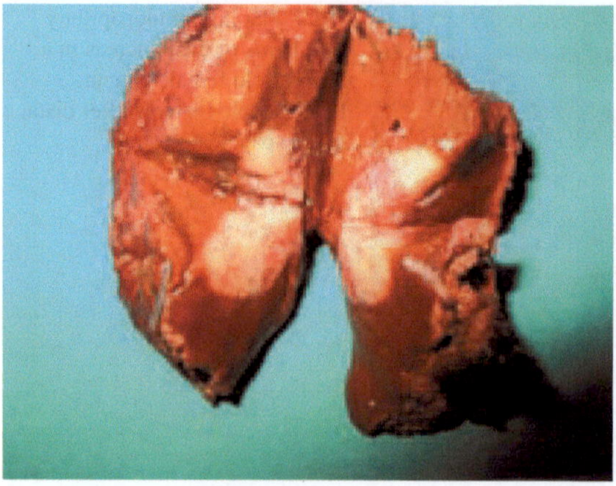

Fig. 7.9 Hepatic metastasis in solid pseudopapillary carcinoma of the pancreas in a 26-year-old female patient (macroscopic features after hepatic resection)

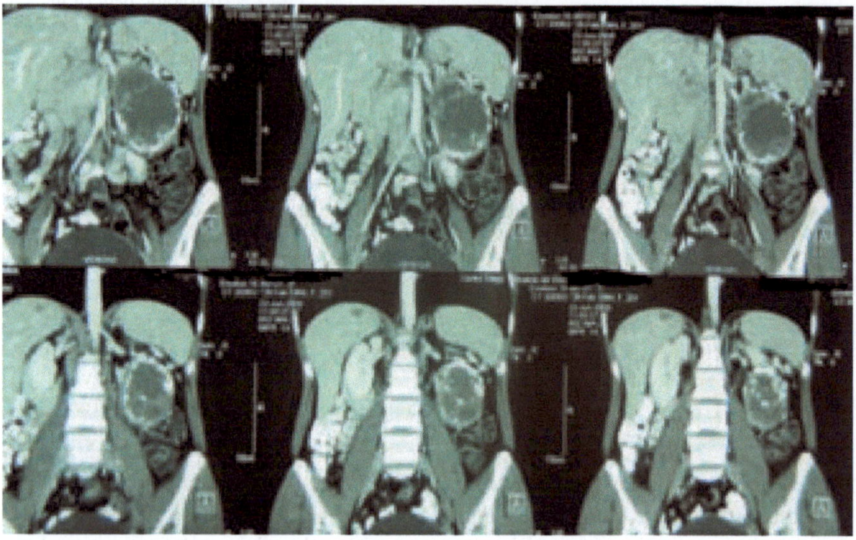

Fig. 7.10 Coronal CT of a solid pseudopapillary carcinoma of the pancreas in a 26-year-old female patient. A hepatic metastatic lesion is visible in segment VIII

Such tumors are usually found in females aged <30 years. Hence, to improve postoperative quality of life, limiting the resection to preserve normal pancreatic tissue and to maintain its functional structure is important. Lymph-node metastasis is uncommon, so lymph-node dissection is not usually necessary. Standard resection with tumor-free margins confirmed by intraoperative frozen sections is recommended if a SPN with malignant potential is found, such as distant metastasis, local lymph-node metastasis, or invasion of adjacent organs. Long-term survival after resection is reported for most patients (even for cases with metastatic disease). Martin et al. reported 4 patients with synchronous liver metastasis who underwent resection of the primary and liver lesions [29] Two of these 4 patients were alive without evidence of disease at 6 months and 11 years, respectively. Conversely, 1 patient died of progression of metastatic disease at 8 months, and the remaining patient was alive with recurrence in the liver at 6 years. In this study, another patient with a tumor of the head of the pancreas with invasion into the colon was described. This patient underwent pancreaticoduodenectomy plus partial transverse colectomy, and was alive without evidence of recurrence after 22 months of follow-up. Therefore, local invasion and metastasis are not surgical contraindications for patients with SPNs, and even recurrence of SPNs is associated with a good prognosis after resection of the recurrent lesion.

7.6 Acinar Cell Cystoadenoma (ACA) and Cystoadenocarcinoma

ACA is a benign lesion more common in adult females, and is usually discovered incidentally [2]. Multicentricity is common, and sometimes large masses are capsulated. Microscopically, the cysts are lined by one to several layers of cytological band acinar cells with round eosinonophilic cytoplasm. The tumor expresses CK7, which is usually negative in normal acinar cells. The cystic form of acinar cell carcinoma is extremely uncommon. The lesions are very large (mean diameter, 24 cm) with cystic lesions ranging from a few millimeters to several centimeters. Metastases are also common at the time of diagnosis.

References

1. Spence RAJ, Dasari B, Love M, Kelly B, Taylor M (2011) Overview of the investigation and management of cystic neoplasms of the pancreas. Dig Surg 28:386-397
2. Basturk O, Coban I, Adsay NV (2009) Pancreatic Cysts. Pathological classification, differential diagnosis and clinical implication. Arch Pathol Lab Med 133:423-438
3. Iftimia N, Yoon WJ, Brugge WR (2012) Cystic lesions of the pancreas: more riable differentiation with in situ high-resolution optical imaging? Expert Rev Gastroenterol Hepatol 6:125-127
4. Compagno J, Oertel JE (1978) Mucinous cystic neoplasms of the pancreas with overt and latent malignancy (cystoadenocarcinoma and cystoadenoma). A clinicopathologic study of 41 cases. Am J Clin Pathol 69:573-80
5. Bosman FT, Carneiro F, Hruban RH et al (2010) World Health Organization classification of tumours of the digestive system, 4th edn. IARC, Lyon
6. Brugge WR, Lauwers GY,Sahani D, Fernandez-del Castillo C, Warshaw AL (2004) Cystic neoplasms of the pancreas. N Engl J Med 351:1218-1226
7. Degan L, Wiesner W, Beglinger C (2007) Cystic and solid lesions of the pancreas. In: Tytgat G (ed) Clincal gastroenterology. Elsevier, pp 91-103
8. Tseng JF, Fernandez-del Castillo C, Warshaw AL (2000) Cystic neoplasms of the pancreas. In: Blumgart H, Fong Y (eds) Surgery of the liver and biliary tract. WB Saunders, pp 858-866
9. Malleo G, Zamboni G., Paini M, Marchegiani G, Manfredi R (2012) Serous Cystic Neoplasms. In: Pederzoli P, Bassi C (eds) Uncommon pancreatic neoplasms (Updates in Surgery Series) Springer-Verlag, Milan, pp 5-13

10. Visser BC, Muthusamay VR, Mulvihill SJ, Coakley F (2004) Diagnostic imaging of cystic pancreatic neoplasms. Surg Oncol 13:27-39
11. Harper AE, Eckhauser FE, Mulholland MW (2002) Resectional therapy for cystic neoplasms of the pancreas. Am Surg 68(4):353-7
12. Zamboni G, Scarpa A, Bogina G et al (1999) Mucinous Cystic tumors of the pancreas: clinicopathological features, prognosis and relationship to other mucinous cystic tumors. Am J Surg Pathol 23:410-422
13. Warshaw AL, Rattner DW, Fernández-del Castillo C, Z'graggen K (1998) Middle segment pancreatectomy: a novel technique for conserving pancreatic tissue. Arch Surg 133:327–331
14. Warshaw AL (1988) Conservation of the spleen with distal pancreatectomy. Arch Surg 123:550–553
15. Crippa S, Bassi C, Salvia R, Falconi M, Butturini G, Pederzoli P (2007) Enucleation of pancreatic neoplasms. Br J Surg 94:1254–1259
16. Fernández-Cruz L, Martínez I, Gilabert R, Cesar-Borges G, Astudillo E, Navarro S (2004) Laparoscopic distal pancreatectomy combined with preservation of the spleen for cystic neoplasms of the pancreas. J Gastrointest Surg 8:493–501
17. Abu Hilal M, Peiris L, Salvia R (2008) Intraductal papillary mucinous neoplasms of th pancreas. In: Taylor I, Johnson C (eds) Recent Advances in Surgery. Royal society of medicine Press Ltd, pp 83-97
18. Frigerio I, Zamboni G, Manfredi R, Pea A, Pennacchio S, Lim E, Salvia R (2012) Intraductal papillary Mucinous Neoplasms. In: Pederzoli P, Bassi C (eds) Uncommon pancreatic neoplasms (Updates in Surgery Series) Springer-Verlag, Milan, pp 33-52
19. Hwang DW, Jang JY, Lim CS et al (2011) Determination of malignant and invasive predictors in branch duct type intraductal papillary mucinous neoplasms of the pancreas: a suggested scoring formula. J Korean Med Sci 26:740-746
20. Tanaka M, Chiari S, Adsay V et al (2006) international consensus guidelines for management of intraductal papillary mucinous neoplasms and mucinous cystic neoplasms of the pancreas. Pancreatology 6:17-32
21. Hawes RH, Clancy J, Hasan MK (2012) Endoscopic ultrasound-guided fine needle aspiration in cystic pancreatic lesions. Clin Endosc 45:128-131
22. Brugge WR, Lewandrowski K, Lee-Lewandrowsky E, centeno BA Szydlo T, Regan S et al (2004) Diagnosis of pancreatic cystic neoplasms: a report of the cooperative pancreatic cyst study. Gastroenterology 126:1330-1336
23. Linder JD, Geenen JE, Catalano MF (2006) Cyst fluid analysis obtained by EUS-guided FNA in the evaluation of discrete cystic neoplasms of the pancreas: a prospective single-center experience. Gastrointest Endosc 64:697-702
24. Kucera S, Centeno BA, Springett G, Malafa MP, Chen YA, Weber J, Klapaman J (2012) Cyst fluid carcino embryonic antigen level is not predictive of invasive cancer in patients with intraductal papillary mucinous neoplasms of the pancreas. J Pancreas 13:409-413
25. Bassi C et al (2008) Natural history of intraductal papillary mucinous neoplasms (IPMN): current evidence and implications for management. J Gastrointest Surg 12:645–650
26. Klimstra DS, Wening BM, Heffess CS (2000) Solid-pseudopapillary tuomor of the pancreas: a typically cystic tumor of low malignant potential. Semin Diagn Pathol 17:66-81
27. Moholkar S, Sebire NJ, Roebuck DJ (2005) Solid pseudopapillary neoplasm of the pancreas: radiological-pathological correlation. Pediatr Radiol 35:819-82
28. Bardales H, Centeno B, Mallery JS, Lai R, Pochapin M, Guiter G, Stanley MW (2004) Endoscopic ultrasound guided-fine needle aspiration cytology diagnosis of solid pseudopapillary tumor of the pancreas. A rare neoplasm of elusive origin but characteristic cytomorphologic features. Am J Clin Pathol 121:654-662
29. Martin RC, Klimstra DS, Brennan MF, Conlon KC (2002) Solid pseudopapillary tumour of the pancreas: a surgical enigma? Ann Surg Oncol 9:35–40
30. Nagri S, Abdu A, Anand S, Krishnaiah M, Arya V (2007) Liver metastasis four years after Whipple's resection for solid-pseudopapillary tumour of the pancreas. JOP J Pancreas (Online) 8:223–227

Gastrointestinal Stromal Tumors: Surgical and Medical Therapy

8

Alessandro Comandone, Silvia Gasperoni, Roberto Manetti and Pietro Tonelli

8.1 Introduction

Gastrointestinal stromal tumors (GISTs) are rare neoplasms, with an estimated incidence of 14.2 cases/million/year in northen Italy [1]. However, they are the most common mesenchymal neoplasms of the gastrointestinal (GI) tract [2]. With a slight male predominance, most GISTs are found in adults >40 years of age, with a median age of 60–65 years. GISTs are nearly all sporadic, but a small subset of GISTs (≤5%) occurs in familial or idiopathic multitumor syndrome. In decreasing order of frequency, the four most important GIST syndromes are: type-1 neurofibromatosis (wild-type GISTs located predominantly in the small bowel and possibly multicentric); Carney triad (gastric GIST, pulmonary chondroma, and extra-adrenal paraganglioma); familial GIST syndromes resulting from germline mutations in c-Kit/PDGFRA; and Carney–Stratakis syndrome (hereditary GIST paraganglioma caused by germline mutations in the mitochondrial tumor suppressor gene pathway involving the succinate dehydrogenase subunits SDHD, SDHC, and SDHB). GISTs are submucosal tumors that arise in the digestive tract. Stomach (60%) and small intestine (30%) are the most common primary sites, the duodenum (5%), colon and rectum (<5%), esophagus and appendix (<1%) are the less common primary sites. Rarely, GISTs develop within the mesentery, omentum, or retroperitoneum [2].

A. Comandone (✉)
Oncology, Presidio Sanitario Gradenigo, Turin, Italy
e-mail: alessandro.comandone@gradenigo.it

S. Gasperoni · R. Manetti
Oncology, Careggi Hospital, Florence, Italy

P. Tonelli
Emergency Surgery, Careggi Hospital, Florence, Italy

A. Valeri et al. (eds.), *What's New in Surgical Oncology*,
DOI: 10.1007/978-88-470-5310-6_8, © Springer-Verlag Italia 2013

8.2 Diagnosis

Clinical presentation can be indolent. Most patients have non-specific symptoms such as nausea, constipation or diarrhea, abdominal discomfort, occult GI bleeding, weight loss, or worsening general condition. Most of these tumors are identified incidentally during endoscopy, ultrasound, computed tomography (CT), or even at laparotomy undertaken for other reasons. Although acute hemorrhage, perforation, or obstruction may lead to an emergency presentation, GISTs usually grow insidiously as extraluminal masses from their submucosal origin in a non-invasive manner, pushing adjacent organs away from the expanding mass. Liver metastases and peritoneal dissemination are the most common signs of malignancy. Between 15% and 50% of GISTs are metastatic at the time of the diagnosis [3].

Endoscopic ultrasonography (EUS) is a useful tool for the diagnosis of GISTs (especially for small esophageal or duodenal nodules <2 cm) because it can visualize the structures of the wall of the digestive tract and harvest tumor samples by endoscopic ultrasonography-guided fine-needle aspiration biopsy (EUS-FNAB) for histological examination using immunohistochemistry (CD117 and/or DOG1) and for mutational analyses. Mutational analyses for known mutations involving KIT and PDGFRA genes can confirm the diagnosis of GIST if there is doubt (particularly in CD117/DOG1-negative suspect GIST), and may predict response to therapy with tyrosine kinase inhibitors (TKIs). However, even if biopsy is useful for the diagnosis and planning the best therapy, percutaneous or laparoscopic biopsies of tumors that cannot be examined by endoscopic means should be avoided for the risk of tumor-cell seeding. Biopsy may also be proposed for suspected sites of metastatic disease.

For GISTs without metastases, risk classification based on mitotic count (expressed as the number of mitoses per 50 high-power fields on a total area of 10 mm^2), tumor size (expressed in centimeters), and tumor site (stomach better than small intestine and rectum) is recommended. Risk classification allows one to distinguish GISTs in very low-, low-, intermediate- and high-risk categories, and to identify patients who may be able to take advantage of adjuvant therapy with imatinib mesylate (imatinib) after radical surgery [4, 5]. "Very low-risk" and "low-risk" categories have a very favorable prognosis, the "high-risk" category has an unfavorable prognosis, and the "intermediate-risk" category cannot be used to discriminate between patients with favorable and unfavorable prognoses.

For staging of the disease, contrast-enhanced CT of the abdomen and pelvis is the main examination because GISTs metastasize to the liver and peritoneum. Magnetic resonance imaging (MRI) or contrast-enhanced ultrasound may be alternatives. MRI provides better preoperative information for rectal GISTs. CT or radiography of the chest and routine laboratory tests complete the staging work-up. ^{18}F-fluorodeoxyglucose (^{18}F-FDG) positron emission tomography (PET) is not employed for initial staging of the disease, but for assessing response to adjuvant therapies.

The decision-making for optimal treatment involves a multidisciplinary team (pathologist, diagnostic radiologist, medical oncologist, surgical oncologist), possibly in reference centers.

8.3 Surgical Therapy

8.3.1 Surgical Therapy of Primary Localized GISTs

The treatment of GISTs has had a radical change with the introduction of the TKI imatinib. This agent has demonstrated exceptional efficacy in GIST treatment, improving the survival of patients with metastatic, recurrent, and advanced-stage disease [6, 7]. Surgery is the "gold standard" for primary localized (≥2 cm) GISTs that are potentially resectable with a low risk of morbidity.

At surgery, careful exploration of abdomen is essential to exclude liver and peritoneal metastases. If a tumor is present and resectable, surgery may be radical, and otherwise supports subsequent treatment with imatinib. The primary therapy is a complete resection, which requires macroscopically negative resection margins, (gross safety margins of 1–2 cm are sufficient). Given its friability, every effort to preserve intact the pseudocapsule of the tumor must be made, and spontaneous or surgical rupture of the tumor must be recorded because a GIST becomes high-risk independent of any other prognostic factor [8]. GISTs metastasize by the hematogenous route and nodal metastases have a low incidence with the exception of syndromic GISTs, which can cause nodal metastases in 20% of cases [9]. Therefore, lymphoadenectomy is not necessary and systemic or prophylactic lymph-node dissection does not improve the prognosis. In case of suspected metastatic lymph nodes, a pick-up dissection is considered sufficient. If the resection margin is macroscopically positive, a re-resection should be considered if: the site(s) of positive margin can be located precisely; the residual tumor is completely resectable; dissemination or serosal invasion is not present; and morbidity is acceptably low. If the site(s) of positive margin is/are uncertain and/or the risk of morbidity is high, the patient should be placed under observation. With the patient's consent, both options are valid with almost similar survival. Re-operation is not indicated if resection margins are microscopically positive on final pathology. According to these oncologic principles, wedge resection is considered sufficient for gastric GISTs as is limited duodenal resection for duodenal GISTs. Enucleation may be undertaken for esophageal leiomyoma because of its favorable prognosis and functional outcomes, but is not indicated for GISTs at other sites.

Treatment decision-making can be different if small (<2 cm) esophago-gastric or duodenal nodules are detected, and EUS-FNAB feasible. In these cases, although standard treatment is surgical excision, the multidisciplinary team can decide with the patient to follow-up the lesion with EUS if the GIST is low-risk, or in case of major surgical morbidity. In the presence of small (<2 cm) rectal nodules, the approach is biopsy and excision because the risk at this site is higher, as well as for small intestinal nodules. However, the management of incidentally discovered GISTs <2 cm is controversial because their natural history remains unknown [10].

Preoperative multidisciplinary planning must carefully consider a course of preoperative imatinib therapy [10] if a GIST is poorly situated. Examples of such poorly situated GISTs are: a GIST at the esophago-gastric junction requiring a esophago-gastric resection; gastric GIST requiring total gastrectomy; duodenal GIST requiring pancreatoduodenectomy; low rectal GIST requiring abdominoperineal resection; or even in patients with GISTs that are resectable with negative margins but associated with significant surgical morbidity. Several case reports have demonstrated that preoperative imatinib may spare multi-visceral resection or preserve organ function if radical treatment is employed [10]. This option may also be adopted if the surgeon believes that a preoperative cytoreduction may reduce the risk of bleeding and pseudocapsule rupture during surgery. In all of these cases, rapid assessment of tumor response by PET or PET CT/MRI is necessary because surgery must not be delayed in the presence of a non-responding resectable GIST. Otherwise, surgery is undertaken after maximal tumor response (which is defined as no further improvement between two successive CT scans, generally after 6–12 months [11]). Imatinib must be suspended a few days prior to surgery, does not affect surgical morbidity, and must be started again as soon as possible after surgery. However, if at surgery the tumor is strongly adherent to or invades adjacent organs, or if the pseudocapsule might injure by separating the tumor from adjacent organs, *en bloc* resection is recommended to prevent tumor cells seeding into the peritoneal cavity. In particular cases (such as if surgery implies major functional consequences, preoperative imatinib does not reduce tumor mass, and the GIST is a low-risk lesion), the multidisciplinary team may propose to the patient a partial resection. According to patient acceptance, this strategy may not imply worse overall survival, especially if the tumor is low risk [8]. Nevertheless, for complete resection, recurrences are common, occurring 18–24 months from the time of the index procedure, and 5-year survival after resection of a localized tumor is ≈50% [12].

Recently, the possibility of endoscopic excision of endoluminal gastric GISTs of small dimensions [13] has been reported. However, any endoscopic treatment should be considered investigational in the context of a clinical trial.

Urgent surgery may be required for GISTs causing acute hemorrhage, perforation, or obstruction. In these circumstances, radical surgery may not be able to be carried out because of the size and site of the tumor, metastases, tumor dissemination after spontaneous rupture of the tumor, or a compromised general condition of the patient. Such instances may be managed by partial resection followed by imatinib. In the case of incidental discovery of a GIST during surgical procedures carried out for other diseases, the GIST should be removed, if possible.

8.3.2 Laparoscopic Surgery

Laparoscopic resection may be considered for GISTs in favorable anatomic locations (e.g., greater curvature or anterior wall of the stomach, jejunum, and ileum) and for GISTs of diameter ≤5 cm [14, 15]. As regards size, there has been a progressive increase in the diameters of the lesions that can be removed. Thus, there is no real limit for laparoscopic resection, even if GISTs >5 cm may require greater mastery of the laparoscopic approach. Surgeons must be skilful in the laparoscopic method and follow the oncologic principles of GIST resection, in particular, avoiding pseudocapsule injury and tumor spillage [14, 16]. The tumor should not be held with forceps. Resection specimens must be removed from the abdomen in a plastic bag to prevent spillage or seeding of port sites (though there are very few cases of GIST recurrence at the port site [17]). With respect to oncologic principles, laparoscopic surgery may not only reduce operating time, blood loss, and duration of hospital stay, but also is associated with low morbidity and low recurrence rates [14, 15]. In gastric GISTs, a combined laparoscopic–endoscopic procedure may be necessary to identify the site of the tumor, and to ensure its complete removal. Laparoscopic surgery may also be carried out because it is safe and has a short operating time. Careful evaluation for laparoscopic treatment must be done if the GIST appears to be highly vascularized, fragile on preoperative imaging, and is high risk at histological examination or EUS imaging (irregular border, cystic space, ulceration, echogenic foci, and heterogeneity).

8.3.3 Surgical Therapy for Locally Advanced Inoperable, Metastatic, or Recurrent GISTs

Imatinib is the standard treatment for locally advanced inoperable, metastatic, or recurrent GISTs. Surgery alone gives poor results in metastatic disease [12], but imatinib has improved overall survival (from 26% in the pre-imatinib era to 76% after 2 years of imatinib treatment [10]), and its efficacy in terms of progression-free survival (PFS) and disease-specific survival (DSS) has been demonstrated widely [18–20]. Nevertheless, secondary progression with imatinib occurs after a median time of 2 years because of secondary mutations that confer drug resistance, and because of pharmacokinetic alterations [21]. Thus, many centers have carried out surgery upon best clinical response to imatinib to ameliorate PFS and DSS. The surgical *rationale* was to remove tumor bulk before secondary resistance develops or to resect lesions that had already developed secondary resistance. The outcome of this strategy was not good. In a study of 80 patients with metastatic GISTs who underwent surgery after imatinib treatment and divided in two groups (group A, n=49, underwent surgery upon best clinical response; group B, n=31, underwent surgery at focal progression), PFS was 64.4% in group A, and 9.7% in group B after 2 years, whereas DSS from the time of imatinib onset was not reached in either group. The conclusions of this study were that surgery for focal progressive disease has a limited benefit in terms of disease control, and does not seem to prevent generalized progression in most patients. Post-imatinib surgery may be considered as part of the second–third-line armamentarium in selected cases [22]. Two other considerations must be added to this conclusion: (i) there may be a discrepancy between disease extension at preoperative diagnostic imaging and that found at surgery which does not allow radical surgery; and (ii) postoperative complications are not minimal for these often complex procedures [22–24]. Furthermore, Blank et al. demonstrated, in 943 patients with advanced GISTs, that many objective responses evolved slowly (in 25% of patients after 5.3 to 39 months), and that one-third of patients with the bulkiest GISTs were long-term survivors [20]. In these cases, imatinib needs to be continued as long as there is no progressive disease according to Response Evaluation Criteria in Solid Tumors (RECIST) criteria [25]. Although a prospective randomized trial on the role of surgery on this issue has not been completed, evidence seems to suggest that medical therapy with a dose escalation of imatinib is better than surgery for patients with recurrent and metastatic GISTs that develop progression. Surgery has a role in the emergency setting as well as in selected cases.

In conclusion, surgery is not recommended for multifocal progression. Surgery is not effective for focal progression owing to a lack of randomized trials, and may be proposed in a multidisciplinary setting on a case-by-case basis. Resection of metastases if a patient is responding to imatinib is not useful [26].

8.4 Medical Therapy

In 1988, the description of the activating mutation in the KIT gene (found in 70–80% of GISTs) and in the PDGRFA gene defined the drivers of tumor progression, and gave two perfect targets for molecular therapy [27, 28].

8.4.1 Pharmacological Profiles of Active Drugs

The TKI imatinib is the first and most active agent against this disease. Originally it was conceived to inhibit abnormal tyrosine kinase encoded by the Philadelphia chromosome (BCR Abl) in chronic myelogenous leukemia, thereby preventing cell proliferation. In GISTs, it is active against the receptor tyrosine kinases cKIT and PDGFRA. Its pharmacokinetic profile is well known: absorbed after oral administration with 98% bioavailability, it reaches a maximum concentration 2 h after dosing, with 95% binding to plasma proteins. Its principal metabolite is N-desmetylimatinib, metabolism is in the liver *via* CYP450 3A4 with a half-life of 18-40 h, and >80% of the dose is eliminated in 7 days, mainly *via* the fecal route (68%) and 13% through the urinary tract. Imatinib has a well defined role in adjuvant therapy as well as in advanced or metastatic disease. The standard dose is 400 mg/day in adjuvant or metastatic settings. There are some suggestions of major activity in GIST exon 9 mutated after a double dose (800 mg/day), along with some problems of patient compliance. In the case of progressive disease, before sunitinib therapy, the drug dose may be increased to 800 mg/day. The toxicity profile is acceptable: edema and fluid retention, and mild neutropenia (grade 1 and 2). Severe toxicities are rare: hepatic dysfunction with increases in transaminase levels, severe cardiac failure, hypothyroidism, dermatologic reactions, bleeding or GI perforation after GIST shrinkage.

Sunitinib is the second drug approved for GIST therapy but only as second-line therapy or in case of imatinib intolerance. The drug has multiple anti-tyrosine kinase activities (KIT, PDGFRA, FLT3, CSF 1R, RET) and anti-angiogenic activity. There are two dosing schedules: (i) 50 mg day, 4 weeks on and 2 weeks off or (ii) 37.5 mg/day continuously. After oral ingestion, the maximum plasma concentration is reached in 6–12 h. Protein binding is 90–95% and sunitinib is metabolized in the liver by CP450 CYP 3A4. The terminal half-life is 40–60 h and the elimination is by the gastrointestinal tract. Toxicities are: hypertension, cardiac failure, thyroid dysfunction (hypo- or hyperthyroidism), asthenia, hemorrhage, skin rashes or discoloration.

Recently, regorafenib was approved by the US Food and Drug Administration (FDA) as third-line therapy for metastatic GIST. Regorafenib (BAY 73-4506) is a novel, orally active, diphenylureamultikinase inhibitor of VEGFR1-3, c-KIT, TIE-2, PDGFR-β, FGFR-1, RET, RAF-1, BRAF and p38 MAP kinase. Two large, randomized Phase III pivotal registration studies in patients with GIST and colorectal cancer (CRC), respectively, lead to the FDA approval. Patients received oral regorafenib 60–220 mg daily (160 mg daily in the extension cohort) in cycles of 21-days on, 7-days off treatment. The most common treatment-related toxicities were hand–foot skin reaction, fatigue, voice change and rash.

8.4.2 Oncogenic Mutation in GISTs and Therapeutic Aspects

Mutation of KIT and PDGFRA results in independent kinase activation and in uncontrolled cell proliferation. Most (>90%) KIT mutations affect exon 11, which encodes the juxtamembrane domain of the receptor. Seven percent to 10% of GISTs have mutations in KIT exon 9, which determines changes in the extracellular portion of the receptor. This mutation is more common in small bowel tumors. Less common mutations are in exon 17 (activation loop) and exon 13 (juxtamembrane domain). Ten percent of GISTs have activating mutations in PDGFRA, which exclude KIT activation. Most PDGFRA mutations occur in exon 18, thereby modifying the loop of the kinase.

About 10–15% of GISTs are wild-type because no KIT or PDGFRA mutations have been found. This subgroup of GISTs is not sensitive to TKIs and alternative oncogenic drivers, such as BRAF V600E and SDH loss of function, are probably responsible for cell activation [29].

8.4.3 Adjuvant Therapy

Risk stratification systems have practical relevance for distinguishing between patients who are likely to be cured by surgery alone and those who could benefit from post-surgery treatment. The first adjuvant randomized controlled trial (RCT) was planned in the USA and published in 2009. The ACOSOG Z 9001 trial was a randomized Phase III study investigating imatinib *vs* placebo in patients with radically resected GISTs of diameter ≥3 cm in diameter and positive for KIT protein. Seven-hundred and thirteen patients were randomized to receive imatinib 400 mg/day for 1 year or placebo. The primary endpoint was PFS. After a median follow-up of 19.7 months, 70 patients of 354 (20%) who received placebo had a recurrence, as compared with 30/359 (8%) in the imatinib arm. One-year PFS was 98% in the imatinib arm and 83% in the placebo arm. Overall survival at 48 months was identical in both arms [30].

A later analysis on the mutation subtypes showed significant PFS at 2 years for GIST exon 11 and PDGFRA mutations, but not for exon 9 and wild-type GIST [31].

In 2012, a German/Scandinavian research team published the results of a smaller study, involving 400 patients, randomized for 3 years *vs* 1 year of imatinib adjuvant therapy. The daily dose of the drug was 400 mg. After 54-month follow-up, only 25% of those who had 36-month therapy had a relapse compared with 42% of patients who received 12-month therapy; 93% of patients in the 12-month arm and 85.4% in the 36-month arm had GISTs that were positive for KIT expression. The primary endpoint was RFS interval, and it was significantly better in the 36-month arm (50 events) than in 12-month arm (84 events). Twenty-five deaths were recorded in the 12-month arm and 12 in the 36-month arm, demonstrating the superiority of a longer period of imatinib therapy [32]. As a consequence of those results, imatinib was approved for adjuvant therapy in intermediate and high-risk GISTs by the FDA and the European Medicines Agency (EMA).

The fundamental questions are: which patients should be treated and for how long? There is no definitive answer, only expert suggestions [33]. Postoperative imatinib administration should be considered in GISTs with a >50% chance of relapse according to the Gold nomogram [34]. Wild-type GISTs or PDGFRA D824V should be excluded because they are insensitive. Patients who suffered GIST rupture should be treated as if they had metastatic disease. In the adjuvant setting, all patients should start the therapy ≤3 months after surgery with a standard dose of 400 mg/day even in exon 9 mutations. In intermediate-risk disease, the length of therapy is 12 months; in high- and very-high-risk disease, 36-month treatment should be the standard [33]. The European Organisation for Research and Treatment of Cancer (EORTC) study is anxiously awaited to add information about intermediate-risk patients.

8.4.4 Therapy in Advanced Disease

Until 2001, there was no active therapy for metastatic GISTs. Chemotherapy was inactive with objective responses <5% and time to progression (TTP) <3 months, and reiterated surgical interventions were the unique alternative with very poor results and death occurring in 6 months time [12]. In 2001, the situation changed dramatically, altered by the first case report by Joensuu et al., [35] who administered imatinib in a single patient with widely metastatic disease. The extraordinary tumor response lead to a Phase I study by the EORTC sarcoma group. In this study, 36 patients with metastatic GISTs were treated with imatinib in escalating doses from 400 mg to 800 mg. Thirty-two patients had an objective response [36]. This result started two contemporary Phase II trials: the first in Europe and the second a USA–Finnish study. Both studies compared doses of 400 mg with 600 mg of imatinib: 87% in the USA–Finnish and 89% in the EORTC study had a partial response or stable disease [20].

Subsequently, two Phase III studies were planned comparing 400 mg *vs* 800 mg daily of imatinib. In the EORTC study, only 18% of patients had progressive disease, whereas in the S0033 study 26% of patients had progressive disease [19, 37]. The metastatic GISTs of those studies showed that in exon 9 GISTs a dose of 800 mg/daily of imatinib gave a better PFS than standard dose [37]. Unfortunately, despite those results, metastatic GISTs often progress within few months. Only 18% of patients did not show progression of GIST at 10 years [38]. Therapy must be continued because discontinuation of imatinib causes disease progression in all patients [39].

Imatinib resistance is a well-known phenomenon and can be divided into two groups: primary resistance (≈10% of patients who never respond to therapy), and secondary resistance (progression of disease after a variable time of continuous treatment). Primary resistance is related to wild-type tumors or intrinsically resistant tumors (PDGFRA mutation D842V; KIT exon 9). Secondary resistance is due to the expansion of GIST cells with secondary mutations. The secondary mutation occurs on the same allele of the leading and primitive allele. The KIT exon 11 mutation is the most common, so this one probably develops a secondary mutation. Secondary resistance develops in the activation loop (exons 17 and 18) and in ATP pockets (exons 13 and 14). The secondary mutation gives a very high resistance to all TKI drugs [40].

8.4.5 Second and Further Lines of Therapy

If disease progression is recorded, the re-biopsy of GISTs is advisable. The biopsy determines which type of mutation has become the new driver in the disease. It may be useful to define the second line of treatment [40]. The suggested intervention is redoubling the dose of imatinib from 400 mg/day to 800 mg/day. About 15–20% of the patients may have a response or stabilization of the disease for several months [33]. Unfortunately, most patients do not benefit from this dose increase and need a different, second line of therapy. After one Phase III study, sunitinib is the approved second-line drug. In this study, patients treated with 50 mg of sunitinib 4 weeks on and 2 weeks off had a TTP of 27.3 weeks compared with 6.4 weeks for the placebo arm. A Phase II trial using sunitinib in a continuous daily dose of 37.5 mg offered the same results [41]. Sunitinib is very active against the secondary mutations on exon 13 and 14, but it is inactive against exon 17 and 18 mutations [42].

If GIST progresses upon sunitinib treatment, the next step is to introduce the patient into a clinical study with an investigational agent [33]. Many agents have been tested to target KIT or KIT signaling (PI3K MEK) or other intracellular events (histone deacetylase inhibitors, heat shock protein, mTOR pathway). Nilotinib and dasatinib failed to restore the sensitivity of GIST [43]. Sorafenib, after an initial positive study, has not been developed further [44]. At the 2012 meeting of the American Society of Clinical Oncology (ASCO), the results of a randomized study with regorafenib *vs* placebo as third-line therapy were presented [45]. Patients were randomized at a ratio of 2:1 to receive best supportive care plus regorafenib (160 mg, p.o.) once daily (3 weeks on/1 week off) or placebo. The primary endpoint was PFS: 234 patients were screened; 199 were randomized (regorafenib 133; placebo

66). Baseline characteristics were balanced between the two arms. The primary endpoint was met: median PFS was 4.8 months for regorafenib *vs* 0.9 months for placebo. The hazard ratio for PFS was 0.27 (95% confidence interval (CI), 0.18–0.39), p<0.0001. PFS rates at 3 months and 6 months were 60% and 38% for regorafenib *vs* 11% and 0% for placebo, respectively.

Lacking an alternative therapy, re-challenge with imatinib as third-line therapy can be considered because several experts believe that GISTs have clones that are sensitive to TKIs even in heavily pre-treated patients, and that continuation of imatinib or sunitinib should be considered to be lifelong [46].

8.4.6 Conclusion

Medical therapy for GISTs has been a great advance in long-term control of the disease. Adjuvant therapy needs longer-term follow-up as well as new studies to define if prolonged postoperative therapy can eradicate the disease. In the metastatic setting, imatinib is the most active drug and can effectively change the natural history of the tumor. After progression on imatinib, sunitinib can improve TTP by several months. The optimal third-line therapy is unclear. New drugs and new studies are needed urgently.

References

1. Mucciarini C, Rossi G, Bertolini F, et al (2007) Incidence and clinicopathologic features of gastrointestinal stromal tumors. A population-based study. BMC Cancer 7:230
2. Miettinen M, Lasota J (2006) Gastrointestinal stromal tumors: review on morphology, molecular pathology, prognosis, and differential diagnosis. Arch Pathol Lab Med 130:1466-1478
3. Roberts PJ, Eisenberg B (2002) Clinical presentation of gastrointestinal stromal tumors and treatment of operable disease. Eur J Cancer 38:S37–S38
4. Fletcher CD, Berman JJ, Corless C, et al (2002) Diagnosis of gastrointestinal stromal tumors: a consensus approach. Hum Pathol 33:459-465
5. Miettinen M, Lasota J (2006) Gastrointestinal stromal tumors: pathology and prognosis at different sites. Semin Diagn Pathol 23:70-83
6. Demetri GD, von Mehren M, Blanke CD, et al (2002) Efficacy and safety of imatinibmesylate in advanced gastrointestinal stromal tumors. N Engl J Med 347:472-480
7. Blackstein ME, Blay JY, Corless C, et al (2006) Gastrointestinal stromal tumors: consensus statement on diagnosis and treatment. Can J Gastroenterol 20:157-163
8. Casali PG, Blay J-Y (2010) Gastrointestinal stromal tumors: ESMO Clinical Practice Guidelines for diagnosis, treatment and follow-up. Ann Oncol 21:v98-v102
9. Agaimy A, Hartmann A (2010) Hereditary and non-hereditary syndromic gastrointestinal stromal tumors. Pathologe 31:430-437
10. Demetri GD, von Mehren M, Antonescu C et al (2010) NCCN Task Force report: update on the management of patients with gastrointestinal stromal tumors. J Natl Compr Canc Netw 8:S1-41
11. Bonvalot S, Eldweny H, Pechoux CL et al (2006) Impact of surgery on advanced gastrointestinal stromal tumors (GIST) in the imatinib era. Ann Surg Oncol 13:1596-1603
12. DeMatteo RP, Lewis JJ, Leung D et al (2000) Two hundred gastrointestinal stromal tumors: recurrence patterns and prognostic factors for survival. Ann Surg 231:51-58

13. Jeong IH, Kim JH, Lee SR et al (2012) Minimally invasive treatment of gastric gastrointestinal stromal tumors: laparoscopic and endoscopic approach. Surg Laparosc Endosc Percutan Tech 22:244-50
14. Novitsky YW, MD, Kercher KW, Sing RF et al (2006) Long-term outcomes of laparoscopic resection of gastric gastrointestinal stromal tumors. Ann Surg 243:738–747
15. Nishimura J, Nakajima K, Omori T et al (2007) Surgical strategy for gastric gastrointestinal stromal tumors: laparoscopic vs open resection. Surg Endosc 21:875-878
16. Pucci MJ, Berger AC, Lim PW, et al (2012) Laparoscopic approaches to gastric gastrointestinal stromal tumors: an institutional review of 57 cases. Surg Endosc 26:3509-3514
17. Furukawa M, Izumi S, Asano H et al (2012) Late umbilical port-site recurrence of a gastrointestinal stromal tumor with an acquired PDGFRα mutation after laparoscopic resection: report of a case. Surg Laparosc Endosc Percutan Tech 22:e109-111
18. Blay JY, Bonvalot S, Casali P et al (2005) Consensus meeting for the management of gastrointestinal stromal tumors: report of the GIST Consensus Conference of 20-21 March 2004, under the auspices of ESMO. Ann Oncol 16:566-578
19. Verweij J, Casali PG, Zalcberg J et al (2004) Progression-free survival in gastrointestinal stromal tumors with high-dose imatinib: randomized trial. Lancet 364:1127-1134
20. Blanke CD, Demetri GD, von Mehren M et al (2008) Long-term results from a randomized phase II trial of standard- versus high-dose imatinibmesylate for patients with unresectable or metastatic gastrointestinal stromal tumors expressing KIT. J Clin Oncol 26:620-625
21. Van Glabbeke M, Verweij J, Casali PG et al (2005) Initial and late resistance to imatinib in advanced gastrointestinal stromal tumors are predicted by different prognostic factors: a European Organisation for Research and Treatment of Cancer – Italian Sarcoma Group – Australian Gastrointestinal Trials Group Study. J Clin Oncol 23:5795-5804
22. Mussi C, Ronellenfitsch U, Jacob J et al (2009) Post-imatinib surgery in advanced/metastatic GIST. Is it worthwhile in all patients? Ann Oncol 21:403-408
23. Raut CP, Posner M, Desai J et al (2006) Surgical management of advanced gastrointestinal stromal tumors after treatment with targeted systemic therapy using kinase inhibitors. J Clin Oncol 24:2325-2331
24. DeMatteo RP, Maki RG, Singer S et al (2007) Results of tyrosine kinase inhibitor therapy followed by surgical resection for metastatic gastrointestinal stromal tumor. Ann Surg 245:347-352
25. Le Cesne A, van Glabbeke M, Verweij J et al (2009) Absence of progression as assessed by response evaluation criteria in solid tumors predicts survival in advanced GI stromal tumors treated with imatinibmesylate: the intergroup EORTC-ISG-AGITG phase III trial. J Clin Oncol 20:3969-3974
26. Reichardt P, Blay J-Y, von Mehren M (2010) Towards global consensus in the treatment of gastrointestinal stromal tumor. Expert Rev Anticancer Ther 10:221-232
27. Hirota S, Isozaki K, Moriyama Y et al (1998) Gain-of-function mutation of c-kit in human gastrointestinal stromal tumors. Science 279:577-580
28. VanGlabbeke M, Verweij J, Blay JY et al (2012) Gastrointestinal Stromal Tumor Meta-Analysis Group (MetaGIST). Comparison of two doses of imatinib for the treatment of unresectable or metastatic gastrointestinal stromal tumors: A meta-analysis of 1640 patients. J Clin Oncol 28:1247-1253
29. Corless CL, Barnett CM, Heinrich MC (2011) Gastrointestinal stromal tumors: origin and molecular oncology. Nat Rev Cancer 11:865-878
30. Dematteo RP, Ballman KV, Antonescu CR et al (2009) Adjuvant imatinibmesylate after resection of localised, primary gastrointestinal stromal tumor: a randomised, double-blind, placebo-controlled trial. Lancet 373:1097-1104
31. Corless CL,Ballman KY, Antonescu C et al (2010) Relation of tumor pathologic and molecular features to outcome after surgical resection of localized primary gastrointestinal stromal tumor (GIST). Results of the Intergroup Phase III trial ACOSOG Z9001. J Clin Oncol 28(suppl; abstr 1006)
32. Joensuu H, Eriksson M, Sundby Hall K et al (2012) One vs three years of adjuvant imatinib

for operable gastrointestinal stromal tumor: a randomized trial. JAMA 307:1265-1272
33. Consensus Panel ESMO Guidelines 2012 (2012) Gastrointestinal stromal tumors: ESMO Clinical Practice Guidelines for diagnosis, treatment and follow-up. Ann Oncol 23:49-55
34. Gold JS, Gonen M, Gutierrez A et al (2009) Development and validation of a prognostic nomogram for recurrence-free survival after complete surgical resection of localised primary gastrointestinal stromal tumor: a retrospective analysis. Lancet Oncol 10:1045-1052
35. Joensuu H, Roberts PJ, Sarlomo-Rikala M et al (2001) Effect of the tyrosine kinase inhibitor STI571 in a patient with a metastatic gastrointestinal stromal tumor. NEJM 344:1052-1056
36. Van Oosterom AT, Judson I, Verweij J et al (2001) Safety and efficacy of imatinib(STI571) in metastatic gastrointestinal stromal tumors: a phase I study. Lancet 358:1421-1423
37. Gastrointestinal Stromal Tumor Meta-Analysis Group (MetaGIST) (2010) Comparison of two doses of imatinib for the treatment of unresectable or metastatic gastrointestinal stromal tumors: a metanalysis of 1640 patients. J Clin Oncol 28:1247-1253
38. Von Mehren M, Heinrich MC, Joensuu H et al (2011) Follow-up results after 9 years (yrs) of the ongoing, phase II B2222 trial of imatinibmesylate (IM) in patients (pts) with metastatic or unresectable KIT+ gastrointestinal stromal tumors (GIST). J Clin Oncol 29 (suppl; abstr 10016)
39. Le Cesne A, Ray-Coquard I, Bui BN et al (2010) Discontinuation of imatinib in patients with advanced gastrointestinal stromal tumors after 3 years of treatment: an open-label multicentre randomised phase 3 trial. Lancet Oncol 11:942-949
40. Antonescu CR, Besmer P, Guo T et al (2005) Acquired resistance to imatinib in gastrointestinal stromal tumors occurs through secondary gene mutation. Clin Cancer Res 11:4182-4190
41. Demetri GD, van Oosterom AT, Garrett CR et al (2008) Efficacy and safety of Sunitinibmalate in patients with advanced gastrointestinal stromal tumor after failure of imatinib: a randomized controlled trial. Lancet 368:1329-1338
42. George S, Blay JY, Casali PG et al (2009) Clinical evaluation of continuous daily dosing of sunitinib malate in patients with advanced gastrointestinal stromal tumors after imatinib failure. Eur J Cancer 45:1959-1968
43. Reichardt P, Blay JY, Gelderbrom H et al (2010) Phase III trial of nilotinib inpatients with advanced gastrointestinal stromal tumor (GIST). First results from ERNEST g3. J Clin Oncol 28 (suppl; abstr 10017)
44. Kindler HL, Campbell K, Wroblewski R et al (2011) Sorafenib (SOR) in patients (pts) with imatinib (IM) and sunitinib (SU)-resistant (RES) gastrointestinal stromal tumors (GIST): final results od a University of Chicago phase II consortium trial. J Clin Oncol 29:607s (suppl; abstr 10009)
45. Demetri GD et al (2012) Randomized phase III trial of regorafenib in patients (pts) with metastatic and/or unresectable gastrointestinal stromal tumor (GIST) progressing despite prior treatment with at least imatinib (IM) and sunitinib (SU): GRID trial. ASCO 2012 Annual Meeting. J Clin Oncol 30:2401-2407
46. Fumagalli E, Coco P, Morosi C et al (2010) Sunitinib rechallenge in two advanced GIST patients after third-line anti-tyrosine kinase therapy. J Clin Oncol 28 (suppl; abstr e20519)

New Knowledge in the Diagnosis and Medical Treatment of Pancreatic Neuroendocrine Tumors

9

Lorenzo Antonuzzo, Luca Messerini, Camilla Comin, Giulia Meoni, Elisa Lucherini and Francesco Di Costanzo

9.1 Introduction

Gastroenteropancreatic neuroendocrine tumors (GEP-NETs) represent a rare and heterogeneous group of neoplasms that arise from the diffuse neuroendocrine system within the pancreas and gastrointestinal tract [1, 2]. Pancreatic neuroendocrine tumors (pNET), a sub-group of GEP-NETs, are characterized by specific tumor genetics, biology and clinicopathological features. These characteristics influence therapeutic decision-making [3–7]. Recently, the incidence of pNET increased by two-to-threefold to reach 2.2/1,000,000, whereas the incidence of pancreatic adenocarcinoma has remained stable [3, 8]. Probably, this observation reflects an improvement in diagnotic procedures because of the introduction of new methods (e.g., spiral computed tomography and ecoendoscopy) rather than a real increase in pNET incidence.

Whilst 50–80% of pNETs are non-functional, 20–50% are defined as "functional" because they produce hormones leading to different syndromes associated with an excess of that specific hormone [1, 2]. There is evidence that patients with functional tumors survive longer than those affected by non-functional tumors, with median overall survival (OS) 54 months *vs* 26 months, respectively [8]. Insulinoma and gastrinoma represent the two most common functional pNETs. Vasoactive intestinal polypeptide-producing tumor (VIPoma), glucagonoma, somatostatinoma, pancreatic polypeptide-producing

L. Antonuzzo (✉) · E. Lucherini · F. Di Costanzo · G. Meoni
Department of Oncology, Careggi Hospital, Florence, Italy
e-mail: lorenzo.antonuzzo@gmail.com

L. Messerini · C. Comin
Division of Pathological Anatomy, Department of Critical Care Medicine and Surgery
University of Florence, Italy

A. Valeri et al. (eds.), *What's New in Surgical Oncology*,
DOI: 10.1007/978-88-470-5310-6_9, © Springer-Verlag Italia 2013

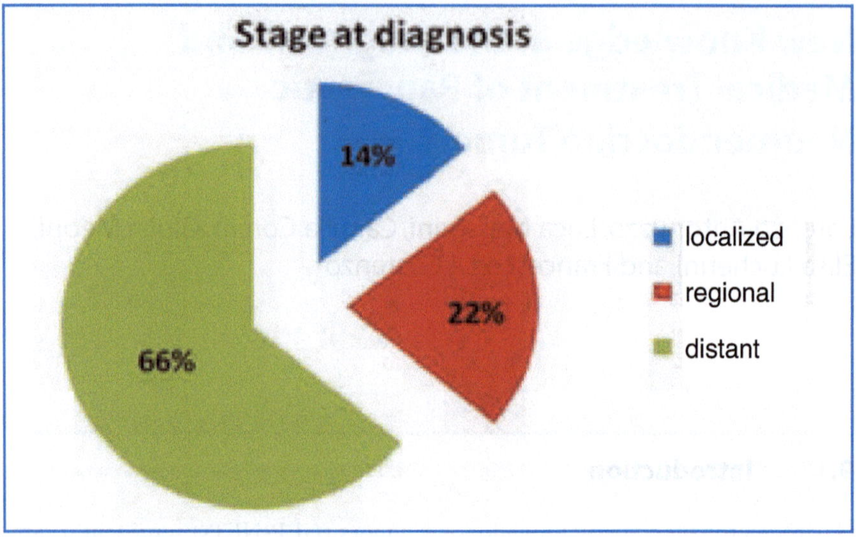

Fig. 9.1 Pancreatic neuroendocrine tumors: stage at diagnosis

tumor (PPoma), adrenocorticotropic hormone-producing tumor (ACTHoma), growth hormone-releasing factor-producing tumor (GRFoma), calcitonin-producing tumor, and parathyroid hormone-related peptide-producing tumor are extremely rare (9). Most pNETs have a sporadic origin, but 15–20% may be associated with familiar disorders such as multiple endocrine neoplasia type 1 (MEN type 1), von Hippel–Lindau (VHL) disease, neurofibromatosis 1 (NF-1) and tuberous sclerosis (TSC) [10, 11]. pNETs show localized disease at diagnosis in only 14% of cases, regional spread and distant metastasis are present in 22% and 64% of patients respectively (Fig. 9.1) [12].

9.2 Histological Features and World Health Organization (WHO) Classification 2010

Neuroendocrine tumors (NETs) are considered to be epithelial neoplasms with neuroendocrine differentiation. However, for many years, these tumors were defined as "carcinoid" since Siegfried Oberndorfer in 1907 coined, for the first time, the term "karzinoide" ("cancer-like") for a tumor in the small intestine. NETs can arise in many organs, but most NETs arise from the gut or bronchopulmonary system. GEP-NETs represent a heterogeneous group of relatively uncommon neoplasms originating from the pancreas or gastrointestinal tract: gastrointestinal neuroendocrine tumors (GI-NETs). The clinical outcome of these tumors is extremely variable, ranging from indolent disease to highly aggressive disease. Despite appreciable behavioral differences, pNETs and GI-NETs, are considered to belong to the same family of tumors (NETs) because they both express neuroendocrine markers.

The diagnosis of NET is based primarily on morphology and immunohistochemical expression of the general markers of neuroendocrine differentiation. Cytological features vary from round-to-ovoid cells with slightly granular cytoplasm and nuclei with dispersed chromatin ("salt and pepper") to small or large neuroendocrine cells. The former are typical of less aggressive tumors; the latter are associated with an adverse outcome. The more common architectural features of NETs are trabecular, nested, glandular or mixed. These patterns are frequently found in less aggressive NETs, whereas aggressive NETs show irregular patterns with areas of necrosis. Among the several immunohistochemical markers of neuroendocrine differentiation available, synaptophysin (a small-vesicle-associated marker) and chromogranin (a large secretory granule-associated marker) are considered to be more useful for the diagnosis of NETs.

The clinical behavior of NETs is related to several characteristics: anatomic location as well as the grading and stage of disease. In 2000, the WHO proposed a clinicopathological classification to stratify NETs according to malignant potential, i.e., well differentiated (benign or with uncertain malignant potential); well-differentiated (low-grade malignant); or poorly differentiated (high-grade malignant). This categorization was based on: tumor size, extent of organ-specific invasion, lymph node or distant metastases, angio-invasion, functional status, and proliferation index. This classification showed NETs arising at different anatomical sites with different biological and clinical behavior. This statement was confirmed and clearly defined by the European Neuroendocrine Tumor Society (ENETS) that in 2006 and 2007 proposed a site-specific tumor/node/metastasis (TNM) staging system for NETs.

Moreover, ENETS proposed a histological grading system based on mitotic activity and the proliferation index that was applicable for all anatomic sites of the digestive system. The same histological grading system for NETs was adopted in 2010 by the WHO [3–14]. Therefore, at the present time, neuroendocrine neoplasms (NENs) of the pancreas are classified by histology based on the same criteria established for NENs arising at other sites by ENETS and WHO. Two main categories can be identified: NETs and neuroendocrine carcinoma (NEC). NETs are well or moderately differentiated tumors that are divided into two grades: G1 or low-grade (mitoses <2 per10 high power fields and/or Ki-67 labeling index ≤2%) and G2 or intermediate grade (mitoses of 2–20 per 10 high

Table 9.1 Grading system for neuroendocrine tumors of the pancreas by the European Neuroendocrine Tumor Society (ENETS) and World Health Organization (WHO)

ENETS/WHO Grade	Mitotic Count (10 HPF)	Ki-67 Index (%)	Clinical Behavior
Low (G1)	<2	≤ 2	Variable
Intermediate (G2)	2-20	3-20	Variable
High (G3)	>20	>20	Highly aggressive

Table 9.2 Comparison of the definition for the T category in the European Neuroendocrine Tumor Society (ENETS) and World Health Organization (WHO) Tumor/Node/Metastasis (TNM) staging systems

Extent of Tumor	TNM for ENETS	TNM for WHO
T1	Confined to the pancreas, <2 cm	Confined to the pancreas, <2 cm
T2	Confined to the pancreas, 2–4 cm	Confined to the pancreas, >2 cm
T3	Confined to the pancreas, >4 cm, or invasion of duodenum or bile duct	Tumor extends beyond the pancreas
T4	Invasion of adjacent organs or major vessels	Tumor involves the celiac axis or superior mesenteric artery

power fields and/or Ki-67 labeling index of 3–20%). NECs are poorly differentiated tumors (mitoses >20 per 10 high power fields and/or Ki-67 labeling index >20%). NECs are highly aggressive tumors that rapidly metastasize, whereas NETs can present with indolent or highly malignant behavior (Table 9.1).

However, other cutoff values have been proposed as prognostic indicators. For p-NETs, it has been demonstrated to be a Ki-67 index >5% (15). Although several cutoff values have been proposed, two parallel systems for the staging of p-NETs are available, i.e., the staging system by the ENETS and the WHO. These systems are different given the fact that, although they use the same TNM terminology, they refer to different extents of disease. This can lead to confusion and limits the possibility of comparing the results of clinical trials (Table 9.2). Recently, a large international cohort study compared the accuracy and the usefulness of the TNM staging systems set by ENETS and WHO in a series of 1,072 NENs of the pancreas. This study demonstrated that the ENETS TNM staging system was more accurate and superior in performance than that set by the WHO TNM staging system [16].

9.3 Treatment

The management of pNETs requires a multidisciplinary approach. Moreover, given the rarity of these tumors, patients should be treated at highly specialized centers. A recent analysis showed a significant difference in survival between two population based-studies (Surveillance, Epidemiology and End Results program (SEER) and National Cancer Data Base (NCDB)) and two institutional databases of centers with experience in the treatment of NETs. Among stage-IV patients, 5-year survival rates were 15% and 19% in the SEER and NCDB *vs* 55% and 57% in the two institutional databases, respectively (Table 9.3). It seems reasonable to suggest that this significant difference in survival could be due to the better care of patients treated in specialized centers [17]. Resection remains the mainstay for the treatment of early-stage disease and hepatic metastasis in selected cases. Medical treatment has a key role in the manage-

Table 9.3 Discrepancies in the survival of patients with neuroendocrine tumors across studies

TNM Stage	Institutional Analysis (US)	Population Database (SEER)
I	100%	62%
II	88%	–
III	85%	53%
IV	57%	20%

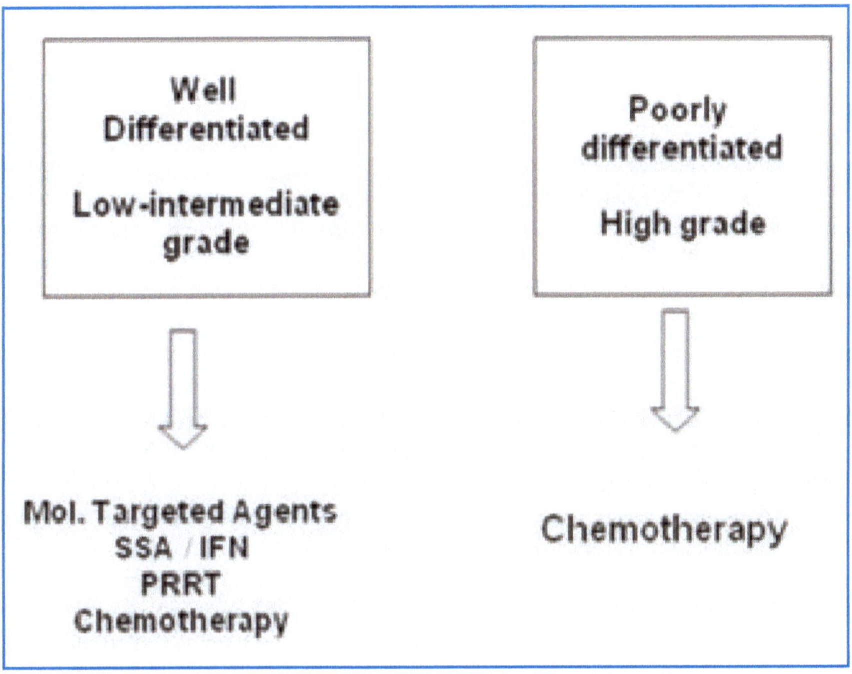

Fig. 9.2 WHO classification 2010 and treatment options

ment of advanced-stage pNETs, allowing symptom control and tumor-mass reduction.

Non-surgical therapeutic approaches include medical treatments, interventional radiology methods and radiotherapy. Medical approaches are represented by chemotherapy (CT), molecular-targeted agents (everolimus and sunitinib), hormonal therapy (somatostatin analogs (SSAs)) and immunomodulating agents (interferon (INF)). Interventional radiology methods include: radiofrequency ablation, transarterial chemoembolization, transarterial radioembolization and nuclear medicine methods (e.g., polypeptide radionuclide receptor therapy (PPRT)). External beam radiotherapy has a palliative role, especially in the treatment of bone metastasis (Fig. 9.2).

9.3.1 SSAs and INF

The neuropeptide somatostatin is one of the major regulatory peptides in the central nervous system and digestive tract. Somatostatin acts by inhibiting the secretion of various hormones and peptides. For this reason, SSAs remain the mainstay of treatment of symptomatic GEP-NETs. Due to their short half-life (<2 min), native SSAs are not currently used. Nevertheless, the SSAs long-acting octreotide and lanreotide autogel are characterized by long-acting formulations which allow monthly administration. Long-acting octreotide and lanreotide autogel bind mainly to the somastostatin receptor subtypes 2 (SSTR2) and 5 (SSTR5) and provide symptomatic as well as biochemical responses in ≤75% of patients [18]. Recently, pasireotide (a SSA with high affinity for all types of SSTRs) was approved for acromegaly treatment. Although early data suggest that this drug is effective in patients affected by NETs not responsive to currently available SSAs, the treatment of NETs with pasireotide is restricted in clinical trials [19]. SSAs are safe, well-tolerated and easy to use. In retrospective experiences, SSAs provided a 5% partial response (PR) and 50% stable disease (SD).

Rinke et al. randomized 85 treatment-naïve patients with metastatic well-differentiated tumors in the midgut to receive placebo or octreotide LAR 30 mg monthly until tumor progression. The primary endpoints were time to progression (TTP) and response rate (RR). The study was designed for the enrollment of 162 patients in 18 academic centers in Germany, but it was stopped early after the enrollment of 85 patients (43 received octreotide LAR 30 mg and 42 received placebo) due to the results of the interim analysis. In fact, median TTP was 15.6 months in the octreotide LAR group *vs* 5.9 months in the placebo group (hazard ratio (HR) 0.34; 95% confidence interval (CI), 20–0.59; p=0.000072) [20]. The authors demonstrated, in a preplanned subgroup analysis, that patients with low (0% to 10%) liver involvement and resected primary tumor benefited most from the treatment (HR, 0.17; 95% CI, 0.08–0.40; and HR, 0.16; 95% CI, 0.07–0.36, respectively). This prospective trial suggested an anti-tumor activity of SSAs in patients with well-differentiated midgut tumors. There is no prospective evidence supporting the anti-tumor activity of SSAs in pNETs but, in our opinion, the first-line treatment of patients affected by well- or moderately differentiated, low proliferating pNETs should consist of SSAs rather then chemotherapy. The Study of Lanreotide Autogel in Non-functioning Entero-pancreatic Endocrine Tumors (CLARINET) is an ongoing randomized trial which aims to define this issue. In this study, patients with G1 and G2 non-functioning pNETs and midgut NETs are randomized to lanreotide autogel (120 mg) monthly or to placebo. The primary endpoint is TTP. The enrolment is complete and data are expected within the next months.

INFα monotherapy has revealed similar efficacy to SSAs for controlling symptoms and inducing biochemical responses (80% of patients). Nevertheless, INFα has a different tolerability profile, with more frequent high-grade toxicity, such as flu-like syndrome, fatigue, weight loss, polyneuropathy, myositis, thrombocytopenia, anemia, leukopenia and hepatotoxicity as well as other side effects [21]. There is evidence that combination therapy (interferon alpha plus SSAs) does not increase RR but leads to a significantly lower risk of progression compared with SSAs alone [22].

9.3.2 Chemotherapy

The role of chemotherapy in the treatment of pNET is controversial. Based on retrospective studies, systemic chemotherapy with cisplatin and etoposide is the standard of care for poorly differentiated NECs with Ki-67 >20% (Fig. 9.1). This platinum-based combination provides a high RR, but the prognosis of this group of patients is poor (median survival, ≈20 months) [23, 24]. The recently published NORDIC NEC study retrospectively analyzed 305 patients affected by metastatic GI-NECs or unknown primary tumor with gastrointestinal metastases [25]. In this large retrospective study, patients with Ki-67 <55% were less responsive to platinum-based chemotherapy but survived longer than patients with Ki-67 >55%. The authors concluded that Ki-67 <55% represents a favorable prognostic factor and a negative predictive factor for the efficacy of platinum-based chemotherapy. Therefore, different from the present WHO classification, we should not consider GI-NECs as a single disease.

Several studies suggest that pNETs are responsive to chemotherapy (Tables 9.4 and 9.5).

Streptozotocin is an alkylating agent that has been studied in combination with 5-Fluorouracil (5FU) and doxorubicin in well-differentiated NETs. Notably, randomized trials comparing first-line chemotherapy *vs* best supportive care (BSC) are lacking. In a randomized trial, streptozotocin plus doxorubicin compared with streptozotocin plus 5FU significantly improved the RR (69% *vs* 45%), progression-free survival (PFS) (20 months *vs* 6.9 months) and

Table 9.4 Chemotherapy in pancreatic neuroendocrine tumors: randomized clinical trials

Regimen	Tumor Type	N	RR %	TTP months	OS months	Reference
Streptozocin/5FU streprozocin/cyfaxan	Mixed carcinoid and pancreas	42 47	33 26	– –	– –	Moertel et al., 1979
Adriamicina/ streprozocin/5FU	Mixed	86 86	21 22	6 7	12 16	Engstrom et al., 1984
Streptozocin/ doxorubicin *vs* streprozocin/5FU	Pancreas only	36 33	69* 45	20* 6.9	26.4* 16.8	Moertel et al., 1992
Streptozocin/5FU *vs* doxorubicina/5FU	Mixed carcinoid and pancreas	88 88	16 15.9	5.3 4.5	24.3* 15.7	Sun et al., 2005

*Statistically significant

Table 9.5 Chemotherapy in pancreatic neuroendocrine tumors: selected non-randomized trials

Regimen	Tumor Type	N	RR %	TTP mo	OS mo	Reference
5FU/doxorubicin/ CDDP	Mixed	74	15	–	–	Rougier et al. [56]
Carboplatin	Mixed	42	5	–	–	Saltz et al. [57]
DTIC/5FU/ epirubicina	Mixed	38	18	5	–	Di Bartolomeo et al. [58]
5FU/DTIC	Mixed	82	24	21	38	Bajetta et al. [59]
Capecitabine/ oxaliplatin	Mixed	40	28	18	32	Bajetta et al. [60]
Temozolomide/ thalidomide	Mixed	79	25	13.5	–	Kulke et al. [32]
Temozolomide	Mixed	36	14	7	16	Ekeblad et al. [31]
Temozolomide/ capecitabine	Pancreas	30	70	18.0	–	Strosberg et al. [33]

OS (26 months *vs* 18 months) [26]. On the basis of these results, streptozotocin was approved by the US Food and Drug Administration (FDA) for the treatment of pNETs. Nevertheless, the authors of this trial used non-standard criteria for response evaluation, and assessed biochemical response rather than objective tumor response as defined by Response Evaluation Criteria in Solid Tumors (RECIST) criteria. Moreover, in two retrospective analyses, streptozotocin plus doxorubicin showed mild anti-tumor activity with a RR of 10% [27, 28]. Dacarbazine monotherapy has been evaluated in a Phase II study enrolling 50 patients with pNETs. In this trial, dacarbazine provided a RR of 34% and OS of 19.3 months [29]. Nevertheless, due to its toxicity profile, dacarbazine is not frequently used in the treatment of pNETs. Temozolomide is an alkylating agent developed as an oral and less toxic alternative to dacarbazine [30]. In a retrospective analysis, Ekeblad et al. evaluated the efficacy and toxicity of temozolamide monotherapy in advanced NETs. The RR was 14% and SD was noted in 53% with a global disease control rate (DCR) of 67% [31]. The median TTP was 7 months. With respect to RR, 1 patient among the 14 affected by GI-NETs and 5 patients among the 11 affected by pNETs showed a radiological response. This observation supports the fact that well-differentiated pNETs are more responsive to systemic chemotherapy than NETs arising from the stomach, small intestine and large intestine. Temozolamide has been studied in patients affected by advanced NETs in combination with different anti-cancer drugs such as thalidomide, capecitabine and bevacizumab. In a Phase II trial, 41 patients affected by well-differentiated NETs were treated with a temozolamide plus thalidomide combination. In this trial, the authors observed a 45% RR (including 1 complete response (CR)) among the 11 patients affected by pNET [32]. The capecitabine and temozolamide combination is also effective in pNETs. In a single-institution retrospective experience, 30 patients with unresectable/metastatic pNETs were treated with capecitabine and temozolamide. The authors observed a RR of 59% and a CR in 6% [33].

In conclusion, there is no evidence strongly supporting the use of chemotherapy in well-differentiated pNETs. Streptozotocin is the only drug approved by FDA for the treatment of this disease, but its toxicity profile and limited availability inhibit wider use. Based on a retrospective analysis of 30 patients, temozolamide-based regimens are widely used in the treatment of advanced pNETs. Nevertheless, this evidence should be confirmed in randomized Phase III trials.

9.3.3 Targeted Therapy

Bevacizumab is a monoclonal antibody directed against vascular endothelial growth factor (VEGF) and has anti-angiogenic activity. Bevacizumab plus cytotoxic chemotherapy improves PFS in solid tumors such as colorectal, breast and non-small-cell lung cancer. Bevacizumab has been evaluated in combination with temozolamide in 29 patients affected by NETs [34]. In this Phase II study, RR was observed in 4/17 (24%) patients with pNET and in 0/12 (0%) patients with well-differentiated GI-NETs. Chemotherapy was inactive in non-pancreatic well-differentiated GI-NETs, even in combination with bevacizumab.

Recently, two pivotal trials led to the FDA approval of everolimus and sunitinib in unresectable/metastatic pNETs. Sunitinib is an oral tyrosine kinase inhibitor (TKI) that targets platelet-derived growth factor receptors (PDGFRs), vascular endothelial growth factor receptors (VEGFRs), the stem cell factor receptor (KIT), FMS-like tyrosine kinase-3 (FLT3), the macrophage colony-stimulating factor receptor (CSF-1R), and the glial cell line-derived neurotrophic factor receptor (RET) [35, 36].

Sunitinib is the standard of care in renal cell carcinoma and gastrointestinal stromal tumors (GISTs) after imatinib failure. Sunitinib was demonstrated to be active in advanced NETs, including patients with pNET and carcinoids [37]. In a Phase II study, 107 patients (pNET, n=66; carcinoid, n=41) were treated with sunitinib (50 mg/day) in a 4-weeks-on and 2-weeks-off regimen. The overall response rate (ORR) in pNET patients was 16.7%, moreover 68% of patients had SD, resulting in a DCR of 84.7%. Among carcinoid patients, the ORR was 2.4% with 83% SD. Median TTP was 7.7 months among patients with pNETs and 10.2 months among carcinoid patients. One-year survival was similar: 81.1% in pNET patients and 83.4% in carcinoid patients [37].

On the basis of these interesting data, the activity of sunitinib has been tested in a randomized double-blind, placebo-controlled, Phase III trial. In this study, patients with advanced progressive pNETs were randomized to sunitinib 37.5 mg/day continuous monotherapy *vs* placebo [38]. A total of 171 patients were randomized (86 received sunitinib and 85 received placebo). Patients with progressive disease receiving placebo were allowed to enroll in a separate open-label sunitinib extension protocol. This Phase III study was discontinued early in 2009 because an independent Data and Safety Monitoring Board undertook an unplanned analysis and found a statistically significant difference in PFS favoring the sunitinib arm [38]. Treatment with sunitinib improved median PFS by 5.9 months compared with placebo (11.4 months *vs* 5.5 months), with an HR of 0.42 (95% CI, 0.26–0.66); $p<0.001$). The ORR was 9.3% (95% CI, 3.2–15.4) with sunitinib [37]. Adverse events (AEs) were more frequently grade 1/2 and manageable. The most common treatment-related grade 3/4 AEs were neutropenia (12%), hypertension (10%), palmar–plantar erythrodysesthesia (6%), diarrhea (5%), asthenia (5%), abdominal pain (5%), stomatitis (4%) and thrombocytopenia (4%).

Mammalian target of rapamycin (mTOR) is a serine/threonine protein kinase that regulates the growth, proliferation and motility of cells as well as the transcription and translation of proteins [39]. Mutations in specific tumor suppressor genes known to regulate the mTOR pathway are associated with an increased risk of developing pNETs. These regulatory genes include phosphatase and tensin homolog (PTEN) [40, 41], the tuberous sclerosis complex 2 gene (TSC2) [42–44] and NF-1 gene [43, 44]. Additionally, patients affected by pNETs carrying mutated mTOR pathway genes (including PTEN and TSC2) have worse prognosis than patients with other common mutations [46].

Temsirolimus and everolimus are the two mTOR inhibitors tested in the treatment of NETs. In a Phase II trial, 37 patients with advanced NECs were treated with temsirolimus. The RR was 5.6% and DCR was 63.9%. Median TTP was 6 months and 1-year PFS was 40.1%. These data suggest a modest clinical activity of temsirolimus in NECs [47]. The rapamycin analog everolimus acts by blocking the signaling pathway downstream of insulin-like growth factor (IGF)-1, VEGF through mTOR inhibition. These combined actions lead to decrease in cell proliferation, angiogenesis and glucose uptake [48].

In a single-institution experience, Yao et al. reported a RR of 20% and a median PFS of 60 weeks in 60 NETs patients receiving 5 mg or 10 mg everolimus in combination with ocreotide LAR 30 mg monthly [49]. Moreover, the activity of everolimus was studied in the Phase II RAD001 In Advanced Neuroendocrine Tumors (RADIANT)-1 trial. This study evaluated everolimus activity in patients with advanced pNETs with progressive disease after chemotherapy [50]. In this study, 160 patients were treated with everolimus (10 mg daily dose). The study population was stratified as follows: stratum 1 (115 patients) received everolimus monotherapy and stratum 2 (45 patients) received combination therapy of everolimus plus octreotide LAR. The DCR was 82% *vs* 77% and the ORR was 9.6% *vs* 4.4% in the combination therapy stratum *vs* monotherapy stratum, respectively. PFS was 9.7 months *vs* 16.7 months and median OS was 24.9 months *vs* value not yet reached in strata 1 and 2, respectively. The most common AEs of everolimus were stomatitis, rash and diarrhea. Due to the study design, we cannot assume with strong evidence that the combination therapy of everolimus plus octreotide LAR is superior to everolimus monotherapy in the treatment of advanced NETs.

RADIANT-3 is a randomized, double-blind, placebo-controlled, Phase III trial that enrolled 410 patients with progressive, unresectable/metastatic pNETs. Patients were randomized to receive everolimus 10 mg/day plus BSC (n=207) or BSC alone (n=203) [51]. Notably, this is the largest trial ever conducted for NETs. The primary endpoint was PFS. Patients randomized to the placebo group were allowed to crossover to open-label everolimus at disease progression [52]. Baseline characteristics were well balanced in the two groups. After a median follow-up of 17 months, treatment with everolimus led to a statistically significant 6.4-month improvement in median PFS compared with placebo [52]. Patients reached 11.0 months PFS (95% CI, 8.4–13.9) with everolimus and 4.6 months PFS (95% CI, 3.1–5.4) with placebo with a HR of 0.35 (95% CI. 0.27–0.45; P<0.001). Confirmed ORR with everolimus was 5%. Treatment-related AEs of everolimus were more frequently grade 1/2 and manageable. The most common treatment-related grade 3/4 AEs were stomatitis (7%), anemia (6%), hyperglycemia (5%), and thrombocytopenia (4%) [52]. On the basis of these impressive data, the FDA and European Medicines Agency (EMEA) approved everolimus for the treatment of pNETs.

9.3.4 Other Biological Agents

Recently, new agents have been evaluated in clinical trials. AMG 479 is a fully human monoclonal antibody directed against the insulin-like growth factor type-I receptor (IGF-IR). Kulke et al. treated 60 patients (30 carcinoid and 30 pNETs) with AMG479 in a Phase II study [53]. There were no objective responses according to RECIST criteria. Median PFS was 10.5 months for carcinoid patients and 4.2 months for pNET patients. The treatment was well tolerated; grade 3/4 toxicity consisted of hyperglycemia (4%), neutropenia (4%) and thrombocytopenia (4%). AMG479 single-agent was not found to result in major tumor response in patients with low–intermediate-grade carcinoid or pNETs [53].

Pazopanib is an oral TKI of the VEGFR, PDGFR and KIT that has demonstrated clinical activity in NETs. In the Pazopanib as a Sequencing Treatment in Progressive Metastatic Neuroendocrine Tumors (PAZONET) Phase II trial, 33 patients with locally advanced or metastatic GI-NETs or pNETs previously treated with at least one anti-angiogenetic or mTOR inhibitor drug received pazopanib (800 mg) daily [54]. At 6 months, the clinical benefit rate (CR plus PR plus SD) was 85%. The clinical benefit rate was 100% in patients with no previous targeted therapy (7 patients), 89% in subjects with previous mTOR inhibitor therapy (9 patients), 83% in individuals with previous anti-angiogenic treatment (12 patients) and 60% in patients with previous anti-angiogenic and mTOR inhibitor therapies (5 patients). Median PFS was reached only in the subgroup of patients previously treated with anti-angiogenic and mTOR inhibitors (20.6 weeks; 95% CI, 10.4–30.8). More frequent toxicities of any grade were asthenia (75%), diarrhea (63%) and nausea (42%). The activity of pazopanib in advanced NETs is promising regardless of previous treatment with other targeted therapies. Phase III randomized clinical trials are needed to confirm these data.

Pertuzumab is a recombinant humanized monoclonal antibody that targets the extracellular dimerization domain (subdomain II) of the human epidermal growth factor receptor (HER)2. It blocks ligand-dependent heterodimerization of HER2 with other HER family members, including EGFR, HER3, and HER4.

Firdaus et al. treated 43 patients with well-differentiated NETs in a Phase II trial with bevacizumab (15 mg/kg) plus pertuzumab (420 mg) after a loading dose of 840 mg as well as Octreotide LAR (30 mg) every 28 days [55]. The ORR for carcinoid patients was 15.6% with a median PFS of 8.5 months (95% CI, 6.3–not applicable). Treatment-related grade-3 toxicities included: hypertension (28%), left ventricular ejection fraction (LVEF) dysfunction (9%; reversible with trial drug hold) and diarrhea (7%). Grade 4 toxicity was not reported. Median treatment duration was 38 weeks (range: 0–76 weeks). The ORR of the combination in carcinoid patients was encouraging and appeared higher than for historical data.

BEZ235 is a potent, specific oral mTOR inhibitor (mTORC1 and 2) and pan-class PI3K inhibitor. Everolimus provides clinical benefit for patients with pNET but *de novo* and acquired resistance to this agent has been noted. A potential mechanism for resis tance tmTOR inhibitors has been identified in activation of the PI3K/AKT pathway. A trial that evaluates if BEZ235 can overcome this mechanism of resistance by targeting PI3K and mTORC1 and 2 in patients with progressive pNET after everolimus treatment is in progress.

9.4 Conclusions

Recently, new agents have been introduced for the medical treatment of pNETs. These agents, characterized by high activity and favorable tolerability profiles, improve the outcome of patients with pNETs.

Patients affected by pNETs should be referred to medical centers with specific experience in the treatment of these rare tumors and who work in dedicated multidisciplinary teams. The goal of a multidisciplinary team is to decide a "treatment strategy" rather than a sequence of single treatments. The therapeutic strategy should be highly individualized based on the different ranges of tumor burden and symptoms. The best therapeutic approach for each patient depends on whether the goal of treatment is to slow tumor growth, to reach resectability (conversion therapy) or to improve symptoms by inhibition of the secretion of bioactive agents. In patients with resectable pNETs, resection of the primary tumor and metastases remains the main (and the only) curative option. In patients with borderline-resectable disease, the aim of the treatment is to reduce tumor burden and make resectable the disease. In this case, chemotherapy provides a better RR. In patients with unresectable disease, the aim of the treatment is to stabilize the disease as long as possible and, in the case of functional tumors, to control syndromes by using SSAs, biotherapy, targeted therapies and chemotherapy in the best sequence for each patient.

References

1. Yalcin S, Oyan B, Bayraktar Y (2007) Current medical treatment of pancreatic neuroendocrine tumors. Hepatogastroenterology 54:278–84
2. Ehehalt F, Saeger HD, Schmidt CM, Grutzman R (2009) Neuroendocrine tumors of the pancreas. Oncologist 14:454–67
3. Yao JC, Hassan M, Phan A et al (2008) One hundred years after "carcinoid": epidemiology of and prognostic factors for neuroendocrine tumors in 35, 825 cases in the United States. J Clin Oncol 26:3063–72
4. Vortmeyer AO, Huang S, Lubensky I, Zhuang Z (2004) Non-islet origin of pancreatic islet cell tumors. J Clin Endocrinol Metab 89:1934–1938
5. Burnik FS, Yalcin S (2009) NF-kappa gene polymorphism in NET. Chemotherapy 2009. Chemotherapy 55:381–5
6. Panzuto F, Nasoni S, Falconi M et al (2005) Prognostic factors and survival in endocrine tumor patients: comparison between gastrointestinal and pancreatic localization. Endocr Relat Cancer 12:1083–92
7. Zikusoka MN, Kidd M, Eick G et al (2005) The molecular genetics of gastroenteropancreatic neuroendocrine tumors. Cancer 104:2292–309
8. Halfdanarson TR, Rabe KG, Rubin J et al (2008) Pancreatic neuroendocrine tumors (PNET): incidence, prognosis and recent trend toward improved survival. Ann Oncol 19:1727–33
9. Kimura W, Kuroda A, Morioka Y (1991) Clinical pathology of endocrine tumors of the pancreas. Analysis of autopsy cases. Dig Dis Sci 36:933–42
10. Zikusoka MN, Kidd M, Eick G et al (2005) The molecular genetics of gastroenteropancreatic neuroendocrine tumors. Cancer 104:2292–309
11. Klöppel G, Perren A, Heitz PU The gastroenteropancreatic neuroendocrine cell system and its tumors. Ann NY Acad Sci 1014:13-27
12. Yao JC, Hassan M, Phan A et al (2008) One hundred years after "carcinoid": epidemiology of and prognostic factors for neuroendocrine tumors in 35, 825 cases in the United States. J Clin Oncol 26:3063–72
13. Rindi G, Kloppel G, Alhman H et al (2006) TNM staging of foregut (neuro)endocrine tumors: a consensus proposal including a grading system. Virchows Arch 449:395-401
14. Rindi G, Arnold R, Bosman FT et al (2010) Nomenclature and classification of neuroendocrine neoplasms of the digestive system. In Bosman FT, Carneiro F, Hruban RH, Theise ND (eds) WHO classification of tumours of the digestive system. IARC Lyon, pp 13-14
15. Scarpa A, Mantovani W, Capelli P et al (2010) Pancreatic endocrine tumors: improved TNM staging and histopathological grading permit a clinically efficient prognostic stratification of patients. Mod Pathol 23.824-833
16. Rindi G, Falconi M, Klersy C et al (2012) TNM staging of neoplasms of endocrine pancreas: results from a large international cohort study. J Natl Cancer Inst 104:764-777
17. Strosberg TR (2011) Survival analyses of pancreatic neuroendocrine tumors: Contrasting institutional databases with population-based studies. J Clin Oncol 29:(suppl 4; abstr 186)

18. Ben-Shlomo A, Melmed S (2007) Pasireotide a somatostatin analog for the potential treatment of acromegaly, neuroendocrine tumora and Cushing's disease. Drugs 10:885-895
19. Bruns C, Lewis I, Briner U et al (2002) SOM230: a novel somatostatin peptidomimetic with broad somatotropin release inhibiting factor (SRIF) receptor binding and a unique antisecretory profile. Eur J Endocrinol 146:707–16
20. Rinke A, Muller HH, Schade-Brittinger C et al (2009) Placebo-controlled, doubleblind, prospective, randomized study on the effect of octreotide LAR in the control of tumor growth in patients with metastatic neuroendocrine midgut tumors: a report from the PROMID Study Group. J Clin Oncol 27:4656–63
21. Pavel ME, Baum U, Hahn EG et al (2006) Efficacy and tolerability of pegylated IFNalpha in patients with neuroendocrine gastroenteropancreatic carcinomas. J Interferon Cytokine Res 26:8–13
22. Kolby L, Persson G, Franzen S, Ahren B (2003) Randomized clinical trial of the eff ect of interferon alpha on survival in patients with disseminated midgut carcinoid tumours. Br J Surg 90: 687–93
23. Mortel CG (1991) Treatment of Neuroendocrine Carcinomas with Combined Etoposide and Cisplatin. Cancer 68:227-232
24. Mitry E (1999) Treatment of poorly differentiated neuroendocrine tumours with etoposide and cisplatin. Br J Cancer 81(8):1351-1355
25. Sorbye H, Welin S, Langer SW et al (2013) Predictive and prognostic factors for treatment and survival in 305 patients with advanced gastrointestinal neuroendocrine carcinoma (WHO G3): The NORDIC NEC study. Ann Oncol 24(1):152-160
26. Moertel CG, Lefkopoulo M, Lipsitz S et al (1992) Streptozotocin-doxorubicin, streptozotocin-fluorouracil or chlorozotocin in the treatment of advanced islet cell carcinoma. N Engl J Med 326:519–23
27. Cheng P, Saltz L (1999) Failure to confirm major objective antitumor activity of streptozocin and doxorubicin in the treatment of patients with advanced islet cell carcinoma . Cancer 86:944-948
28. McCollum AD, Kulke MH, Ryan DP et al (2004) Lack of efficacy of streptozocin and doxorubicin in patients with advanced pancreatic endocrine tumors. Am J Clin Oncol 27:485-488
29. Ramanathan RK, Cnaan A, Hahn RG, Carbone PP, Haller DG (2001) Phase II trial ofdacarbazine (DTIC) in advanced pancreatic islet cell carcinoma. Study of the Eastern Cooperative Oncology Group-E6282. Ann Oncol 12:1139-1143
30. Stevens MF, Hickman JA, Langdon SP et al (1987) Antitumor activity and pharmacokinetics in mice of 8-carbamoyl-3-methyl-imidazo [5,1-D]-1,2,3,5-tetrazin-4(3H)-one (CCRG 81045; M&B 39831), a novel drug with potential as an alternative to dacarbazine. Cancer Res 47:5846-5852
31. Ekeblad S, Sundin A, Janson ET et al (2007) Temozolomide as monotherapy is effective in treatment of advanced malignant neuroendocrine tumors. Clin Cancer Res 13:2896–991
32. Kulke MH, Stuart K, Enzinger PC et al (2006) Phase II study of temozolomide and thalidomide in patients with metastaticneu roendocrine tumors. J Clin Oncol 24:401–6
33. Strosberg JR, Fine R.L,Choi J et al (2011) First-Line Chemotherapy With Capecitabine and Temozolomide in Patients With Metastatic Pancreatic Endocrine Carcinomas. Cancer 117:268–75
34. Kulke MH, Stuart K, Earle CC (2006) A phase II study of temozolomide and bevacizumab in patients with advanced neuroendocrine tumors. ASCO annual meeting proceedings, part I. J Clin Oncol 24:18S
35. Sutent (Sunitinib malate) capsules, oral [prescribing information]. New York, NY: Pfizer Inc; May 2011
36. Raymond E, Dahan L, Raoul JL et al (2011) Sunitinib malate for the treatment of pancreatic neuroendocrine tumors. N Engl J Med 364:501–13
37. Kulke MH, Lens H, Meropol NJ et al (2008) Activity of Sunitinib in patients with advanced neuroendocrine tumors. J Clin Oncol 26:3403–10
38. Raymond E, Dahan L, Raoul JL, et al (2011) Sunitinib malate for the treatment of pancreatic neuroendocrine tumors. N Engl J Med 364:501–13

39. Tokunaga C, Yoshino K, Yonezawa K (2004) mTOR integrates amino acid- and energysensing pathways. Biochem Biophys Res Commun 313:443–6
40. Perren A, Komminoth P, Saremaslani P et al (2000) Mutation and expression analyses reveal differential subcellular compartmentalization of PTEN in endocrine pancreatic tumors compared to normal islet cells. Am J Pathol 157:1097–1103
41. Wang L, Ignat A, Axiotis CA (2002) Differential expression of the PTEN tumor suppressor protein in fetal and adult neuroendocrine tissues and tumors: progressive loss of PTEN expression in poorly differentiated neuroendocrine neoplasms. Appl Immunohistochem Mol Morphol 10:139–146
42. Dworakowska D, Grossman AB (2009) Are neuroendocrine tumours a feature of tuberous sclerosis? A systematic review. Endocr Relat Cancer 16:45–58
43. Francalanci P, Omedi-Camassei F, Purificato C et al (2009) Malignant pancreatic endocrine tumor in a child with tuberous sclerosis. Am J Surg Pathol 27:1386–1389
44. Merritt JL, Davis DM, Pittelkow MR, Babovic-Vuksanovic D (2006) Extensive acrochordons and pancreatic islet-cell tumors in tuberous sclerosis associated with TSC2 mutations. Am J Med Genet A 140:1669–1672
45. Johannessen CM, Reczek EE, James MF et al (2005) The NF1 tumor suppressor critically regulates TSC2 and mTOR. Proc Natl Acad Sci USA 102:8573–8578
46. Perren A, Wiesli P, Schmid S et al (2006) Pancreatic endocrine tumors are a rare manifestation of the neurofibromatosis type 1 phenotype: molecular analysis of a malignant insulinoma in a NF-1 patient. Am J Surg Pathol 30:1047–1051
47. Jiao Y, Shi C, Edil BH et al (2011) DAXX/ATRX, MEN1, and mTOR pathway genes are frequently altered in pancreatic neuroendocrine tumors. Science 331:1199–203
48. Duran I, Kortmansky J, Singh D et al (2006) A phase II clinical and pharmacodynamic study of temsirolimus in advanced neuroendocrine carcinomas. Brit J Cancer 95:1148–54
49. Afinitor (Everolimus) tablets for oral administration [prescribing information]. East Hanover, NJ: Novartis Pharmaceuticals Corporation; May 2011
50. Yao JC, Phan AT, Chang DZ et al (2008) Efficacy of RAD001 (Everolimus) and octreotide LAR in advanced low- to intermediate-grade neuroendocrine tumors: results of a phase II study. J Clin Oncol 26:4311–8
51. Yao JC, Lombard-Bohas C, Baudin E et al (2010) Daily oral Everolimus activity in patients with metastatic pancreatic neuroendocrine tumors after failure of cytotoxic chemotherapy: a phase II trial. J Clin Oncol 28:69–76
52. Yao JC, Shah MH, Ito T et al (2011) Everolimus for advanced pancreatic neuroendocrine tumors. N Engl J Med 364:514–23
53. Kulke M, Chan JA, Ryan D et al (2012) A multi-institutional phase II open-label study of AMG 479 in advanced carcinoid and pancreatic neuroendocrine tumors. J Clin Oncol 30 (suppl; abstr 4125)
54. Pulido EG, Castellano DE, Garcia Carbonero R et al (2012) PAZONET: Results of a phase II trial of Pazopanib as a sequencing treatment in progressive metastatic neuroendocrine tumors (NETs) patients, on behalf of the Spanish task force for NETs (GETNE)—NCT01280201. J Clin Oncol 30 (suppl; abstr 4119)
55. Firdaus I, Shih K.C, Zakari A et al (2012) Bevacizumab, pertuzumab, and sandostatin for patients (pts) with advanced neuroendocrine cancers (NET). J Clin Oncol 30 (suppl; abstr 4127)
56. Rougier P, Oliveira J, Ducreux M et al (1991) Metastatic carcinoid and islet cell tumours of the pancreas: a phase II trial of the efficacy of combination chemotherapy with 5-fluorouracil, doxorubicin and cisplatin. Eur J Cancer 27:1380-1382
57. Saltz L, Lauwers G, Wiseberg J et al (1993) A phase II trial of carboplatin in patients with advanced APUD tumors. Cancer 15,72:619-622
58. Di Bartolomeo M, Bajetta E, Bochicchio AM (1995) A phase II trial of dacarbazine, fluorouracil and epirubicin in patients with neuroendocrine tumours. A study by the Italian Trials in Medical Oncology (I.T.M.O.) Group. Ann Oncol 6:77-79
59. Bajetta E, Ferrari L, Procopio G et al (2002) Efficacy of a chemotherapy combination for the treatment of metastatic neuroendocrine tumours. Ann Oncol 13(4):614-21

Adrenal Tumors

10

Carlo Bergamini, Jacopo Martellucci, Tatiana Bargellini, Ancuta Leahu, Domenico Capizzi, Alfredo Miseri and Andrea Valeri

10.1 Introduction and Epidemiology

Adrenocortical tumors (ACTs) are common, with an estimated prevalence of 7.3% in autopsy cases [1]. A computed tomography (CT) study reported an overall prevalence of 4.4% of adrenal lesions in a population aged >50 years [2]. In contrast, adrenocortical cancer (ACC) is a rare malignancy with an estimated incidence of 4–12 per million population and a variable (but generally poor) prognosis. Women are more often affected than men (ratio 1.5:1) [3]. An exceptionally high annual incidence of ACC has been reported for children in southern Brazil (3.4–4.2 per million children *vs* an estimated worldwide incidence of 0.3 per million children younger than 15 years) and is related to a mutation in the TP53 tumor suppressor gene. The age distribution is reported to be bimodal with a first peak in childhood and a second higher peak in the fourth and fifth decade.

10.2 Pathogenesis and Genetics

10.2.1 Hereditary Tumor Syndromes

ACTs can arise from several hereditary tumor syndromes. The causative genes in these syndromes have also been found to be involved in the tumorigenesis of some sporadic ACTs. Table 10.1 summarizes these hereditary tumor syndromes and the gene/chromosomal loci involved.

C. Bergamini (✉) · J. Martellucci · T. Bargellini · A. Leahu · A. Valeri
General, Emergency and Minimally Invasive Surgery
Careggi Hospital, Florence, Italy
e-mail: drcarlobergamini@gmail.com

D. Capizzi · A. Miseri
General Surgery, Gorizia Hospital, Gorizia, Italy

A. Valeri et al. (eds.), *What's New in Surgical Oncology*,
DOI: 10.1007/978-88-470-5310-6_10, © Springer-Verlag Italia 2013

Table 10.1 Hereditary tumor syndromes associated with adrenocortical tumors

Hereditary Tumor Syndrome	Manifestation of Tumor		
	Gene (chromosomal locus)	Syndrome	Prevalence of ACT
Li–Fraumeni	TP53 (17p13), hCHK2 (22q12.1), lq23	Soft tissue sarcoma, osteosarcoma, breast cancer, brain tumor, leukemia, ACC	ACC, 3%
Beckwith–Wiede mann	IGF2, H19, CDKN1C, KCNQ1 (11p15)	Exomphalos macroglossia, gigantism, ACC, nephroblastoma, hepatoblastoma, rhabdomyosarcoma	ACC, 5%
Carney complex	PRKAR1A (17q23-q24) 2P16	Cardiac, endocrine, cutaneous and neural myxomatous tumors, and pigmented lesions of the skin and mucosa	PNAD 90–100%
MEN1	MEN1 (11Q13)	Parathyroid, pancreatic islet cell, anterior pituitary and ACTs	ACT, 55%; ACC, rare
Congenital adrenal	CYP21B (6P21.3)	Adrenal hyperplasia, virilization, salt wasting	ACT, 82%; hyperplasia, hyperplasia 100%

ACT Adrenocortical tumor, *ACC* adrenocortical cancer

10.2.1.1 Li–Fraumeni Syndrome (LFS)

LFS is an autosomal dominant familial disease characterized by the early onset of tumors and multiple tumors in affected individuals. ACCs have been reported to occur in 3–4% of patients with LFS [4]. Seventy percent of LFS cases are a result of a germline mutation in the *TP53* gene [5]. A second variant is caused by a heterozygous germline mutation in the *hCHK2* gene [6].

10.2.1.2 Beckwith–Wiedemann Syndrome (BWS)

BWS is a congenital overgrowth syndrome characterized by exomphalos, macroglossia, and gigantism in the neonate as well as the development of childhood tumors. About 15% of cases with BWS are familial, with the remainder being sporadic. BWS is linked to the 11p15 chromosomal locus. Genes located at 11p15 and implicated in the pathogenesis of BWS are the insulin-like growth factor 2 (*IGF2*), H19, and cyclin-dependent kinase inhibitor 1C genes [7].

10.2.1.3 Carney Complex (CNC)

CNC is a dominantly inherited syndrome characterized by cardiac, endocrine, cutaneous, and neural myxomatous tumors, as well as pigmented lesions of the skin and mucosa [8]. Primary pigmented nodular adrenocortical disease (PPNAD), a main feature of CNC, is a rare cause of adrenocorticotropic hormone (ACTH)-independent Cushing's syndrome, seen usually in children and young adults.

10.2.1.4 Multiple Endocrine Neoplasia 1 (MEN1)

MEN1 is an autosomal dominant syndrome characterized by parathyroid, pancreatic islet cell, and anterior pituitary tumors. ACCs have been reported only rarely with MEN1. The *MEN1* gene, located on 11q13, encodes the menin protein. Although the function of menin is not known, mutations have resulted in the loss of its function, suggesting that menin has suppressor activities [9].

10.2.1.5 Congenital Adrenal Hyperplasia (CAH)

CAH is an autosomal recessive disorder resulting from an enzyme deficiency in the cortisol synthesis pathway. Typically, the enzyme 21-hydroxylase, which is encoded by cytochrome P450, family 21, subfamily B (*CYP21B*), is deficient. A lack of this enzyme leads to compensatory stimulation of the adrenal cortex by corticotrophin-releasing hormone and ACTH with consequent adrenal hyperplasia and overproduction of cortisol precursors, engendering higher levels of androgens. Rarely, ACCs have been described in CAH [10].

10.2.2 Genetics of Sporadic ACC (Table 10.2)

10.2.2.1 TP53 Gene

The *TP53* gene is a tumor suppressor gene that is most frequently mutated in human cancers [11]. The p53 protein is a transcription factor in regulation of

Table 10.2 Evidence of genes involved in sporadic ACTs

Gene (Chromosomal Locus)	Evidence of Involvement in Sporadic ACTs
TP53 (17p13)	Mutation of TP53 in 20–27% of ACCs and 0–6% of ACAs; 17p13 LOH occurs in ≤87.5% of ACCs and ≤30% of ACAs
IGF2 (11p15)	Overexpression of IGF2 mRNA in ACCs compared with ACAs. 11p15 LOH occurs in ≤83% of ACCs and 34% of ACAs
PRKAR1A (17q23-q24)	LOH of 17 q23-q24 occurs in 53% of ACCs and 23% of ACAs; mutation of PRKAR1A occurs in 10% of ACAs but not in ACCs
MEN1 (11q13)	LOH of 11q13 occurs in 100% of ACCs and 25% of ACAs; MEN1 mutation occurs in 7% of and ACAs
GNAS (20q13.2)	Mutation of GNAS occurs in ACAs and tumors of patients with adrenocorticotropic hormone-independent macronodular hyperplasia

LOH, loss of heterozigosity

the cell cycle, causing cell-cycle arrest or cell death in response to DNA-damaging agents such as radiation and viruses. *TP53* mutation is thought to be a late event in the evolution of malignant transformation in sporadic ACTs. Mutations in exons 5– 8 of *TP53* have been found in 20–27% of sporadic ACCs and 0–6% of sporadic adrenocortical adenomas (ACAs).

10.2.2.2 IGF2, p57^{kip2} (CDKN1C), and H19 Genes

Rearrangements, loss of heterozygosity (LOH; loss of one of two alleles of a gene), and abnormal imprinting of the 11p15.5 locus result in low p57^{kip2} and H19 and elevated IGF2 mRNA expression, and have been reported in sporadic ACCs. Higher *IGF2* expression is associated with a more malignant phenotype, and over-expression of *IGF2* is associated with a higher risk of ACC recurrence. Furthermore, LOH of the 11p15 locus has been demonstrated more frequently in ACCs than in ACAs (in 67% of ACCs *vs* 13% of ACAs) [12].

10.2.2.3 MEN1 Gene

Because LOH of 11q13 occurs in ≈20% of sporadic ACTs, and adrenal tumors occur in ≤40% of patients from MEN1 kindreds, *MEN1* was considered to be a prime candidate gene in the pathogenesis of these lesions. However, on basis of other studies, at present it is unlikely that the *MEN1* gene plays a prominent part in the pathogenesis of sporadic ACTs [13].

10.2.2.4 RKAR1A Gene

PRKAR1A is the main mediator of cyclic adenosine monophosphate (cAMP) signaling. One study found LOH of 17q22–24 (the locus for *PRKAR1A*) in 23% of ACAs and 53% of ACCs [14].

10.2.2.5 ACTH–cAMP–PKA Pathway

The binding of ACTH to its receptor (a member of the G protein-coupled receptor family) results in the dissociation of the heterotrimeric Gs, causing the stimulation of adenylate cyclase, which in turn leads to the production of cAMP from ATP. The ACTH–adenylate cyclase signaling pathway has been implicated in the pathogenesis of ACTs in many ways. First, activating mutations of components of the adenylate cyclase pathway have been found in other human endocrine disorders, including toxic thyroid adenomas and acromegaly. Second, there is a correlation between circulating ACTH levels and the size of the adrenal cortex, as seen in patients with CAH or Cushing's disease [15].

10.2.2.6 Wnt Pathway

The Wnt family comprises a group of highly conserved growth factors with similar amino-acid sequences, which have roles in developmental and homeostatic processes. The central event in the canonical Wnt signaling pathway is accumulation of beta-catenin in the cytoplasm with subsequent translocation into the nucleus. The Wnt pathway has been implicated in the pathogenesis of several cancers, particularly in patients with familial adenomatous polyposis and in the development of colorectal carcinomas. Because beta-catenin mutations have been found in ACAs and ACCs, it may be an early step in a common multistep pathogenesis of ACAs and ACCs [16].

10.2.3 Molecular Markers in ACC (Table 10.3)

Several studies have assessed the use of immunoistochemical (IHC) molecular markers for discriminating ACCs from ACAs. The markers studied have included insulin-like growth factor (IGF)2, Ki-67/MIB1, p53, murine double minute 2, p21, p27, cyclin D1, Bcl-2, topoisomerase II, human epidermal growth factor receptor 2/neu, E-cadherin, and the retinoblastoma gene product. Many of these molecular markers, however, lack specificity to achieve discrimination between ACCs and ACAs.

Combining IGF2 and MIB1 (a mouse monoclonal antibody that recognizes a formalin-fixation resistant epitope on the cell proliferation-associated antigen Ki-67), IHC analyses yielded a sensitivity of 100% and a specificity of 95.5% for differentiating ACCs from ACAs [17].

Table 10.3 Molecular markers for adrenocortical carcinoma

Marker	Feature
IGF2/MIBI1	Yields a sensitivity of 100% and a specificity of 95.5% for differentiating ACCs from ACAs
Ki-67/MIB1	Poor sensitivity and specificity
p53	Poor sensitivity and specificity
Murine double minute 2	Poor sensitivity and specificity
p21	Poor sensitivity and specificity
p27	Poor sensitivity and specificity
cyclin D1	Poor sensitivity and specificity
Bcl-2	Poor sensitivity and specificity
Topoisomerase II	Poor sensitivity and specificity
Human epidermal growth factor receptor 2/neu	Poor sensitivity and specificity
E-cadherin	Poor sensitivity and specificity
Retinoblastoma gene product	Poor sensitivity and specificity
SF1 (transcription factor)	Can distinguish between primary and secondary ACC
GATA6 (transcription factor)	ACTs with a Weiss score of 4–9 are lower than the others
VEGF	Not yet in clinical use

Transcription factors have also been used as possible molecular markers to differentiate ACCs from ACAs. A member of the nuclear receptor family of transcription factors, steroidogenic factor 1 (SF1) maps to 9q33.3. IHC analyses with SF1 have not been shown to differentiate between ACCs and ACAs, but are useful for distinguishing between primary ACC and metastasis from other sites [18].

GATA6 is from the GATA family of transcription factors, which is characterized by binding to the DNA consensus sequence (A/T)GA T A(A/G). GATA6 has a role in the maturation and differentiation of cells. GATA6 protein expression has been found to be significantly lower in ACCs than in ACAs upon IHC anlyses. Accordingly, ACTs with Weiss scores of 4–9 had a significantly lower GATA6 level than ACTs with Weiss scores of 1–3 [19].

Vascular endothelial growth factor (VEGF) plays a pivotal part in the regulation of normal and tumor angiogenesis. Angiogenesis is critical for tumor growth and metastasis. VEGF has been found to be increased in most cancers and is associated with a worse outcome. Serum VEGF levels have also been assessed in patients with ACCs *vs* patients with ACAs, and they were not found to be significantly different between the two groups. VEGF, however, as a molecular marker for ACC, has not been integrated into clinical practice [20].

In conclusion, progress into the elucidation of the genes and pathways involved in the pathogenesis of ACC has been slow largely because of the rarity of this tumor. The *TP53, IGF2, H19,* $p57^{kip2}$, and *MEN1* genes are involved in adrenocortical carcinogenesis, as are the ACTH–cAMP–PKA and Wnt pathways.

10.3 Clinical Presentation (Table 10.4)

ACCs are functional in ≈60% of cases, more commonly in children (85%) than in adults (15–30%). Unlike ACAs that predominantly secrete cortisol, ACCs secrete various hormones, including androgens, cortisol, estrogens, and aldos-

Table 10.4 Clinical picture of adrenocortical carcinoma

Non-functioning	Clinically silent Abdominal mass at palpation Late appearance of compression signs signs due to metastases paraneoplastic signs
Functional	Cushing syndrome Conn syndrome Virilization (women) Gynecomastia and impotence (men) Feminization and early pseudo-puberty (children)

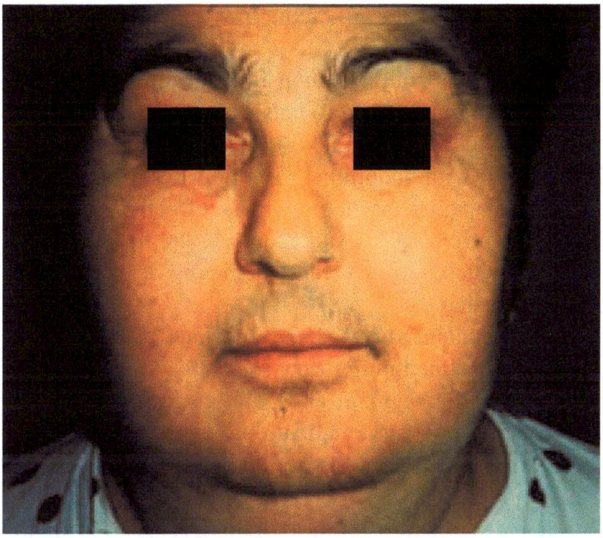

Fig. 10.1 Appearance of virilization in a female patient with an adrenocortical carcinoma

terone. In adult patients with functioning tumors, 30% present with Cushing syndrome, 20% with virilization, and 10–20% with a combination of the two. Feminization and hyperaldosteronism are much rarer, each accounting for ≈2% of ACC cases. The rapid onset of Cushing syndrome, often with virilizing features, is characteristic of ACCs in adults. Although benign adrenocortical tumors tend to secrete a single class of steroid, ACCs can secrete various types contemporarily; co-secretion of cortisol with androgens is a frequent combination and is highly suggestive of malignancy. In children, ACCs can present with virilization, Cushing syndrome, feminization, or Conn syndrome.

The rapid development of hypercortisolism influences its clinical pattern: the main features are profound muscle weakness, skin atrophy, diabetes mellitus and hypertension with hypokalemia (due to activation of mineralocorticoid receptors induced by high levels of cortisol). In patients from the German ACC Registry, autonomous cortisol secretion, either alone or in combination with other steroids, was detectable in 60% of cases in whom hormonal analyses had been unertaken before surgery. However, autonomous cortisol secretion was not clinically suspected in all of these cases. Hypersecretion of adrenal androgens determines virilization in affected women (Fig. 10.1) with amenorrhea, hirsutism, acne and baldness. Estrogen-secreting adrenal tumors in males lead to gynecomastia and testicular atrophy, and are almost invariably malignant. In children, androgen excess determines incomplete iso-sexual precocious puberty in males and incomplete heterosexual precocious puberty in females. In the case of estrogen-secreting ACCs, men suffer from impotence, loss of libido, gynecomastia and testicular atrophy, whereas menstrual disturbances are the main characteristics in fertile women. In children, estrogen excess determines sexual precocity (incomplete hetero- or isosexual precocious puberty in males or females, respectively). Mineralocorticoid-producing ACCs are rare and characterized by hypertension and hypokalemia.

Approximately 65–85% of ACCs in adults are non-functioning, and patients present with a large mass and symptoms related to mass effect (e.g., abdominal or flank pain in 55%) or with a palpable mass (40–50%). Only occasionally do hormonally inactive ACCs present with abdominal discomfort (nausea, vomiting, abdominal fullness) or back pain caused by a mass effect of the large tumor; patients present with fever, weight loss, and anorexia, and it is a remarkable feature of non-cortisol-producing ACCs that wellbeing is often little affected by even a large tumor burden.

Some ACCs are discovered incidentally (0–25%) and tend to be smaller. Due to the late presentation of non-functioning tumors, ≈ 30% of ACC cases present with metastatic disease to the regional and para-aortic lymph nodes, lung, liver, and bone. [21]. In the Italian survey on adrenal incidentaloma, pain was significantly associated with ACCs and was not fully explained by large tumor size *per se* [22].

A high concentration of dehydroepiandrosterone sulfate (DHEA-S) is another clue suggesting ACC, whereas decreased serum DHEA-S concentrations are suggestive of a benign adenoma. Aldosterone-producing ACCs present with hypertension and pronounced hypokalemia. However, severe hypokalemia is more likely caused by grossly elevated cortisol secretion, leading to insufficient inactivation of renal cortisol by 11-hydroxysteroid dehydrogenase type 2 with consecutive activation of the mineralocorticoid receptor. In many patients with a seemingly hormonally inactive ACC, high concentrations of steroid precursors such as androstenedione or 17-hydroxyprogesterone can often be demonstrated, thereby establishing the adrenocortical origin of the tumor.

10.4 Diagnosis and Differential Diagnosis

10.4.1 Hormonal Workup

Careful endocrine assessment is essential before surgery in ACCs (Table 10.5). The pattern of hormone secretion may point to the malignant potential of the lesion (e.g., estradiol in males, high concentration of serum DHEA-S, or secretion of steroid precursors) and may thus affect surgical strategy (open instead of minimally invasive surgery). In addition, autonomous cortisol secretion by the tumor is associated with the risk of postoperative adrenal insufficiency. Due to the variable hypercortisolemia and the rapid development of ACC, the clinical features of Cushing's syndrome are often incomplete or even absent (atypical or subclinical Cushing's syndrome). To establish tumor markers for monitoring tumor recurrence, a thorough hormonal workup is essential. Finally, it is important to exclude a pheochromocytoma before surgery because imaging often cannot reliably differentiate between ACC and pheochromocytoma.

Table 10.5 Recommended hormonal evaluation in suspected or proven adrenocortical carcinoma

Cortisol excess (minimum 3 or 4 tests)
Dexamethasone suppression test (1 mg, 23.00 h)
Urinary free cortisol (24-h urine)
Basal cortisol (serum)
Basal ACTH (plasma)
Sexual steroids and steroid precursors
Dehydroepiandrosterone sulfate (DHEAS) (serum)
Androstenedione (serum)
Testosterone (serum)
17-OH-progesterone
17-beta-estradiol (serum, in men and postmenopausal women)
Mineralocorticoid excess
Potasium (serum)
Aldosterone: reinin ratio (only in patients with arterial hypertension and/or hypokalemia)
Exclusion of pheochromocytoma (minimum 1 or 3 tests)
Catecholamine excretion (24-h urine)
Metanephrine excretion (24-h urine)
Meta- and nor-metanephrine (plasma)

10.4.2 Imaging

10.4.2.1 General Properties

Metastatic disease is definitive of malignancy [23]. However, several imaging features should increase the suspicion of ACC within an adrenal mass [24]: tumor diameter >4 cm, irregular tumor margins, central intratumoral necrosis or hemorrhage, heterogeneous enhancement, invasion into adjacent structures, venous extension (renal vein or inferior vena cava (IVC)), and calcification. ACCs are usually large at presentation, ranging from 2 cm to 25 cm (average size ≈9 cm). Approximately 70% of ACCs are larger than 6 cm. They are bilateral in 2–10% of cases and are slightly more common on the left than on the right. Tumors are frequently hemorrhagic and necrotic, and may contain small areas of intracytoplasmic lipid or fatty regions. Using a logistic regression model, Hussain et al. found tumor size >4 cm and heterogeneous enhancement to be the most important discriminators of malignancy [25]. The existence of intracytoplasmic fat in ACCs has been attributed to cortisol and related fatty precursors in hormonally active tumors. On occasion, pockets of fat may be seen within the mass, indicating coexistent myelolipomatous tissue. Invasion into the IVC has been reported in 9–19% of ACC cases at presentation.

10.4.2.2 CT (Fig. 10.2)

The typical appearance of ACC on unenhanced CT is of a large, inhomogeneous (but well-defined) suprarenal mass that displaces adjacent structures as it grows [26]. Regions of low attenuation correspond to necrosis pathologically. After the intravenous administration of contrast material, there is inhomoge-

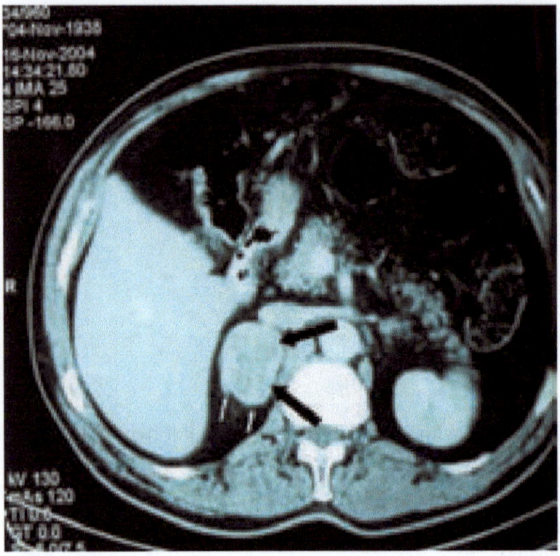

Fig. 10.2 Contrast CT of a right adrenocortical carcinoma. In the arterial phase, an irregularly oblong mass in the right adrenal gland is evident (*thick black arrows*). The neoplasm has a main diameter of 5.8 cm, irregular edges, shares some jagged edges (*thin white arrows*), and a finely irregular structure

neous enhancement of the tumor, typically with greater enhancement seen peripherally and relatively little enhancement seen centrally, because of central necrosis [27]. Measurement of the attenuation of adrenal lesions on unenhanced CT is of great value in distinguishing between benign and malignant masses. Cumulative data obtained for the identification of adrenal adenomas indicate that ACCs rarely have an attenuation <10 Hounsfield units (HU). The specificity of this threshold for the identification of benign adenomas is ≈98%. Equally, ACCs retain intravenous contrast material and have absolute and relative percentage washout of <60% and <40%, respectively, 15 min after contrast administration or <50% and <40%, respectively, at 10 min [28]. Calcification (micro or coarse) is seen on CT in ≈30% of patients with ACC and is usually centrally located (Fig. 10.3). Calcification is rare in adenomas, but is present in ≈10% of pheochromocytomas [29]. Tumor thrombus extending into the IVC at presentation is not rare and is more frequently seen in right-sided tumors. A tumor thrombus within a vein is usually well encapsulated and can often be withdrawn intact from the vein [30]. The cephalad extent of the tumor thrombus can be identified on contrast-enhanced CT or magnetic resonance imaging (MRI).

CT is also of value in showing the local and distant spread of an ACC. Preservation of fat planes around the tumor indicates that there is no local invasion. Where there is a paucity of retroperitoneal fat, it may not be possible to determine if the tumor has invaded adjacent organs. Metastases are frequently found at presentation: regional and para-aortic lymph nodes (25–46%), lungs (45–97%), liver (48–96%), and bone (11–33%) are the common sites. Hepatic metastases tend to be hyper-vascular and are best seen on arterial-phase imaging after intravenous administration of contrast.

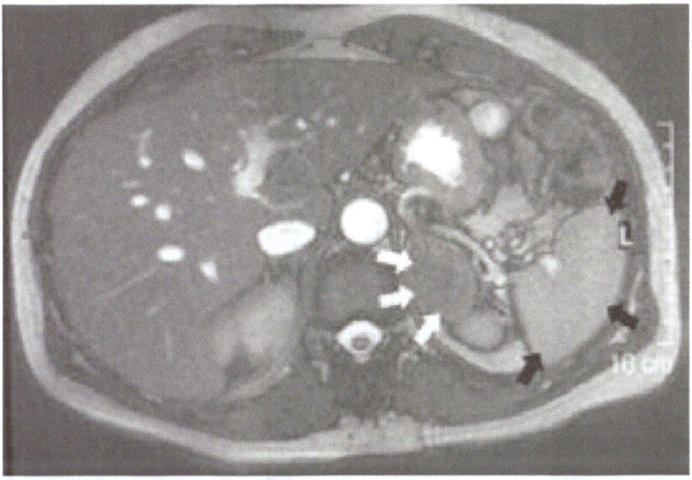

Fig. 10.3 MRI features of adrenal malignancy. This left adrenal neoplasm is big, irregularly oblong, and dark in this MRI "out of phase" acquisition. It presents a finely irregular structure, with a "salt and pepper" aspect (*arrows*) due to necrotic phenomena. All these aspects suggest a malignant adrenal mass

10.4.2.3 MRI (Fig. 10.3)

ACCs are typically heterogeneous in signal intensity on MRI because of hemorrhage and/or necrosis [31]. On T1-weighted imaging, ACCs are typically isointense or slightly hypointense to normal liver parenchyma. However, high T1 signal intensity is often seen because of hemorrhage. On T2-weighted imaging, ACCs are usually hyperintense to liver parenchyma and have a heterogeneous texture because of intratumoral cystic regions and hemorrhage [32]. A functioning ACC can contain small regions of intracytoplasmic lipid, resulting in small non-uniform areas of loss of signal on chemical shift imaging (<30% of the lesion) [33]. Although similar small non-uniform loss can occur in lipid-poor adenomas, the significant uniform signal loss seen in lipid-rich adenomas does not occur.

The results of early studies suggested that proton MR spectroscopy may be useful in differentiating adrenal adenomas and pheochromocytomas from adrenal metastases and ACCs. Faria et al. looked at the spectral traces obtained from 60 patients with adrenal masses. Adenomas and pheochromocytomas could be differentiated from ACCs and metastases using choline:creatine ratios of >1.20 (92% sensitivity and 96% specificity) and choline:lipid ratios of >0.38 (92% sensitivity and 90% specificity). ACCs and pheochromocytomas could be differentiated from adenomas and metastases using a 4.0–4.3 ppm/creatine ratio >1.50 (87% sensitivity and 98% specificity). By combining these two spectral analyses, they could divide adrenal mass lesions into one of four distinct groups: adenoma, pheochromocytoma, ACC, or metastasis [34]. Although there were some criticisms of this study, the method appears to offer potential in helping to distinguish among adrenal mass lesions.

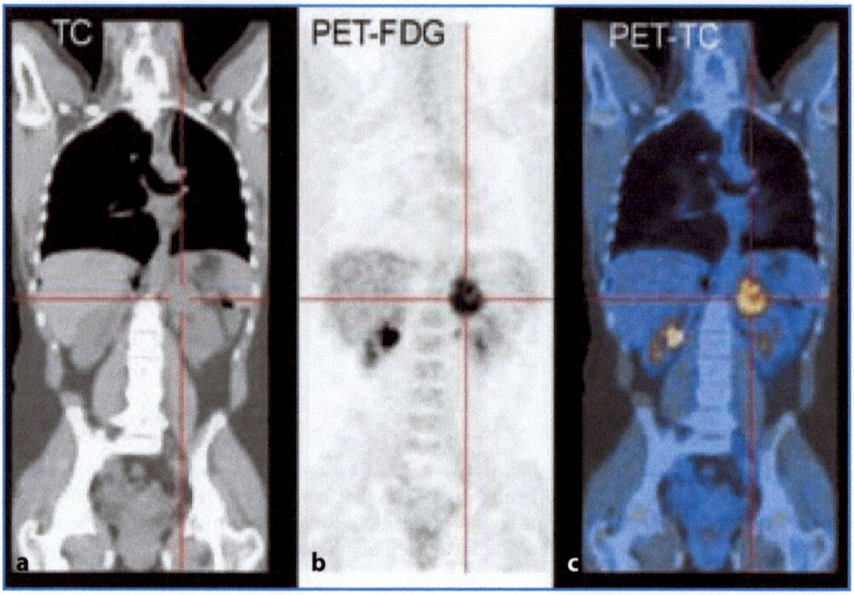

Fig. 10.4 FDG-PET (**b**) and CT-PET (**c**) of adrenocortical carcinoma. PET of a small left adrenal incidentaloma is shown. It was iso-dense at CT (**a**), which is a suspicious criterion of malignancy, so FDG-PET and PET-CT were necessary, even if the mass did not share a dimensional aspect typical of adrenocortical carcinoma (dimension, ≈3.9 cm). The final diagnosis was a small adrenocortical carcinoma at a very early stage (T1 according to the WHO classification)

10.4.2.4 Functional Imaging (Fig. 10.4)

Fluorodeoxyglucose-positron emission tomography (FDG-PET) can be used to identify certain malignant adrenal masses by virtue of their increased metabolic activity; however, if FDG uptake is only modest, the likelihood of benign *vs* malignant is approximately equal [35]. FDG-PET combined with contrast-enhanced CT has a sensitivity of 100% and specificity of 87–97% for identifying malignant adrenal masses. The lower specificity is because a small number of adenomas and other benign lesions mimic malignancy [36]. The novel PET tracer 11C metomidate (a marker of 11β-hydroxylase) is used as a tracer for adrenocortical tissue and is taken up by adenomas and ACCs. This marker differentiates adrenal cortical lesions from pheochromocytomas and metastases, which are uptake-negative [37]. However, the most valuable aspect of PET is its ability to detect distant metastases (one-third of patients with ACCs will have metastatic disease at presentation).

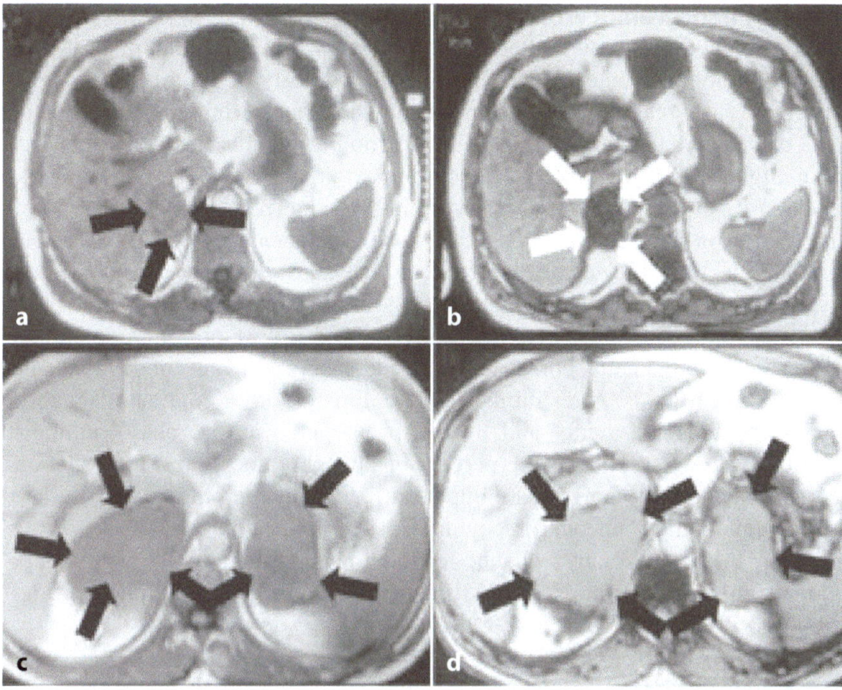

Fig. 10.5 MRI differential diagnosis of adrenocortical adenoma and adrenocortical carcinoma using the "chemical-shift" method. a A left benign neoplasm sharing a positive chemical shift is shown. In the "out of phase" sequences, the signal intensity of the neoplasm (*white arrows*) is typically lower than that of the spleen, different from what happeoccursn in the "in phase" image (b) (*black arrows*), where their grayscale aspect is similar. On the left the mass seems to be darker and it is therefore more readily recognizable. Reduction of signal intensity >20%, is almost pathognomonic of a benign lesion. In c and d, the signal intensity of a bilateral, large adrenal incidentaloma does not significantly change from in phase to out of phase acquisitions. This phenomenon is called a "negative chemical shift" and suggests an adrenocortical carcinoma

10.4.3 Differential Diagnosis and Distinguishing Features

10.4.3.1 Adenoma

Adenomas may be diagnosed with a sensitivity of 75–98% and specificity of 92–100% using the characteristics of CT washouts. However, in some cases, it can be difficult to distinguish benign from malignant lesions. If they measure 3–4 cm in diameter, the pathologic label of "indeterminate malignant potential" is often applied, and if they are >4 cm, and the "chemical shift" imaging is negative (Fig. 10.5) they are generally managed as malignant lesions [38].

10.4.3.2 Pheochromocytoma

Pheochromocytomas may be benign or malignant. Small pheochromocytomas are usually homogeneous in appearance with a density of 40–50 HU on unenhanced CT, whereas larger pheochromocytomas can be inhomogeneous with areas of hemorrhage and necrosis. There is no correlation between tumor size and malignancy [39]. On MRI, pheochromocytomas are typically described as "isointense" or "hyperintense" to liver on T1-weighted imaging and hyperintense to fat on T2-weighted imaging. However, appearances can be variable. For example, only 11% of pheochromocytomas show "typical" T2 hyperintensity, and pheochromocytomas that are only mildly hyperintense to the spleen (34%) or those that are heterogeneous on T2 (39%) are more common. Increasing heterogeneity correlates with increasing amounts of hemorrhage, necrosis, and fibrosis. After intravenous administration of contrast, pheochromocytomas enhance avidly and have a prolonged washout phase, although exceptions do exist. Ninety-one percent of pheochromocytomas are functioning, and biochemical markers are important in establishing the diagnosis.

Non-functioning pheochromocytomas (9%) pose more of a diagnostic dilemma. Although many will be differentiated from ACCs using meta-iodobenzylganidine scintigraphy (MIGB), some non-functioning pheochromocytomas will not be MIBG-avid [40].

10.4.3.3 Lymphoma

The primary pathologic type that involves the adrenal glands is non-Hodgkin diffuse large B-cell lymphoma. It is usually bilateral with enlarged adrenal glands that keep their normal "adeniform" shape [41].

10.4.3.4 Metastases (Fig. 10.6)

Adrenal metastases are found in ≤27% of patients with malignant epithelial tumors at autopsy. This diagnosis should be considered if bilateral adrenal lesions are present and there is a known primary malignancy elsewhere or there is evidence of other metastases. The most common primary site is the lung [42].

10.4.3.5 Ganglioneuroma

Ganglioneuromas are benign neoplasms arising from the sympathetic ganglia. In general, they are large solid lesions on CT with homogeneous to mildly heterogeneous enhancement after intravenous administration of contrast. On MRI they are typically hypointense on T1 and heterogeneously hyperintense on T2 depending on the content of their myxoid stroma [43].

10.4.3.6 Infection

The imaging appearances of infection within the adrenal gland are generally non-specific and can be seen as soft-tissue masses and cystic changes with or without calcification. Tuberculosis and histoplasmosis tend to be bilateral but can be asymmetric and give the appearance of unilateral disease [44].

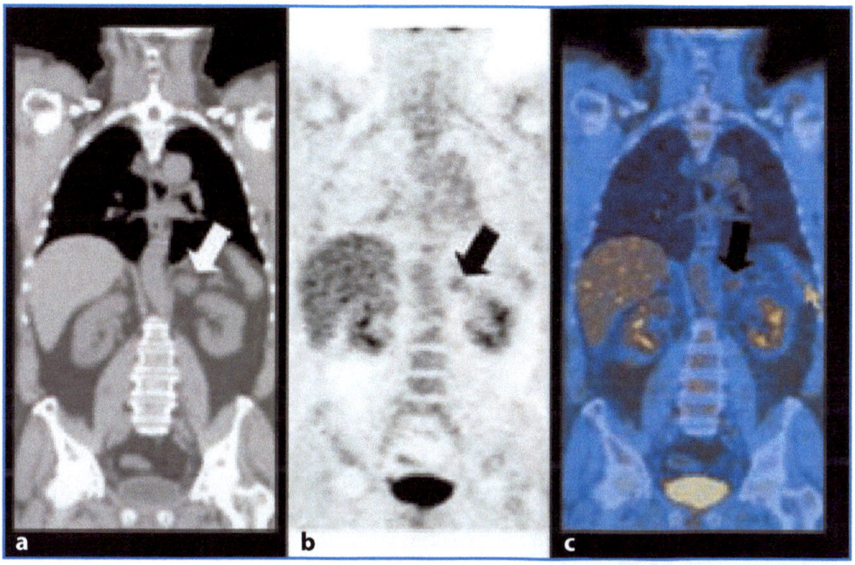

Fig. 10.6 FDG-PET and PET-CT of a bilateral, small, left adrenal recurrence in patient with a history of lung cancer. PET-CT allows one to attribute a malignant nature to the small, left adrenal neoplasm (**b**) (*black arrow*), which had already been identified at CT (**a**) (*white arrow*). PET-CT reconstruction permits identification of a metastasis in the spleen parenchyma (**c**) (*yellow arrow*)

10.4.3.7 Neuroblastoma

Neuroblastomas occur most frequently in children and are rare in the adult population. Calcification is a hallmark of neuroblastoma in children but is rarely seen in adults. Adults with neuroblastoma tend to show a higher rate of metastatic disease at presentation than children [45].

10.4.4 Pathological Assessment

10.4.4.1 Role of Fine-needle Aspiration Cytology (FNAC)

CT or endoscopic ultrasonographic sonography (EUS)-mediated FNAC is an accurate and safe method for sampling left adrenal gland masses. In particular, for patients with lung cancer and an enlarged left adrenal gland, FNA of the left adrenal gland modifies disease stage and treatment strategy in approximately half of patients; it is recommended if a cytopathological result positive for malignancy is likely to change management. No significant procedure-related complications have been reported. The diagnostic yield of EUS-FNAC ranged between 76% and 100% in the largest series published, which involved 2,485 patients [46].

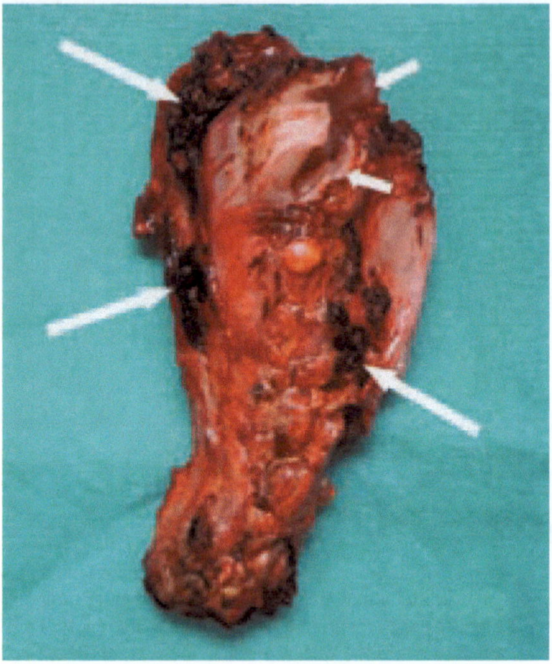

Fig. 10.7 Gross aspect of a surgical specimen of adrenocortical carcinoma. Gross examination of this adrenal mass demonstrates a large volume (15 cm and ≤200 g), absence of a capsule, and an irregular internal surface. This is due to hemorrhagic (*long arrows*) and necrotic zones, together with cystic areas (*short arrows*). In the most aggressive neoplasm, it is possible to macroscopically identify invasion of the middle adrenal veins or renal veins

10.4.4.2 Gross Pathology (Fig. 10.7)

As a rule, malignant tumors are larger than those which are clinically benign, usually weigh >100 g and appear lobulated owing to fibrous bands subdividing the tumour irregularly. Larger tumors often invade surrounding tissues and organs, including the kidney and liver. On cut section, extensive areas of necrosis and hemorrhage may be noted. Most ACCs can therefore be assumed to be malignant at macroscopic examination alone.

10.4.4.3 Microscopic Pathology (Fig. 10.8)

The pathological diagnosis should be carried out by an experienced pathologist. ACCs have alveolar, trabecular, or solid architectures, and admixtures of these patterns of growth are common. Foci of myxoid change, pseudoglandular patterns and spindle cell growth can occasionally be observed, while invasion of the capsule, sinusoids or even large veins is often seen. Necrosis may be abundant.

Most of the tumor cells are relatively lipid-poor with compact eosinophilic cytoplasm, though there may be a limited proportion of vacuolated, lipid-rich

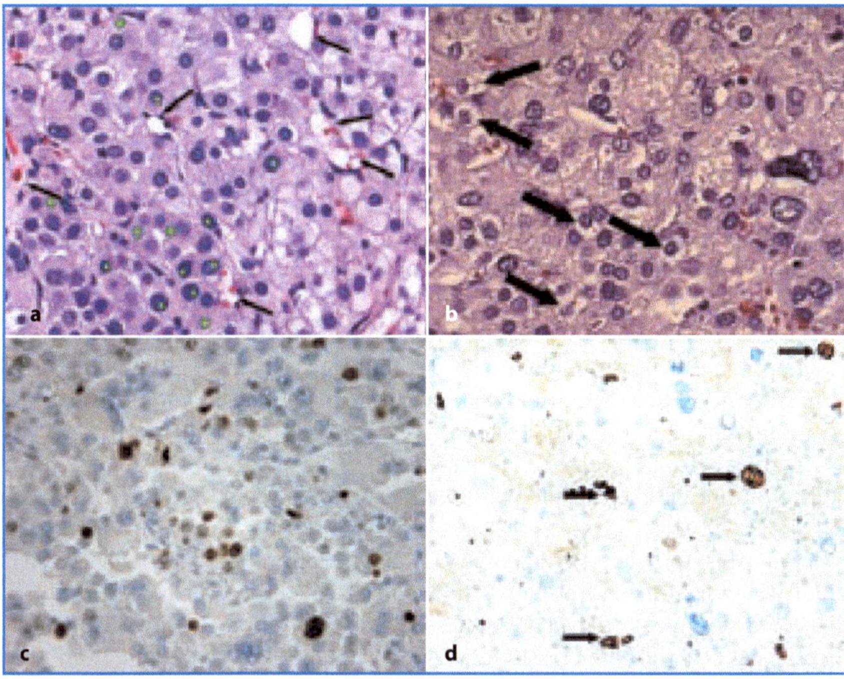

Fig. 10.8 Histological aspect of adrenocortical carcinomas. The adrenocortical carcinoma shares the following microscopic features: hypervascularization (panel **a**, *arrows*); cells with a large amount of eosinophilic cytoplasm (panel **a**, *crosses*), which sometimes assumes a vacuolar aspect (panel **b**, *arrows*); a pinocytotic and polymorphic nucleus with prominent nucleoli (panel **a**, *asterisk*); positive staining for the p53 oncogene in the nucleus (panel **c**, *brown*), and for synaptophysin in the cytoplasm (panel **d**, *arrows*)

cells. A minority of adrenal cortical carcinomas are predominantly composed of oncocytic cells. Nuclear pleomorphism is a constant finding, with occasional multi-nucleated giant cells. Mitotic rate differs widely, from rare to several mitoses per high-power field (HPF), with easily recognizable atypical forms. Nuclear atypia, atypical and frequent mitoses (>5 of 50 HPF), vascular and capsular invasion, and necroses are suggestive of malignancy. In addition, broad fibrous bands are a characteristic feature separating ACCs from benign tumors.

Among the various criteria proposed, the one proposed by Weiss (which requires only histopathological findings) has been most widely employed. The nine histological criteria are:

1. *Nuclear grade:* nuclear grade III and IV based on criteria of Fóhrman;
2. *Mitotic rate*: greater than 5/50 HPF (×40 objective). According to Weiss, mitosis was evaluated by counting 10 random HPF in the area of the greatest numbers of mitotic figures on the five slides with the greatest number of mitoses. If less than five slides were available for a case, a correspondingly greater number of fields per slide were used to make 50 HPF;

3. *Atypical mitotic figures*: mitosis was regarded as atypical if it definitely showed an abnormal distribution of chromosomes or an excessive number of mitotic spindles;
4. *Cytoplasm:* presence of ≤25% clear or vacuolated cells resembling the normal zona fasciculate;
5. *Diffuse architecture:* diffuse architecture was present if greater than one-third of the tumor formed patternless sheets of cells. Trabecular, columnar, alveolar or nesting organizations were regarded as non-diffuse patterns;
6. *Necrosis* was regarded as present if occurring in at least confluent nests of cells;
7. *Venous invasion*: Weiss defined a vein as an "endothelial-lined vessel with smooth muscle as a component of the wall";
8. *Sinusoid invasion*: a sinusoid was defined as an "endothelial-lined vessel in the adrenal gland with little supportive tissues";
9. *Invasion of tumor capsule* was accepted if nests or cords of tumor extended into or through the capsule, with a corresponding stroma reaction.

Each Weiss criterion was scored 0 if absent and 1 if present. Thus, each tumor was graded from 0 to 9 to produce a total Weiss score. Tumors with ≤3 of these histological criteria were classified as ACAs; those with ≥4 of these histological criteria were classified as ACCs. All the slides were reviewed by a pathologist who was blinded to clinical features and gross findings.

As well as distinguishing ACAs from ACCs, the Weiss system (adopted by pathologists worldwide) may also supply useful information regarding disease-free survival, local relapse and distant metastasis. The modification of the Weiss system accomplished by Aubert et al. has simplified the Weiss criteria. The diagnostic value of the modified Weiss system for evaluating malignancy in adrenal cortical neoplasms has been confirmed in a recent study, which also proved a significant correlation of this scoring system with time of survival in ACC patients.

In diagnostic practice, IHC analyses are most commonly applied in the differential diagnosis of ACCs from renal cell and hepatocellular carcinomas as well as adrenal medullary and metastatic tumors. Several studies have demonstrated the value of Ki-67 staining in differentiating benign from malignant lesions. In addition, Ki-67 expression may be of prognostic relevance because high expression (10%) has been associated with poor survival. Most ACCs exhibit a high Ki-67 labelling index with MIB-1 antibody. However, labelling indeces may overlap with those observed in ACAs and consequently MIB-1 immunoreactivity is of limited value in differentiating between benign and malignant adrenal cortical tumors. Nevertheless, increased Ki-67 immunoreactivity has been significantly associated with shortened disease-free survival and death from disease.

Immunoreactivity for alpha-inhibin, as well as for the anti-melan-A antibody, is a useful tool for the identification of ACCs. Unlike other epithelial tumors, ACCs are reported to be from negative to weakly positive for cytoker-

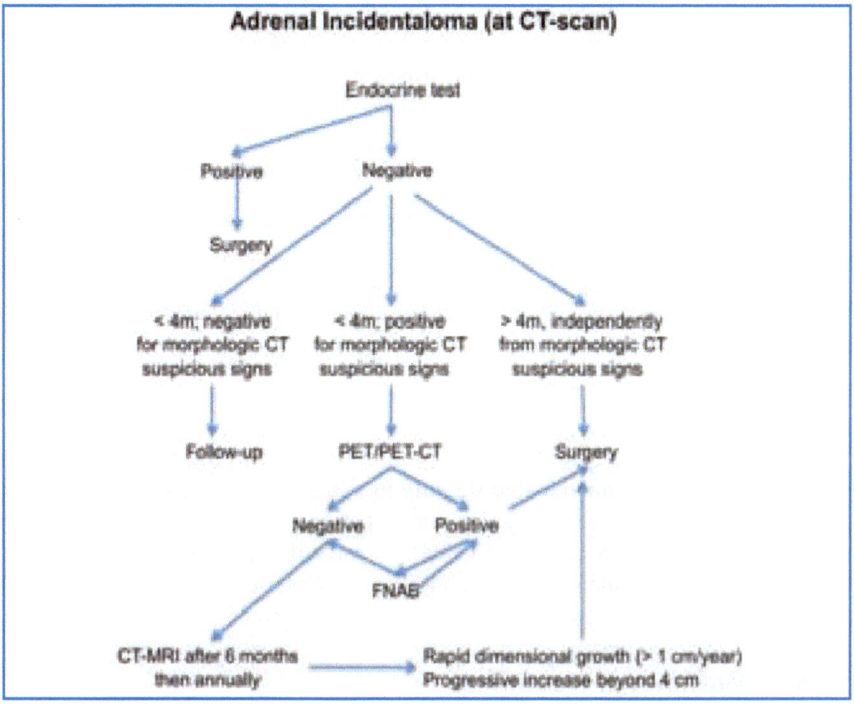

Fig. 10.9 Diagnostic algorithm for adrenal incidentalomas with malignant potential

atin and negative for epithelial membrane antigen (EMA). They also stain negative for chromogranin A, which is the most reliable marker of adrenal medullary neoplasms. Other markers such as D11 and chromogranin A are helpful to define or exclude the adrenocortical origin of the tumor [47]. Several new markers (LOH at 17p13, IGF-II overexpression, cyclin E) have been proposed to separate benign from malignant adrenal lesions. A possible diagnostic algorithm of ACCs, from the occasional evidence of an adrenal incidentaloma, is shown in Fig. 10.9.

10.4.5 Staging (Table 10.6)

Until 2004, no official tumor/node/metastasis (TNM) classification was available for ACCs, and different staging systems were used, most often the Sullivan modification of the Macfarlane system. Accordingly, the new Union for International Cancer Control (UICC) staging system published by the World Health Organization (WHO) in 2004 is based on this classification. Stages I and II describe localized tumors ≤5 cm or ≥5 cm, respectively. Locally invasive tumors or tumors with regional lymph-node metastases are classified as stage III, whereas stage IV consists of tumors invading adjacent organs or prsenting

Table 10.6 Staging for adrenocortical carcinoma

Stage	TNM	Feature
I	T1, N0, M0	Diameter <5 cm, within adrenal capsule
II	T2, N0, M0	Diameter >5 cm, within adrenal capsule
III	T1 pr T2, N1, M0	Within adrenal capsule, with lymphatic involvement
	T3, N0, M0	Beyond the adrenal capsule, without lymphatic involvement
IV	T3 or T4, N1, M0	Beyond the adrenal capsule or invasion of adjacent organs, with lymphatic involvement
	T1, 2, 3, 4 M1	Distant metastases

with distant metastases. However, the prognostic value of the different staging systems has never been compared directly in a large series of patients. Because one of the major objectives of staging classifications is to facilitate the exchange of information between treatment centers, we recommend the use of the new WHO system until evidence that a modification is needed becomes available.

10.5 Multimodal Treatment

The management of patients with ACCs requires a multidisciplinary approach. Despite recent advances in terms of adjuvant treatment, including mitotane and chemotherapy protocols, complete local excision has, until now, been the only curative treatment. Adjuvant medical therapy or irradiation may also be considered. Systematic therapies for advanced ACCs are limited. In recurrent disease, repeat resection can positively affect patient outcome [48].

10.5.1 Surgical Indications and Methods

Resection should be considered for tumors that demonstrate size >4 cm, functionality and specific imaging characteristics. On CT or MRI, ACCs usually appear heterogeneous, with irregular borders and focal areas of hemorrhage and necrosis. Most ACCs are >6 cm in diameter. Imaging can also detect local invasion, regional lymph nodes, and metastases.

Complete surgical excision is the only curative treatment for ACCs and should include the adrenal gland and periadrenal fat. It should be extended (if required) to include *en bloc* resection of macroscopically invaded surrounding tissues: liver, IVC, kidney, pancreas, spleen, stomach and colon.

The role of lymph-node dissection is not clear. Periadrenal lymph nodes have been routinely excised by some surgical teams in patients with stage I/II ACCs, and carried out only in the case of proven invasion (stage III) by other surgical teams. There is no precise definition of locoregional lymph-node dissection in the management of ACCs; moreover, routine lymph-node excision does not improve oncological outcome. In contrast, there is a general agreement with respect to the oncological principles of R0 resection *en bloc* for tumors large enough for complete excision, without grasping, fragmentation or rupture of the tumor capsule [49].

ACCs (stage I–II) can be treated with curative intent with laparoscopy or open surgery. For lesions <10–12 cm, an open anterior approach using a unilateral or bilateral subcostal incision is usually recommend because it permits access to sites of potential invasion and metastatic spread. Laparoscopic adrenalectomy was done by Gagner in 1992, and rapidly became the "gold standard" method for the resection of functioning and non-functioning adrenal disease [50]. With increasing experience, larger tumors have been removed safely using a laparoscopic approach. The advantages of laparoscopic adrenalectomy are known and well documented. These benefits have been shown in institutional studies comparing open with laparoscopic adrenalectomy. The role of laparoscopy in the management of ACCs remains controversial. In recent years, the potential for the increased risk of local recurrence, peritoneal carcinomatosis and port-site seeding after laparoscopic surgery for ACCs has led to strong recommendations in support of open adrenalectomy.

More recent and larger comparative series have shown that oncological outcomes after laparoscopic resection of ACCs are similar to those seen after open resection for ACCs in stage I–II disease if oncological principles are followed and complete R0 local resection is achieved. The authors interpreted previous reports of poor outcomes with laparoscopy as being due to technical problems such as non-radical resection, capsule rupture or laparoscopic adrenalectomy for ACCs undertaken before referral to a tertiary center. However, surgeons are expanding their indications for metastatic disease to the adrenal glands and ACC [51].

In patients with stage I–II ACCs, laparoscopic adrenalectomy is not inferior to open adrenalectomy in terms of oncological outcome if it is carried out by experienced surgeons respecting the principles of radical R0 resection. Conversion to the open approach is recommended in cases if signs of local invasion are found or the dissection is difficult, and implies the risk of rupture of the tumor capsule. Open adrenalectomy is essential in cases of preoperative or intraoperative evidence of invasion into adjacent organs and lymph-node involvement or distant metastases [52]. Preoperative CT and MRI is important for indicating the laparoscopic approach. Preservation of fat planes between the adrenal gland, kidney, aorta and IVC suggests the absence of an extra-tumoral entity. Stage-III ACCs with radiological evidence of lymph-node involvement, invasion of surrounding tissues or venous thrombosis are a contraindication to laparoscopy. In doubtful cases with signs of local invasion and if the principles of oncological radical surgery cannot be met, laparoscopic exploration with eventual conversion to open surgery is possible [53–56].

In conclusion, the results from comparisons of oncological outcomes in

ACC between open and laparoscopic approaches are equivocal: increased risk of local recurrence and peritoneal carcinomatosis by the laparoscopic route, as well as identical results between the two approaches in terms of survival, and recurrence and peritoneal carcinomatosis. An open approach is recommended in case of local invasion, with a view to achieving an R0 resection. Laparoscopic resection of ACCs/potentially malignant tumors, which involves removal of surrounding periadrenal fat and results in an R0 resection without rupture of the tumor capsule, may be carried out for preoperative and intraoperative stage I–II ACCs and tumors with diameter <10 cm.

The role of robot-assisted minimally invasive surgery in the treatment of ACCs is not well established. It was recently shown that robot-assisted adrenalectomy, compared with the laparoscopic method, is safe and effective if done in highly specialized centers. Robot-assisted surgery requires a very long learning curve, longer operating time, and implies a substantial increase in costs [57].

Posterior retroperitoneal adrenalectomy is another minimally invasive approach. However, it does not seem to be indicated for patients who show clear signs of malignancy or who have a tumor diameter >8 cm [1].

10.5.2 Percutaneous Ablation

Percutaneous ablation methods such as radiofrequency ablation (RFA), cryoablation, microwave ablation, or chemical ablation with ethanol or acetic acid can be used in the treatment of adrenal neoplasms. In general, ablation is carried out under the guidance of ultrasound or CT.

RFA has been shown to be effective for the short-term local control of ACCs <5 cm in diameter. RFA is used in the treatment of primary tumors and metastatic lesions which are unresectable, in patients who refuse surgery (even though this method is feasible) and if surgery is not recommended due to poor physical status. Percutaneous ablation can also be used in the treatment of functional adenomas, pheochromocytomas and adrenal metastases. It is a safe method, effective, easy to apply and gives immediate results that are quite verifiable by TC as early as 1 week after treatment. Ablation of adrenal tumors leads to excessive release of hormones in the blood that can trigger a hypertensive crisis, adverse cardiac events or ischemic stroke. Some authors believe that it is useful to pretreat patients undergoing ablation with a lytic agent. Other studies have reported variable outcomes and adverse effects, including bleeding, infection, and injury to adjacent structures [58].

10.5.3 Management of Hormonal Excess

Hormonal excess causes significant morbidity in patients with advanced ACCs. Although mitotane reduces steroidogenesis, its slow onset of action often necessitates the introduction of alternative adrenostatic drugs. Adrenal insufficiency is a potentially life-threatening risk of these therapies. Ketoconazole is an antifungal agent that inhibits multiple adrenal steroidogenic enzymes, and may also act as a glucocorticoid receptor antagonist. The use of ketoconazole is limited by hepatotoxicity and gastrointestinal side effects.

10.5.4 Medical Therapy

Adrenal cancer often occurs at the time of diagnosis at an advanced or metastatic stage. Therapies do not provide real benefits, so it is essential to use systemic chemotherapy agents that can offer guarantees, especially in the case of advanced-stage adrenal cancer and those forms treated surgically with curative intent that carry a high risk of local recurrence (R1). For many decades, mitotane has been the principal systemic drug specific for the adrenal cancer even though it is burdened by poor tolerability, limited efficacy and toxicity.

Mitotane is an isomer of a pesticide. Its toxic actions are directed towards adrenal cells; it inhibits the synthesis of steroids of the adrenal cortex. After complete removal of the tumor with curative intent, relapse is observed in a very high percentage of patients, thereby justifying the use of adjuvant therapy with mitotane. Use of advanced forms of this drug induces a 5–30% reduction in tumor mass and, in rare cases, leads to a total regression of the tumor. Approximately 80% of patients with hormonally active tumors who undergo mitotane treatment have clinically significant decreases in hormone production. After radical surgical excision, mitotane can prolong the time interval between surgery and reappearance of the disease (disease-free survival (DFS)), so it does not seem to have a real influence on overall survival (OS). Patients taking mitotane for prolonged periods often suffer from gastrointestinal and neurologic toxicities, and these side effects (diarrhea, vomiting, depression, ataxia) are usually the limiting factor in the use of mitotane.

Mitotane treatment is limited to patients with distant metastases and residual tumors after adrenalectomy. Use of mitotane in conjunction with other chemotherapeutic agents (cisplatin, etoposide, doxorubicin) has been proposed for advanced-stage and metastatic ACCs; the results are promising but the role of these chemotherapeutic agents in patients with ACC remains unresolved.

Recent studies have highlighted that some drugs may have a specific action towards tumorigenesis, such as inhibition of the IGF1 receptor, epidermal growth factor receptor (EGFR) and tyrosine kinase. It seems that the association with mitotane may yield promising results.

10.5.5 Radiotherapy (RT)

The efficacy of RT for adrenal tumors is controversial. These neoplasms have been considered to be radio-resistant for a long time. Many authors have noticed poor results in patients subject to RT after surgical removal of the adrenal mass due to the proximity of the adrenals to radiosensitive structures. Older series concluded that ACC was a radio-resistant tumor.

RT has also been used as palliative care treatment; it should be considered for patients with surgically unresectable disease and in ACC cases associated with bone metastases. It seems that treatment with ionizing radiation can reduce the size of metastases and symptoms. RT as an adjuvant therapeutic option has been described to significantly reduce recurrence rate, thereby suggesting a significant therapeutic potential. In particular, RT is recommended if microscopic tumor residues are detectable after surgery for incomplete removal of the tumor (R1). These patients exhibit macroscopically visible residual tumors (R2) that cannot be removed surgically. RT is also suitable if residual tumor dimensions are not known (RX) and if the risk of recurrence is high. Patients with advanced disease and those with stage-III tumors with local lymph-node invasion and no distant metastases may benefit from adjuvant RT. In the case of R0 resection, the need for RT is assessed individually, and is dependent upon large tumors (>8 cm), unfavorable histology, and a high risk of relapse (signs of vascular micro-invasion, intraoperative rupture of the tumor capsule or spillage of necrotic liquid). Combined treatment based on the association between RT and cytotoxic drugs, such as mitotane, is under investigation, and is recommended for patients who undergo R1 and RX resection. For isolated metastatic disease to the adrenal glands, highly focal RT to the metastatic lesion, without including regional lymph nodes, may be an appropriate strategy. Stereotactic body radiation therapy (SBRT) makes use of CT-based planning to deliver high individual doses of radiation with extreme precision [59].

10.5.6 Treatment of Adrenal Metastases

Adrenal metastases are the most common malignant tumors found within the adrenal gland. Lung carcinoma is the most common adrenal metastases; other malignances that commonly metastasize to the adrenal gland are breast, kidney and melanoma. Adrenal metastases usually indicate extensive systemic disease that is treated with chemotherapy rather than surgery. Isolated adrenal metastases can occur in patients with non-small-lung cancer and colorectal cancer. Several authors have advocated resection of these lesions to improve survival. Patients with adrenal metastases are better cared for by a multidisciplinary team, and PET-CT is the imaging of choice. Adrenal biopsy can be reserved for lesions without a conclusive imaging diagnosis. Patients with suspected adrenal metastases should be considered for adrenalectomy if control of extra-adrenal disease has been achieved, or a definitive plan for control is in place, and if metastases are isolated to the adrenal gland. Laparoscopy is a feasible and oncologically safe approach in appropriately selected patients. Systemic chemotherapy and/or RT may be used with real benefit in association with surgery or individually for the palliative treatment of symptoms. Small adrenal metastases can be treated with percutaneous ablative methods or with SBRT [60].

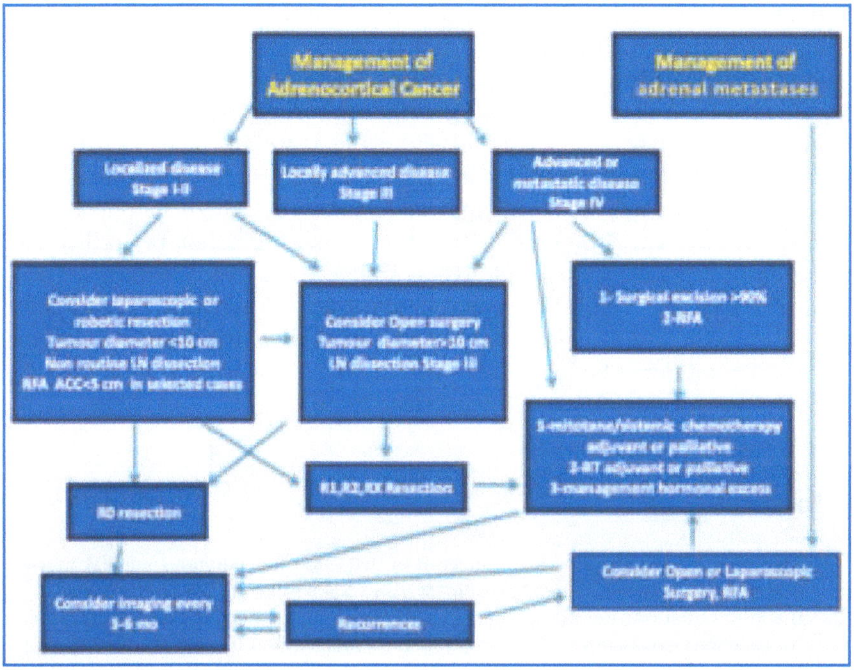

Fig. 10.10 Therapeutic algorithm for adrenocortical carcinoma. *RFA*, radiofrequency ablation; *LN*, lymph node; *ACC*, adrenocortical cancer

10.5.7 Management of Recurrent or Metastatic ACC

Surgery is an effective treatment of locally advanced adrenal cancer. In centers with sufficient experience, consideration should be given to resection recurrences and metastases because this can be accomplished with limited morbidity. Patients undergoing complete resection for recurrences and metastatic disease have a significantly improved median survival. Mitotane, alone or in combination with standard chemotherapy (etoposide, doxorubicin, and cisplatin), remains the standard treatment for unresectable or metastatic ACC. In many patients, advanced disease at presentation precludes resection, whereas chemotherapy is often administered if persistent hormonal excess results in severe sequelae. Ketoconazole, mitotane, metyrapone, and etomidate may be used to alleviate hormonal symptoms [61]. The therapeutic algoritm for ACC is reported in Fig. 10.10.

10.6 Prognosis and Survival

Whereas in older series most patients were diagnosed with advanced disease (stage IV), recent studies have reported the highest percentage of patients in stage II; this most likely reflects improved and more widely available imaging methods. ACCs are characterized by a poor prognosis, with a mean survival at 5 years from diagnosis ranging from 16% to 38%. The poor prognosis of ACCs is strictly related to their biological aggressiveness. In fact, ACCs may precociously metastasize to regional and para-aortic lymph nodes, the lungs, the liver and bones. Metastases in the contralateral gland as well as bilateral ACC may be found in 4% of cases. The prognosis is influenced largely by tumor staging at surgery and certain histopathological features (e.g., high mitotic count). Longer survival is usually seen in younger patients. Secretion of cortisol and androgens is often associated with ACCs; probably less than one-third are non-hypersecretory after careful hormonal investigations. The worse prognosis for cortisol-secreting ACCs may relate to the morbidity of Cushing syndrome and/or different tumor biology. The 5-year survival is 60% for stage I, 58% for stage II, 24% for stage III, and 0% for stage IV [62].

References

1. Abecassis M, McLoughlin MJ, Langer B et al (1985) Serendipitous adrenal masses: Prevalence, significance, and management. Am J Surg 149: 783–788
2. Bovio S, Cataldi A, Reimondo G et al (2006) Prevalence of adrenal incidentaloma in a contemporary computerized tomography series. J Endocrinol Invest 2006;29:298–302
3. NIH state-of-the-science statement on management of the clinically inapparent adrenal mass ("incidentaloma") (2006). NIH Consens State Sci Statements 19:1–25
4. Hisada M, Garber JE, Fung CY et al (1998) Multiple primary cancers in families with Li-Fraumeni syndrome. J Natl Cancer Inst;90:606 – 611
5. Varley JM, McGown G, Thorncroft M et al (1999) Are there low-penetrance TP53 Alleles? Evidence from childhood adrenocortical tumors. Am J Hum Genet 65:995–1006
6. Bell DW, Varley JM, Szydlo TE et al (1999) Heterozygous germ line hCHK2 mutations in Li-Fraumeni syndrome. Science 286:2528 –2531
7. Maher ER, Reik W (2000) Beckwith-Wiedemann syndrome: Imprinting in clus- ters revisited. J Clin Invest 105:247–252
8. Carney JA, Gordon H, Carpenter PC et al (1985) The complex of myxomas, spotty pigmentation, and endocrine overactivity. Medicine (Baltimore) 64:270–283
9. Thakker RV (1998) Multiple endocrine neoplasia—syndromes of the twentieth century. J Clin Endocrinol Metab 83:2617–2620
10. Bauman A, Bauman CG. Virilizing ACC. (1982) Development in a patient with salt-losing congenital adrenal hyperplasia. JAMA 248:3140 –3141
11. Hollstein M, Sidransky D, Vogelstein B et al (1991) p53 mutations in human cancers. Science 253:49–53)
12. Giordano TJ, Thomas DG, Kuick R et al (2003) Distinct transcriptional profiles of adrenocortical tumors uncovered by DNA microarray analysis. Am J Pathol 162:521–531
13. Zwermann O, Beuschlein F, Mora P et al (2000) Multiple endocrine neoplasia type 1 gene expression is normal in sporadic adrenocortical tumors. Eur J Endocrinol 142:689–695
14. Bertherat J, Groussin L, Sandrini F et al (2003) Molecular and functional analysis of PRKAR1A and its locus (17q22–24) in sporadic adrenocortical tumors: 17q losses, somatic mutations, and protein kinase A expression and activity. Cancer Res 63:5308–5319
15. Rosenberg D, Groussin L, Bertagna X et al (2002) cAMP pathway alterations from the cell surface to the nucleus in adrenocortical tumors. Endocr Res 28:765–775

16. Tissier F, Cavard C, Groussin L et al (2005) Mutations of beta-catenin in adre- nocortical tumors: Activation of the Wnt signaling pathway is a frequent event in both benign and malignant adrenocortical tumors Cancer Res 65:7622–7627
17. Schmitt A et al (2006) IGFII and MIB1 immunohistochemistry is helpful for the differentiation of benign from malignant adrenocortical tumours. Histopathology 49:298–307
18. Sasano H, Shizawa S, Suzuki T (1995) Transcription factor adrenal 4 binding protein as a marker of adrenocortical malignancy. Hum Pathol 26:1154–1156
19. Kiiveri S, Liu J, Arola J et al (2005) Transcription factors GATA-6, SF-1, and cell proliferation in human adrenocortical tumors. Mol Cell Endocrinol 233:47–56
20. Kolomecki K, Stepien H, Bartos M et al (2001) Usefulness of VEGF, MMP-2, MMP-3 and TIMP-2 serum level evaluation in patients with adrenal tumours. Endocr Regul 35:9–16
21. Barzon L, Boscaro M (2000) Diagnosis and management of adrenal incidentalomas. J Urol 163:398–407
22. Mantero F, Terzolo M, Arnaldi G et al (2000) A survey on adrenal incidentaloma in Italy. Study Group on Adrenal Tumors of the Italian Society of Endocrinology. (2000) J Clin Endocrinol Metab 85:637– 644
23. Fishman EK, Deutch BM, Hartman DS et al (1987) Primary adrenocortical carcinoma: CT evaluation with clinical correlation. AJR 148:531–535
24. Rockall AG, Babar SA, Sohaib SA, et al (2004) CT and MR imaging of the adrenal glands in ACTH-independent Cushing syndrome. RadioGraphics 24:435–452
25. Hussain S, Belldegrun A, Seltzer SE et al (1985). Differentiation of malignant from benign adrenal masses: predictive indices on computed tomography. AJR 144:61–65
26. Fishman EK, Deutch BM, Hartman DS et al (1987). Primary adrenocortical carcinoma: CT evaluation with clinical correlation. AJR 1987 148:531–535
27. Dunnick NR, Heaston D, Halvorsen R et al (1982) CT appearance of adrenal cortical carcinoma. J Comput Assist Tomogr 6:978–982
28. Slattery JM, Blake MA, Kalra MK et al (2006) Adrenocortical carcinoma: contrast washout characteristics on CT. AJR 187:197
29. Park BK, Kim CK, Kwon GY et al (2007) Re-evaluation of pheochromocytomas on delayed contrast-enhanced CT: washout enhancement and other imaging features. Eur Radiol 17:2804–2809
30. Geelhoed GW, Dunnick NR, Doppman JL (1980) Management of intravenous extensions of endocrine tumors and prognosis after surgical treatment. Am J Surg 139:844–848
31. Schlund JF, Kenney PJ, Brown ED et al (1995) Adrenocortical carcinoma: MR imaging appearance with current techniques. J Magn Reson Imaging 5:171–174
32. Smith SM, Patel SK, Turner DA et al (1989) Magnetic resonance imaging of adrenal cortical carcinoma. Urol Radiol 11:1–6
33. Ferrozzi F, Bova D et al (1995) CT and MR demonstration of fat within an adrenal cortical carcinoma. Abdom Imaging 20:272–274
34. Faria JF, Goldman SM, Szejnfeld J et al (2007) Adrenal masses: characterization with in vivo proton MR spectroscopy—initial experience. Radiology 245:788–797
35. Caoili EM, Korobkin M, Brown RK et al (2007) Differentiating adrenal adenomas from nonadenomas using (18)F-FDG PET/CT: quantitative and qualitative evaluation. Acad Ra- diol 14:468–475
36. Groussin L, Bonardel G, Silvera S et al (2009) 18F-Fluorodeoxyglucose positron emission tomography for the diagnosis of adrenocortical tumors: a prospective study in 77 operated patients. J Clin Endocri- nol Metab 94:1713–1722
37. Hennings J, Lindhe O, Bergstrom M et al (2006) Metomidate positron emission tomography of adrenocortical tumors in correlation with histopathological findings. J Clin Endocrinol Metab 91:1410–1414
38. Haider MA, Ghai S, Jhaveri K et al (2004) Chemical shift MR imaging of hyperattenuating (>10 HU) adrenal masses: does it still have a role? Radiology 2004; 231:711–716

39. Jacques AE, Sahdev A, Sandrasagara M et al (2008) Adrenal phaeochromocytoma: correlation of MRI appearances with histology and function. Eur Radiol 18:2885–2892
40. Bhatia KS, Ismail MM, Sahdev A et al (2008) 123 I-metaiodobenzylguanidine (MIBG) scintigraphy for the detection of adrenal and extra-adrenal phaeo- chromocytomas: CT and MRI correlation. Clin Endocrinol 69:181–188
41. Chua SC, Rozalli FI, O'Connor SR (2009) Imaging features of primary extranodal lymphomas. Clin Radiol 64:574–588
42. Abrams HL, Spiro R, Goldstein N (1950) Metastases in carcinoma: analysis of 1000 autopsied cases. Cancer 3:74–85
43. Johnson GL, Hruban RH, Marshall FF et al (1997) Primary adrenal ganglioneuroma: CT findings in four patients. AJR 169:169–171
44. Wilson DA, Muchmore HG, Tisdal RG et al (1984) Histoplasmosis of the adrenal glands studied by CT. Radiology 150:779–783
45. Gross MD, Korobkin M, Assaly WB et al (2009)Contemporary imaging of incidentally discovered adrenal masses. Nat Rev Urol 6:363–373
46. DeWitt J, Alsatie M, LeBlanc J et al (2007) Endoscopic ultrasound-guided fine needle aspiration of left adrenal gland masses. Endoscopy 39:65-71
47. Allolio B, Fassnacht M (2006) Clinical review: Adrenocortical carcinoma: clinical update. J Clin Endocrinol Metab 91(6):2027-37
48. Stigliano A, Cerquetti L, Sampaoli L et al (2012) Current and emerging therapeutic options in adrenocortical cancer treatment. J Oncol 408131, Epub 2012 Aug 14 PubMed PMID: 22934112
49. Carnaille B (2012) Adrenocortical carcinoma: wich surgical approach? Langenbecks Arch Surg 397:195-199
50. Gagner M, Lacroix A Bolté E (1992) Laparoscopic adrenalectomy in Cushing's syndrome and pheochrocytoma. N.Engl Med 327 (14):1033
51. Wandoloski M, Bussey KJ, Demeure MJ (2009) Adrenocortical cancer. Surg Clin North Am 89:1255-67
52. Miller BS, Ammori JB, Gauger PG et al (2010) Laparoscopic rescection is inappropriate in patients with known or suspected adrenocortical carcinoma. W J Surg 34:1380-1385
53. Bergamini C, Martellucci J, Tozzi F et al (2011) Complications in laparoscopic adrenalectomy: the value of experience. Surg Endosc 25:3845-51
54. Valeri A, Bergamini C (2010) Surgery of the adrenal glands, in the second decade of the century: no more doubts G Chir 31:69-74
55. Valeri A, Bergamini C, Manca G et al (2005) Adrenal incidentaloma: the influence of a decision-making algorithm on the short-term outcome of laparoscopy. J Laparoendosc Adv Surg Tech A 15:451-9
56. Valeri A, Borrelli A, Presenti L et al (2001) Laparoscopic adrenalectomy. Personal experience in 78 patients. G Chir 22:185-9
57. Taskin EH, Berber E (2012) Robotic Adrenalectomy. Journal of Surgical Oncology 106:622-625
58. Venkatesan AM, Locklin J, Dupuy DE et al (2010) Percutaneous ablation of adrenal tumors. Tech Vasc Interv Radiol 13:89-99
59. Polat B, Fassnacht M, Pfreundner L et al (2009) Radiotherapy in Adrenocortical Carcinoma. Cancer 115:2816-23
60. Sancho JJ, Triponz F et al (2012) Surgical management of adrenal metastases. Langenbecks Arch Surg 397:179-194
61. Mawardi M, Al-Judaibi B, Marotta P (2012) Hepatic Metastases from Adrenocortical Carcinoma Fifteen Years after primary resection. The Saudi journal of gastroenterology 18:140-142
62. Libè R, Fratticci A, Bertherat J (2007) Adrenocortical cancer: pathophysiology and clinical management. Endocr Relat Cancer. 14:13-28

Hematologic Malignancies of Surgical Interest and Splenic Tumors

11

Jacopo Martellucci, Carlo Bergamini, Caterina Santi, Riccardo Somigli and Andrea Valeri

11.1 Introduction

According to the theory of Hippocrates (460–370 BC), the spleen was a source of "black bile" and connected to the melancholic Galenic temperament (Fig. 11.1). In the seventeenth century, Blackmore characterized the spleen as an organ to which "hypochondrial and hysterical affections" could be attributed. Historically, the spleen has always been considered to be a locus of conflicting emotions.

Anecdotal reports of splenic surgery began to emerge in the sixteenth century (Zacarello, 1549). Until modern times, however, removal of the spleen usually resulted in death. Most splenectomies were done in patients who had undergone penetrating trauma and with the spleen protruding from the wound. The first elective splenectomy was carried out for portal hypertension in 1826 by Quittenbaum: the patient died. In 1966, Bryant was the first to attempt splenectomy for leukemia. Over the following 15 years, 14 splenectomies were attempted as therapy for leukemia: none of the patients survived. By 1877, only 50 splenectomies had ever been undertaken, with a mortality rate of >70%. In 1908, Johnston reported a mortality of 87.7% in a review of splenectomy for hematologic disorders [1].

With the increased use of automobiles, in the twentieth century splenectomy became more common and the morality rate dropped rapidly. In a 1920 report of the experience with splenectomy of the Mayo Clinic, a mortality rate of 11% was documented [2]. Nowadays, the largest splenectomy series reported mortality rates of <1%.

Moreover, since the first laparoscopic splenectomy (LS) described by

J. Martellucci (✉) · C. Bergamini · C. Santi · R. Somigli · A. Valeri
General, Emergency and Minimally Invasive Surgery
Careggi Hospital, Florence, Italy
e-mail: jamjac64@hotmail.com

A. Valeri et al. (eds.), *What's New in Surgical Oncology*,
DOI: 10.1007/978-88-470-5310-6_11, © Springer-Verlag Italia 2013

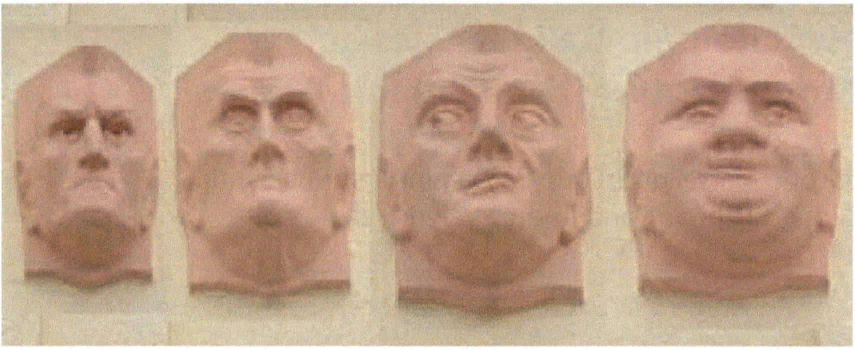

Fig. 11.1 The four temperaments—(*from left to right*) choleric, melancholic, sanguine and phlegmatic—on the wall of a house at the corner of Am Dornbusch and Eschersheimer Landstraße in Dornbusch, Frankfurt am Main, Germany. Artist unknown

Delaître in 1991 [3], numerous case series have shown the feasibility of LS for a large variety of benign and malignant hematologic diseases. Excluding trauma, benign hematologic diseases are now the most common indication for splenectomy. Splenectomy may be indicated as a diagnostic tool and surgical staging or for palliation in patients with malignant hematologic disease. Patients with malignant hematologic diseases are more likely to have massively enlarged spleens (>1,000 g), resulting in significant discomfort and pain. Splenectomy can also provide relief to patients with symptomatic splenomegaly.

11.2 Anatomical and Functional Considerations

Consisting of an encapsulated mass of vascular and lymphoid tissue, the spleen is the largest reticuloendothelial organ in the body. The abdominal surface of the diaphragm separates the spleen from the lower left lung and pleura and the ninth to eleventh ribs. The visceral surface faces the abdominal cavity and contains gastric, colic, renal, and pancreatic impressions (Fig. 11.2).

11.2.1 Size and Dimensions

Spleen size and weight vary with age and pathologic conditions. The average adult spleen is 7 cm to 11 cm in length and weighs 150 g (range, 70 g to 250 g). Splenomegaly is described variably and the surgical literature reflects a lack of consensus. Spleen size is expressed in terms of the maximum interpole length and is generally classified into three categories: normal size (<11 cm), moderate splenomegaly (11 cm to 20 cm or >500 g in weight) and severe or massive splenomegaly (>20 cm or >1,000 g in weight) [4].

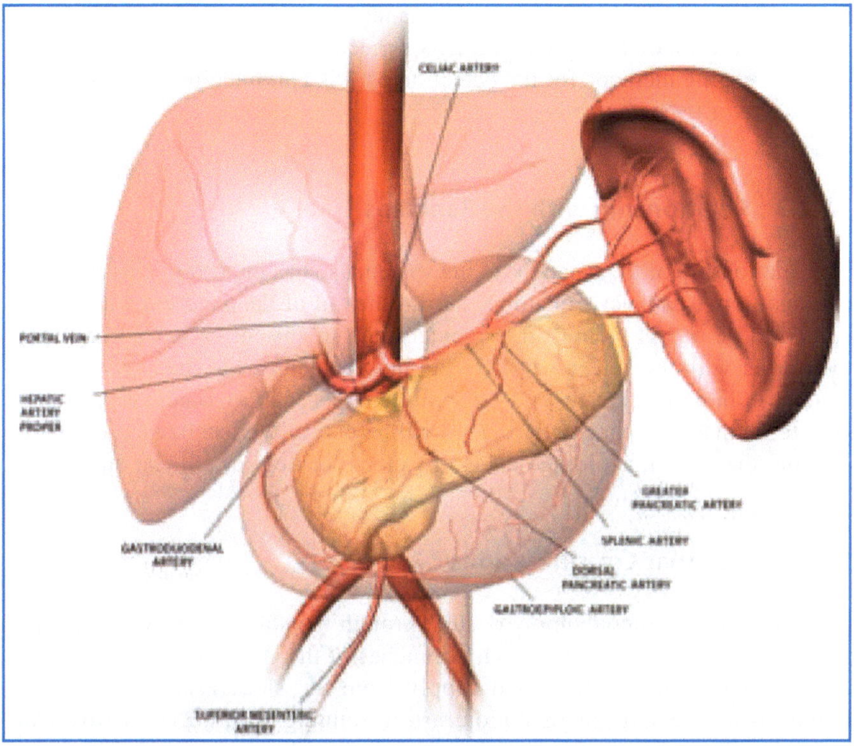

Fig. 11.2 Three-dimensional drawing of the normal anatomy in the upper abdomen shows the main splenic artery and its branches. Reproduced from [25] with permission from the Radiological Society of North America

11.2.2 Anatomical Anomalies

The most common anomaly of splenic embryology is the accessory spleen (AS). Present in ≤20% of the population, one or more ASs may also occur in ≤30% of patients with hematologic disease. More than 80% of ASs are found in the region of the splenic hilum and vascular pedicle. Other locations for ASs (in descending order of frequency) are the gastrocolic ligament, pancreas tail, greater omentum, greater curve of the stomach, splenocolic ligament, small and large bowel mesentery, left broad ligament in women, and left spermatic cord in men [5]. For these reasons, ASs should always be considered, even if the hematologic significance of the presence of AS and the impact of their removal on results are not clear. The role of ASs in failed splenectomy has been studied extensively, and the prevalence of residual splenic tissue (as detected by post-splenectomy scintigraphy) reaches ≤48%, even if the efficacy of accessory splenectomy varies from 27% to 75% [6].

Surprisingly, also after laparoscopic splenectomy, residual splenic tissue was noted in 50% of patients, [7] even if it could be related to the surgical approach. The problem of ASs can be managed by careful videoscopic examination of the abdominal cavity during splenectomy, whereas the use of preoperative imaging methods for the detection of ASs is limited by the insufficient sensitivity of these methods [8].

11.2.3 Relationship with the Pancreas

The relationship of the pancreas to the spleen also has important clinical implications. In one cadaveric anatomic series, the tail of the pancreas was demonstrated to lie within 1 cm of the splenic hilum in 75% of cases and in 30% to the border with the spleen [9]. Considering that injuries to the pancreatic tail can cause important postoperative complications such as pancreatitis or pancreatic fistulas, the pancreatic tail should be carefully visualized and dissected from the spleen, avoiding damage by electrocautery or a linear stapler.

11.2.4 Vascular Considerations

The main arterial blood supply occurs through the splenic artery (the longest and most tortuous of the three main branches of the celiac artery). The spleen also receives some of its blood supply from the short gastric vessels that branch from the left gastroepiploic artery running within the gastrosplenic ligament. The splenic artery can be characterized by the pattern of its terminal branches. The distributed type of splenic artery is the most common (70%) and is distinguished by a short trunk with many long branches entering over three-fourths of the medial surface of the spleen. The less common magistral type of splenic artery (30%) has a long main trunk dividing near the hilum into short terminal branches, and these enter over 25% to 30% of the medial surface of the spleen [10]. Early identification of the type of splenic blood supply can help the surgeon to estimate how difficult the splenectomy is likely to be.

Outside the spleen, the arteries also frequently form transverse anastomoses with each other and, as a consequence, attempts to close a splenic-artery branch by clips or embolization, if undertaken proximal to these anastomosis, may fail to devascularize the corresponding splenic segment. Before division of the splenic trunk, it usually gives few small branches (the most important is the pancreatica magna) to the tail of the pancreas. Occlusion or section of these branches could result in pancreatitis. The main venous drainage is through the splenic vein, which joins the superior mesenteric vein behind the neck of the pancreas to form the portal vein.

11.2.5 Spleen Function

The spleen combines the innate and adaptive immune system in a uniquely organized way. The structure of the spleen enables it to remove older erythrocytes from the circulation and leads to the efficient removal of blood-borne microorganisms and cellular debris. This function, in combination with a highly organized lymphoid compartment, makes the spleen the most important organ for antibacterial and antifungal immune reactivity [11].

The spleen, which has important hematopoietic functions during early fetal development (until the fifth month), has no significant hematopoietic function remaining in adults, but continues to function as a "sophisticated filter" because of the unique circulatory system and lymphoid organization, and it has blood-cell monitoring and management functions as well as important immune functions throughout life. However, under certain pathological conditions (such as myelodysplasia), the spleen can reacquire its hematopoietic function.

Removal of the spleen results in loss of immunologic and filtering functions. It is well established that, after splenectomy, patients are at a significantly higher risk for overwhelming post-splenectomy nfection (OPSI) with fulminant bacteremia, pneumonia, or meningitis, as compared with those with normal splenic function. Asplenic subjects have defective activation of complement by the alternative pathway, leaving them more susceptible to infection. Asplenic patients also have a normal response to re-immunization to an antigen first encountered before splenectomy, but do not have an optimal response to exposure to new antigens, especially if the antigen is administered intravenously.

The spleen is a major site of production of opsonins (molecules that target an antigen for an immune response), properdin (important for initiation of the alternative pathway of complement activation) and tuftsin (a tetrapeptide that enhances the phagocytic activity of polymorphonuclear leukocytes and mononuclear phagocytes). Removal of the spleen results in decreased serum levels of these factors. As a result, neutrophil function is decreased in asplenic patients, and the defect appears to be related to the absence of circulating mediators [12].

For these reasons, it is suggested that splenectomized persons receive the following vaccinations (ideally before planned splenectomy):

- Pneumococcal polysaccharide vaccine (not before 2 years of age);
- *Hemophilus influenzae* type B vaccine (especially if not received in childhood);
- Meningococcal conjugate vaccine (especially if not received in adolescence);
- Influenza vaccine, every winter (to help prevent getting secondary bacterial infection).

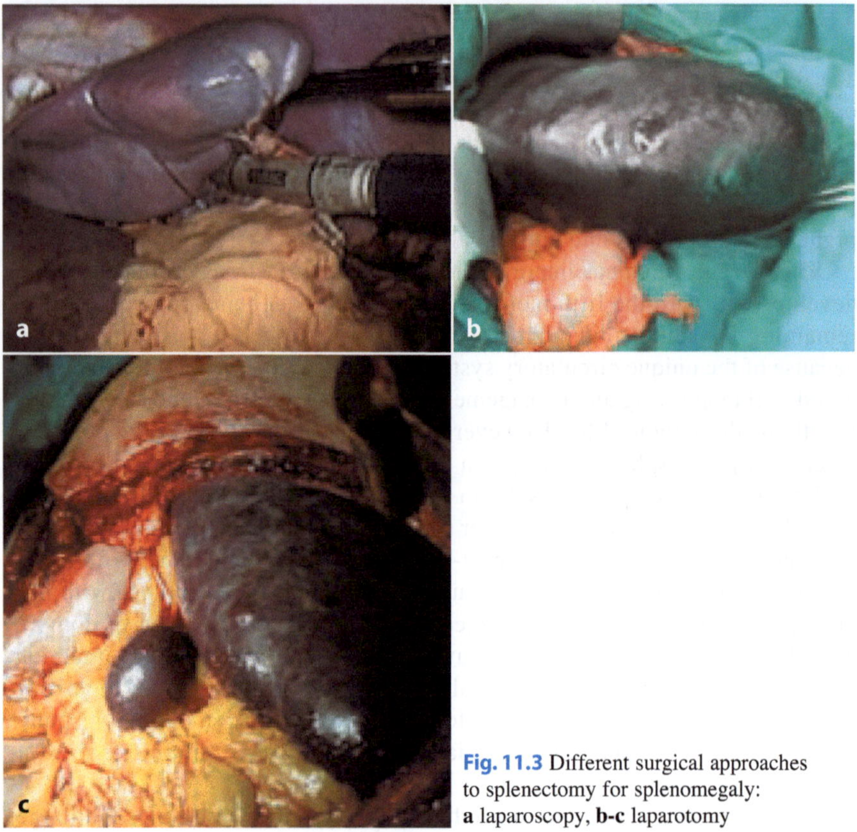

Fig. 11.3 Different surgical approaches to splenectomy for splenomegaly: **a** laparoscopy, **b-c** laparotomy

11.3 Surgical Considerations

11.3.1 Preoperative Evaluation

Currently, we consider all patients evaluated for elective splenectomy to be potential candidates for laparoscopic splenectomy (Fig. 11.3). Large case series and non-randomized comparative trials have consistently reported better outcomes from laparoscopic splenectomy than from open splenectomy. Although operating times were longer among patients who underwent LS, the duration of hospital stay, transfusion requirements, and morbidity and mortality were reduced [13].

Contraindications to a laparoscopic approach include severe portal hypertension, uncorrectable coagulopathy, severe ascites, and most traumatic injuries to the spleen. Extreme splenomegaly also remains a relative contraindication.

Because most patients scheduled for splenectomy have a hematologic disorder, a multidisciplinary treatment protocol should be adapted to each patient, in particular about the use of corticosteroids, gamma-globulins, and platelet transfusion.

Patients undergoing elective splenectomy should be vaccinated preoperatively (or within 30–40 days postoperatively) with pneumococcal, meningococcal, and *Haemophilus* vaccines. Low-molecular-weight heparin (LMWH) prophylaxis for thromboembolism and antibiotics are administered according to standard guidelines (and if there are no hematologic contraindications). Bowel preparation is not routinely necessary. Patients need to be given all the information about the consequences of the asplenic state.

11.3.2 Massive Splenomegaly

The literature reports that, with sufficient experience, even massive spleens can be removed safely using minimally invasive methods [14]. In any case, rather than the absolute size of the spleen, the relationship between the same and amplitude of the laparoscopic chamber is more important [15]. Knowledge of anatomy is essential for preparation of the splenic hilum and liberation of the organ. Moreover, preoperative embolization of the splenic artery and the hand-assisted method allowed extension of the laparoscopic indications for massive splenomegaly [16]. In the process of hand-assisted laparoscopic splenectomy for splenomegaly, tactile senses may help to identify dissection planes, to define ASs, and to prevent splenic capsular injury by trocars and instruments. The hand may function as a retractor to hold the stomach, colon and pancreas moderately while holding the spleen laterally simultaneously. Furthermore, dissection of the splenic hilum could be easier with the tactile sense of the hand combined with a laparoscopic dissector in the other hand even in the setting of a spleen with dense adhesion.

However, because of the larger-sized spleen that narrows the operative space, exposure is limited and the manipulation difficult, LS becomes more technically challenging. The hypervascularization and dense adhesion around the spleen also hampers the procedure. Moreover, once the dissection is completed, extraction of the giant spleen with a totally laparoscopic approach by placing into a retrieval bag followed by morcellation can be difficult, and the procedure time can be longer. LS for splenomegaly has been associated with longer operating time, more blood loss, and higher intraoperative and postoperative complication rates than LS for normal-sized spleens,and with a higher conversion rate [17].

11.3.3 Extraction of Specimens

Spleens removed by an anterior laparoscopic approach are extracted through the umbilical trocar site after fragmentation in a plastic bag. It is rarely necessary to enlarge the incision by >2–3 cm. If the lateral approach is undertaken, extraction is more readily carried out through one of the ports situated anteriorly. This extraction site also requires little or no enlargement. On occasion, for spleens longer than 20 cm, a Pfannenstiel incision should be made or the spleen can be readily extracted through the accessory incision used for hand assistance during hand-assisted laparoscopic surgery.

Special mention should be made for laparoscopic splenectomy in patients with malignant disease. If lymphoma (Hodgking or non-Hodgkin) is suspected, neither preoperative splenic artery embolization nor spleen fragmentation should be performed, for avoid compromising the histological diagnosis. In practice, however, the histological diagnosis was made preoperatively in the majority of the patients, then this measure may not be necessary.

11.3.4 Percutaneous Image-guided Biopsies

Historically, image-guided percutaneous biopsy of the spleen has been approached with trepidation by radiologists because of concerns regarding accessibility and the risk of hemorrhage. This reluctance may be related to an early report of a high rate of major complications (13%) for percutaneous biopsy of the spleen performed with a 14-G needle [18]. Several more recent studies have reported much lower complication rates with smaller needle diameters (≤18 G gauge), similar to that reported for kidney or liver biopsies [19]. Diseases that commonly affect the spleen can pose a diagnostic challenge to the clinician, radiologist, and pathologist. The reported diagnostic accuracy of splenic biopsy varies, ranging between 84% and 90% [20].

For cases in which the spleen is the only abnormal or most accessible organ for biopsy and a tissue diagnosis is required, the use of image-guided percutaneous biopsy of the spleen could be considered a safe alternative to splenectomy with a high overall diagnostic accuracy (but only in experienced hands) [21].

11.3.5 Preoperative Embolization of the Splenic Artery

Preoperative embolization of the splenic artery can reduce the operating time and decrease intraoperative blood loss when compared with laparoscopic or open splenectomy alone [22]. However, besides higher costs, radiation exposure for the patient and the unavailability of the procedure in each hospital, there are other problems related to the angiographic embolization, in particular the higher risk of portal-vein thrombosis (≈15%) and the pain related to ischemic damage [23]. In fact, ≈45% of patients report some degree of pain [24].

As the use of splenic arterial interventions increases in interventional radiology practice, clinicians must be familiar with splenic vascular anatomy, the indications and contraindications for carrying out interventional procedures, the technical considerations involved, and the potential use of other interventional procedures (such as radiofrequency ablation) in combination with splenic arterial interventions. Familiarity with the complications that may result from these interventional procedures, including abscess formation and pancreatitis, is also important [25].

11.4 Splenectomy for Benign Hematologic Disorders

Splenectomy continues to find common therapeutic indications for hematologic disorders in which the spleen has a pathologic role (Table 11.1). Hematologic disorders can be categorized by various criteria, including the origin of the disorder (splenic, peripheral blood cell, bone marrow, genetic) or cell-line abnormality (platelets, red blood cells (RBCs), white blood cells (WBCs), and bone marrow). Therapeutic splenectomy rarely cures the underlying hematologic disease but, in many of these disorders, splenectomy can significantly improve the pathologic effects of splenic sequestration and symptomatic splenomegaly, can correct the hematologic abnormality, and can aid in the diagnosis and staging. Removal of the spleen can play an important part in reducing the morbidity of hematologic conditions [26, 27].

11.4.1 Idiopathic Thrombocytopenic Purpura (ITP)

ITP is the most common indication for elective splenectomy. It is an acquired disorder characterized by splenic production of immunoglobulin (Ig)G that induces splenic sequestration and the destruction of platelets. The hallmarks of this condition are low platelet levels, ecchymoses, purpura, petechiae, and abnormal bleeding.

The management of childhood ITP is different from that for adults, particularly with regard to the role of splenectomy. The condition is often self-limiting in children, with >70% of cases resolving spontaneously. Splenectomy for children is rarely indicated. It is reserved for the rare case of severe, symptomatic thrombocytopenia of >1 year duration that is refractory to medical management (including corticosteroids and intravenous infusion of immunoglobulin (IVIG)).

In adults, the thrombocytopenia associated with ITP is usually more severe and requires medical and surgical intervention. In general, splenectomy is indicated in adults with ITP if the patient does not improve after 8 weeks of corticosteroid therapy or if the thrombocytopenia recurs after the suspension of medical treatment. Intracranial hemorrhage is an indication for emergency IVIG and splenectomy.

The spleen is often not enlarged in ITP, making laparoscopic splenectomy an attractive option for these patients. Because the splenic tissue is the source of the disorder, a key component of the surgcial strategy is thorough inspec-

Table 11.1 Indication and response to splenectomy in hematologic diseases

Disease/Condition	Indications for Splenectomy	Response to Splenectomy
Benign Diseases		
Idiopathic thrombocytopenic purpura	Failure of medical therapy, recurrent disease	75–85% rate of long-term response
Thrombotic thrombocytopenic purpura	Excessive plasma exchange requirement	40% curative rate
Hereditary spherocytosis	Hemolytic anemia, recurrent transfusions, intractable leg ulcers	Improves or eliminates anemia
Pyruvate kinase deficiency	Only in severe cases, recurrent transfusions	Decreased transfusion requirement, palliative only
G6PD deficiency	None	—
Warm-antibody autoimmune hemolytic anemia	Failure of medical (corticosteroid) therapy	60–80% response rate, recurrences common
Sickle cell disease	History of acute sequestration crisis, splenic symptoms or infarction	Palliative, variable response
Thalassemia	Excessive transfusion requirements, symptomatic splenomegaly or infarction	Diminished transfusion requirements, relief of symptoms
Felty's syndrome	Neutropenia	80% durable response rate
Gaucher's disease	Hypersplenism	Improves cytopenias; does not correct underlying disease
Niemann–Pick disease	Symptomatic splenomegaly	Improves symptoms; does not correct underlying disease
Amyloidosis	Symptomatic splenomegaly	Improves symptoms; does not correct underlying disease
Sarcoidosis	Hypersplenism or symptomatic splenomegaly	Improves symptoms and cytopenias; does not correct underlying disease
Malignant Diseases		
Non-Hodgkin's lymphoma	Cytopenias, symptomatic splenomegaly	Improved complete blood count values, relief of symptoms
Hodgkin's disease	Surgical staging in select cases	—
Chronic lymphocytic leukemia	Hypersplenism or symptomatic splenomegaly	Improves symptoms and cytopenias (60–70% response rate)
Hairy cell leukemia	Cytopenias and symptomatic splenomegaly	40–70% response rate
Acute myeloid leukemia	Intolerable symptomatic splenomegaly	Relief of abdominal pain and early satiety
Chronic myeloid leukemia	Symptomatic splenomegaly	Relief of abdominal pain and early satiety

(*cont.*) →

Table 11.1 (*continued*)

Myelofibrosis (AMM)	Severe symptomatic splenomegaly	76% clinical response at 1 year, high risk of hemorrhagic, thrombotic, and infectious complications (26%)
Essential thrombocythemia and polycytemia vera	Only for advanced disease with severe symptomatic splenomegaly	Relief of abdominal pain and early satiety

tion of the abdomen for ASs. In patients who have recurrent symptoms after splenectomy, a ^{99m}Tc-labeled RBC or ^{111}In-labeled platelet scan can be employed to identify the location of the AS and facilitate resection, with removal of the remnant AS typically associated with ITP cure.

Splenectomy results in surgical cure of 75% to 85% of patients with ITP. Petechiae, ecchymosis, and significant bleeding are uncommon even in the remaining 15% to 25% with persistent post-splenectomy thrombocytopenia.

11.4.2 Thrombotic Thrombocytopenic Purpura (TTP)

Is a severe disorder characterized by thrombocytopenia, purpura, fever, microangiopathic hemolytic anemia, neurologic deficits, and renal dysfunction (hematuria or renal failure). Abnormal clumping of platelets occurs in arterioles and capillaries, reducing the lumen of these vessels and predisposing the patient to microvascular thrombotic episodes. The reduced lumen size also causes shearing stresses on erythrocytes, which leads to deformed RBCs being subject to hemolysis. Hemolysis may be due in part to sequestration and destruction of erythrocytes in the spleen.

Plasmapheresis is the first-line therapy for TTP. Mortality is >60% for patients who do not respond to plasmapheresis. Platelet administration in TTP patients is typically avoided because their administration has been associated with clinical deterioration. Splenectomy has a key role for patients who experience relapse or who require multiple plasma exchanges to control symptoms, and generally is well tolerated without significant morbidity, coupled with high-dose corticosteroids [28]. Unfortunately there is only a 40% cure rate with splenectomy for TTP.

11.4.3 Disorders in the RBC Membrane

11.4.3.1 Hereditary Spherocytosis (HS)

HS is the most common congenital anemia for which splenectomy is carried out. Lack of spectrin protein in erythrocyte membranes leads to loss of surface area of the RBC membrane and causes the characteristic shape of HS RBCs, called "spherocytes". These abnormal RBCs are less deformable and have increased osmotic fragility, and therefore cannot easily pass through the splenic pulp and have an increased tendency to be sequestered and destroyed within the spleen. Patients present with anemia, jaundice, and splenomegaly. The splenomegaly develops from the first year of age. By the age of 5 years, many patients with HS have pigmented gallstones. Pigmented gallstones are present in 30% to 60% of HS patients. The diagnosis is made by identification of spherocytes on the peripheral blood smear, an increased reticulocyte count, increased osmotic fragility, and a negative Coombs' test. Although the spherocytes persist, splenectomy decreases the rate of hemolysis and usually leads to resolution of the anemia. Removal of the gallbladder in the same procedure is warranted if the patient has developed gallstones. If possible, the surgeon should try to delay splenectomy until the patient is 4 years old to reduce the risk of overwhelming post-splenectomy infection (OPSI).

Other anemias associated with erythrocyte structural abnormalities include hereditary elliptocytosis, hereditary pyropoikilocytosis, hereditary xerocytosis, and hereditary hydrocytosis. All of these conditions result in abnormalities of the erythrocyte cellular membrane and increased destruction of RBCs. The severity of the anemia is extremely variable, and usually of limited clinical significance in which splenectomy is not indicated. Splenectomy is indicated only for severe hemolytic anemia and can be curative.

11.4.4 Enzyme Deficiencies in RBCs

Enzyme deficiencies in RBCs associated with hemolytic anemia may be classified into two groups: (i) deficiencies of enzymes involved in glycolytic pathways, such as pyruvate kinase (PK) deficiency, and (ii) deficiencies of enzymes needed to maintain a high ratio of reduced to oxidized glutathione in the RBC, protecting it from oxidative damage, such as glucose-6-phosphate dehydrogenase (G6PD) deficiency.

The most common RBC enzyme deficiency that causes congenital chronic hemolytic anemia is PK deficiency. It is an autosomal recessive condition and its pathophysiology is not clear. Manifestations of the disease vary widely, from transfusion-dependent severe anemia in early childhood to well-compensated mild anemia in adolescents or adults. The diagnosis is made by a screening test or by detection of specific mutations at the complementary DNA or genomic level. Splenomegaly is common and, in severe cases, splenectomy can alleviate transfusion requirements.

The most common RBC enzyme deficiency overall is G6PD deficiency (X-linked). Manifestations—chronic hemolytic anemia, acute intermittent hemolytic episodes, or no hemolysis—depend on the variant of G6PD deficiency. The mainstay of therapy is avoidance of drugs known to precipitate hemolysis in patients with G6PD deficiency. Transfusions are given in cases of symptomatic anemia. Splenectomy is not indicated in most patients affected by this disease.

11.4.5 Hereditary Hemolytic Anemias

11.4.5.1 Thalassemias

Thalassemias are inherited disorders of hemoglobin synthesis prevalent among people of Mediterranean extraction and classified according to the hemoglobin chain affected. Most forms of this disorder are inherited in a Mendelian autosomal recessive fashion from asymptomatic carrier parents. The RBCs have intracellular precipitation of excess altered globin chains. These intracellular precipitates lead to the premature destruction of RBCs when they are filtered in the spleen. There are several subtypes, determined on the basis of which globin chain is defective (α, β, γ, or δ). Individuals who are homozygous (thalassemia major) have a more severe presentation, whereas the heterozygous patients (thalassemia minor) can be asymptomatic. Signs of thalassemia major include growth retardation, pallor, ulcers in the extremities, gallstones, bone abnormalities (enlargement of the head), and splenomegaly. Individuals with thalassemia major benefit from splenectomy if they require frequent transfusions (>1 per month), suffer from severe pain caused by splenic infarct, or have severe thrombocytopenia (<20,000 platelets/mm^3).

11.4.5.2 Sickle Cell Anemia

Sickle cell anemia is a hereditary autosomal recessive (with overdominance) hemolytic anemia caused by a single amino-acid substitution on the beta chain of the hemoglobin molecule. It is characterized by RBCs that assume an abnormal, rigid, "sickle" shape. The altered hemoglobin molecule is called hemoglobin S (Hb-S). Because the RBCs are less flexible, they tend to cause infarcts in the microvasculature and be related to severe pain. Although it is rare for subjects with sickle cell anemia to require splenectomy, splenic abscess or acute sequestration may be indications. In most patients, subsequent infarction of the spleen and autosplenectomy can occur [29]. Splenic abscess may complicate splenic infarction, making splenectomy beneficial. Splenectomy does not affect sickling, but elective splenectomy is a consideration after one major acute splenic sequestration crisis to avoid the 40–50% probability of subsequent acute sequestration crises, which can be associated with mortality ≤20%. The prevalence of acute sequestrations in patients with sickle cell anemia is ≈5%, with ≈3% requiring splenectomy. Key perioperative management principles for subjects with sickle cell anemia include adequate hydration and avoidance of hypothermia.

11.4.5.3 Autoimmune Hemolytic Anemias (AIHAs)

AIHAs are characterized by the destruction of RBCs caused by autoantibodies. AIHAs are classified as primary or secondary depending on whether an underlying cause (such as a disease or toxin) is identified. AIHAs can also be divided into "warm" and "cold" categories based on the temperature at which the autoantibodies exert their effect. In cold-agglutinin disease, severe symptoms are uncommon and splenectomy is almost never indicated. However, warm-antibody AIHA has clinical consequences with which the surgeon should be familiar. Warm-antibody AIHA, although occurring primarily in middle age, can affect individuals at all ages. The disorder is more common among women, and half of warm-antibody AIHA cases are idiopathic. Presentation may be acute or gradual. Findings include mild jaundice and the symptoms and signs of anemia. One-third to one-half of patients present with splenomegaly. Treatment of AIHA depends on disease severity and whether it is primary or secondary. Severe symptomatic anemia demands prompt attention, often requiring RBC transfusion. The mainstay of treatment for primary and secondary forms of symptomatic, unstable AIHA is corticosteroids. Favorable responses to splenectomy have been reported in patients with warm-antibody AIHA (≤80%). Unfortunately, transient responses are more common, and many patients could experience new episodes of hemolysis despite splenectomy. The decision regarding splenectomy in the case of AIHA should be individualized based on careful consideration of the clinical history and frank discussion with the patient.

11.4.6 Other Conditions

Felty's syndrome (autoimmune neutropenia) is an uncommon disorder that includes splenomegaly, neutropenia, and rheumatoid arthritis. Subjects with Felty's syndrome can also have thrombocytopenia and anemia. All of these conditions leave patients vulnerable to aggressive infections. Corticosteroids are the main treatment. Splenectomy can be helpful in correcting the neutropenia. In some cases, the neutropenia persists despite splenectomy, but the neutrophil response to infectious agents is improved. Frequent need for transfusion (>1 per month), thrombocytopenia, and recurrent infections are also indications for splenectomy.

Gaucher's disease is a familial disorder in which abnormal storage of glycolipid cerebrosides into reticuloendothelial cells occurs. As a result, it is associated with splenomegaly and lymph-node enlargement. Although splenectomy does not alter the course of Gaucher's disease, it is the procedure of choice if there are signs of hypersplenism (thrombocytopenia that may be associated with anemia and neutropenia). After splenectomy, the thrombocytopenia improves.

Sarcoidosis: Approximately one-quarter of patients with sarcoidosis have granulomatous involvement of the spleen, causing splenomegaly. Of these patients, 20% have hypersplenism in which the enlarged spleen is hyperactive, resulting in thrombocytopenia. This low platelet count generally improves after splenectomy. These patients can also have anemia, neutropenia, and spontaneous splenic rupture. Because of the splenomegaly and hypersplenism, the role of laparoscopic splenectomy for these patients is selective.

11.5 Splenectomy for Malignant Hematologic Disorders

The role of splenectomy in patients with malignant hematologic disorders varies. As for the myelogenous diseases, splenectomy for WBC disorders can be effective for symptomatic splenomegaly and hypersplenism, improving some clinical parameters but generally not altering the course of the underlying disease. Historically, splenectomy has had a role during the surgical staging for Hodgkin's disease, although this practice has become less common with the advent of advanced imaging technologies and less extensive biopsy strategies [30]. Careful consideration of the intended benefits of splenectomy must be weighed against the significant perioperative and post-splenectomy risks in this often complex patient population.

11.5.1 Hodgkin's Disease (HD)

HD is a malignant lymphoma that typically affects young adults in their twenties and thrities. Most patients have asymptomatic lymphadenopathy at the time of diagnosis, and most present with cervical node enlargement. More than 90% of patients with HD present with lymphadenopathy above the diaphragm. A few patients (usually with more advanced disease) may present with constitutional symptoms such as night sweats, weight loss, and pruritus. Lymphadenopathy below the diaphragm is rare upon presentation, but can arise with disease progression. The spleen is often an occult site of spread, but massive splenomegaly is not common. In addition, large spleens do not necessarily signify involvement.

The histologic type, along with location of disease and symptomatology, influence survival for patients with HD. HD can be classified histologically as: lymphocyte predominance type, nodular sclerosis type, mixed cellularity type, and lymphocyte depletion type. The disease is pathologically staged according to the Ann Arbor classification (Table 11.2).

Stage-I disease is limited to one anatomic region. Stage-II disease is defined by two or more contiguous or non-contiguous regions on the same side of the diaphragm. Stage-III disease involves disease on both sides of the diaphragm, but limited to lymph nodes, spleen, and Waldeyer's ring (the ring of lymphoid tissue formed by the lingual, palatine, and nasopharyngeal tonsils). Stage-IV disease includes involvement of the bone marrow, lung, liver, skin, gastrointestinal tract, or any organ or tissue other than the lymph nodes or Waldeyer's ring.

Historically, staging laparotomy including splenectomy provided essential pathologic staging information that was necessary to select appropriate therapy for HD. Staging laparotomy for HD is less commonly undertaken in the current era of minimally invasive surgery and advanced imaging methods. The improved non-surgical staging, along with the use of less toxic systemic chemotherapeutics for earlier stages of HD, has led to a dramatic decrease in the number of patients requiring staging laparotomy. Indications for surgical staging are clinical stage-I or -II disease of the nodular sclerosing type and no symptoms referable to HD. The surgical staging procedures for HD are liver biopsy, splenectomy, and the removal of representative nodes in the retroperitoneum, mesentery, and hepatoduodenal ligament. In general, an iliac marrow biopsy is included. Some studies have concluded that surgical staging has altered clinical staging in as many as 42% of cases [31].

11.5.2 Non-Hodgkin's Disease

Non-Hodgkin's lymphoma (NHL) encompasses all malignancies derived from the lymphoid system except classic HD. A proliferation of any one of the three predominant lymph cell types—natural killer cells, T cells, or B cells—may be included in the category of NHL. The subentities of NHL may be classified into nodal or extranodal, as well as indolent, aggressive, and very aggressive groups. Splenomegaly or hypersplenism is a common occurrence during NHL. Splenectomy is indicated for patients with NHL for treatment of massive splenomegaly when the bulk of the spleen contributes to abdominal pain, fullness, and early satiety. Splenectomy may also be effective in the treatment of patients who develop hypersplenism with associated anemia, thrombocytopenia, and neutropenia [32].

Splenectomy occasionally plays an important part in the diagnosis and staging of patients who present with isolated splenic disease. The most common primary splenic neoplasm is NHL. The spleen is involved in 50% to 80% of NHL patients, but <1% of patients present with splenomegaly without

Table 11.2 Ann Arbor staging system for Hodgkin's lymphoma

Stage	Description
I	Single lymphatic site
II	Lymphatic disease on the same side of the diaphragm
III	Lymphatic disease on both sides of the diaphragm
IV	Multiple extranodal sites (liver, lung, bone marrow)
X	Bulk >10 cm
E	Single or contiguous extralymphatic involvement
A/B	Absence/presence of constitutional symptoms (weight loss >10%, fever, drenching night sweats)
S	Splenic involvement

peripheral lymphadenopathy [33].

Disease that appears clinically confined to the spleen has been called "malignant lymphoma with prominent splenic involvement". Most affected patients have low-grade NHL. There is frequent involvement of the splenic hilar lymph nodes, extrahilar nodes, bone marrow, and liver in these patients. About 75% exhibit clinical evidence of hypersplenism.

One of the most common indications for splenectomy in NHL is the palliation of symptoms, such as pain in the left upper quadrant, early satiety, weakness and fatigue that accompany the marked splenomegaly often seen in this disease. Another common indication for splenectomy is for the treatment of cytopenias resulting from hypersplenism. Data from most series indicate that splenectomy is successful in relieving anemia, thrombocytopenia or leukopenia in 50% to 94% of cases. Response rates appear to be best if splenectomy is carried out before the spleen becomes massively enlarged or before the patient experiences severe or life-threatening symptoms from cytopenia or from the progression of lymphomatous process.

Residual splenomegaly in a patient who has otherwise successfully responded in other sites after chemotherapy for lymphoma is another reason for carrying out a splenectomy. In these cases, the procedure may be done for diagnostic and therapeutic reasons; it can determine if the splenomegaly is due to persistent lymphoma and, should this be true, it can potentially eliminate the focus of residual disease.

Splenectomy can also be indicated in autoimmune cytopenias (in corticosteroid-refractory cases) and in splenic marginal zone lymphoma (for diagnosis and treatment) as reported in the National Comprehensive Cancer Network (NCCN) Guidelines for Non-Hodgkin Lymphoma (version 3.2012) [34].

11.5.3 Hairy Cell Leukemia (HCL)

HCL is an uncommon blood disorder, representing only 2% of all adult leukemias. HCL is characterized by splenomegaly, pancytopenia, and large numbers of abnormal lymphocytes in the peripheral blood and bone marrow. These lymphocytes contain irregular hair-like cytoplasmic projections identifiable on the peripheral smear. Patients are usually elderly males with palpable splenomegaly. Many HCL patients have few symptoms and require no specific therapy. Splenectomy does not correct the underlying disorder but does return cell counts to normal in 40–70% of patients and alleviates the symptoms of splenomegaly [35]. Even if chemotherapy has replaced the role of splenectomy, it is indicated for some patients with massive enlargement of the spleen or with evidence of hypersplenism refractory to medical therapy. The responses to splenectomy usually last for ≥10 years, and about half of patients require no further therapy.

11.5.4 Chronic Lymphocytic Leukemia (CLL)

CLL is a B-cell leukemia characterized by the progressive accumulation of relatively mature (but functionally incompetent) lymphocytes. CLL occurs more frequently in men and usually occurs after 50 years of age. Symptoms of CLL are non-specific and include weakness, fatigue, fever without illness, night sweats, and frequent bacterial and viral infections. The most frequent finding is lymphadenopathy.

The role of splenectomy in the treatment of CLL continues to be for palliation of symptomatic splenomegaly and for treatment of cytopenia related to hypersplenism. Relief of bulk symptoms from splenomegaly is nearly always successful, whereas the hematologic response rates for correction of anemia and thrombocytopenia are between 60% and 70% [36].

11.5.5 Chronic Myelogenous Leukemia (CML)

CML is a myeloproliferative disorder that results from neoplastic transformation of myeloid elements. Ninety percent of patients with CML have the characteristic Philadelphia chromosome—a reciprocal translation between chromosomes 9 and 22 that results in the expression of an abnormal chimeric oncogenic protein called *p210*bcr-abl. The disease is characterized by progressive replacement of the normal diploid elements of the bone marrow with mature-appearing neoplastic myeloid cells. CML may occur from childhood to old age. CML usually presents with an indolent or chronic phase that is asymptomatic. Progression to the accelerated phase is marked by the onset of symptoms such as fever, night sweats, and progressive splenomegaly. However, this phase may also be asymptomatic and detectable only from changes in the peripheral blood or bone marrow. The accelerated phase may give rise to the blastic phase, which is characterized by the symptoms stated above as well as anemia, infectious complications, and bleeding. Splenomegaly with splenic sequestration of blood elements often contributes to these symptoms. Treatment of CML is primarily medical (even if symptomatic splenomegaly is present) and may be palliated effectively by splenectomy.

11.5.6 Myelofibrosis

The term "myelofibrosis" may be used to describe the generic condition of fibrosis of the bone marrow (which may be associated with several benign and malignant disorders) or a specific, chronic, malignant hematologic disease associated with splenomegaly, RBC and WBC progenitors in the bloodstream, marrow fibrosis, and extramedullary hematopoiesis, otherwise known as "agnogenic myeloid metaplasia" (AMM).

Treatment depends on symptoms: asymptomatic patients are followed closely, whereas symptomatic patients undergo therapeutic intervention targeted to their symptoms. Splenomegaly-related symptoms are best treated with splenectomy.

Splenectomy provides durable, effective palliation for nearly all patients with AMM (though postoperative complications are more common in patients with AMM than in those with other hematologic indications). In the postoperative period, these patients are at high risk of developing thrombocytosis and portal-vein thrombosis. In the experience of the Mayo Clinic, 49% of the procedures for AMM were done to alleviate the mechanical symptoms of splenomegaly; the remainder were undertaken to manage anemia, thrombocytopenia, or portal hypertension. Response to splenectomy was 76% at 1 year; the complication rate was 28%, with perioperative deaths in 6.6% [37]. Thrombosis, hemorrhage, and infection complications were common, with preoperative thrombocytopenia an independent predictor of mortality risk. These data underscore the severity of this malignancy and emphasize the need for careful selection of patients when considering splenectomy in AMM.

11.6 Primary Tumors of the Spleen

Vascular neoplasms are the most common primary splenic tumors and include benign and malignant variants. Hemangiomas are usually findings identified in spleens removed for other reasons.

Although primary involvement of the spleen is extremely rare, angiosarcoma is the most common primary non-lymphoid malignant lesion of the spleen. Since the first description of primary splenic angiosarcoma, more than 100 cases have been reported [38]. It is a very aggressive neoplasm with a high metastatic rate and poor prognosis. Metastasis typically involves the liver, lungs, bone, bone marrow and lymphatic system.

Angiosarcomas (or hemangiosarcomas) of the spleen have been associated with environmental exposure to thorium dioxide or monomeric vinyl chloride because of their association with hepatic angiosarcomas, but they most often occur spontaneously. The presentation of splenic angiosarcoma is variable. Patients usually present with left upper abdominal pain, fatigue, weight loss, and anorexia. Left upper abdominal pain is the most common symptom. It occurs in 75% to 83% of patients with splenic angiosarcoma [39]. Patients with these tumors may also present with splenomegaly, hemolytic anemia, ascites, and pleural effusions or with spontaneous splenic rupture. Splenomegaly is the most common finding (in 68% of cases) at physical examination [40].

Cytopenia (91%), leukocytosis (20%), thrombocytosis (5%) and elevated erythrocyte sedimentation rate (15%) are the abnormal laboratory findings [41]. Anemia and thrombocytopenia are detected in 75% to 81% and 14% to 55% of reported cases, respectively.

Primary splenic angiosarcomas are very aggressive neoplasms, with a median survival of 5 months irrespective of treatment. High and early prevalence of metastasis (in 69–100% of cases) has been reported and most often involves the liver (89%), lung (78%), lymph nodes (56%), and bone (44%).

Biopsy is contraindicated in splenic angiosarcoma because of the high risk of rupture. Therefore, histological studies can be made only after splenectomy. The differential diagnosis should include lymphoma, metastatic tumors, and other splenic vascular lesions such as hemangioma. Differentiation between angiosarcoma and these tumors is difficult for radiologists because of overlapping imaging findings. Therefore, a definitive diagnosis can be made only by histopathologic examinations after splenectomy.

Lymphangiomas are usually benign endothelium-lined cysts that may become symptomatic by causing splenomegaly. Splenectomy should be considered for symptomatic splenomegaly or an uncertain diagnosis.

11.7 Metastatic Tumors of the Spleen

In the literature, the frequency of splenic metastases is documented inconsistently. The spleen is a site of metastatic tumors in ≤7% of autopsies of cancer patients but the prevalence ranges from 0% to 34%. These data originate mainly from autopsy studies between 1920 and 1965 [42]. Primary solid tumors that most frequently metastasize to the spleen are carcinomas of the lung, melanoma and breast, accounting for 24.6%, 15.8%, and 12.3% of all spleen metastases respectively, but also ovarian, endometrial, gastric, colonic, and prostate [43]. However, virtually any primary malignancy may metastasize to the spleen. The involvement of the spleen may be a function of the immunologic role of the spleen and its ability to eliminate microscopic metastatic disease.

Different hypotheses describe the rarity of the splenic metastases compared with the metastases rate of other organs. The preferred hypotheses are based on the differences between the lymphatic system, the vessels of the spleen and the rest of the body. Other hypotheses are based on the immune function of the spleen or resistance against metastases. However, it seems clear that the non-gastrointestinal-originating tumors metastasize just as often into the spleen than in other organs, and the reason for the smaller number of metastases could be that the spleen is examined only selectively during autopsy [44]. In fact, if there is a generalized tumor growth, then the spleen is one of the three most frequent sites of metastases [45].

Metastases to the spleen are often asymptomatic but may be associated with symptomatic splenomegaly or even spontaneous splenic rupture, and usually can be a manifestation of disseminated disease and an indicator of a poor prognosis. Splenectomy may provide effective palliation in carefully selected symptomatic patients with splenic metastasis. Splenectomy is acceptable if a thorough workup reveals solitary splenic metastases and the primary tumor is controlled. Splenectomy can also be justified in conjunction with an abdominal debulking procedure for ovarian carcinoma.

References

1. Johnston GB (1908) Splenectomy. Ann Surg 48:50
2. Moynihan B (1920) The surgery of the spleen. Br J Surg 8:307
3. Delaitre B, Maignien B (1991) Splenectomie par voie laparoscopique, 1 observation. Presse Med 20:2263
4. Goerg C, Schwerk WB, Goerg K, Havemann K (1990) Sonographic patterns of the affected spleen in malignant lymphoma. J Clin Ultrasound 18:569-74
5. Poulin EC, Thibault C (1993) The anatomical basis for laparoscopic splenectomy. Can J Surg 36:484
6. Akwari OE, Itani KMF, Coleman RE, Rosse WF (1987) Splenectomy for primary and recurrent immune thrombocytopenic purpura (ITP): current criteria for patient selection and results. Ann Surg; 206:529-541
7. Gigot J-F, Jamar F, Ferrant A et al (1998) Inadequate detection of accessory spleens and splenosis with laparoscopic splenectomy: a shortcoming of the laparoscopic approach in hematologic diseases. Surg Endosc 12:101-106
8. Stanek A, Stefaniak T, Makarewicz W et al (2005) Accessory spleens: preoperative diagnostics limitations and operational strategy in laparoscopic approach to splenectomy in idiopathic thrombocytopenic purpura patients. Langenbecks Arch Surg 390:47-51
9. Baronofsky ID, Walton W, Noble JF (1951) Occult injury to the pancreas following splenectomy. Surgery 29:852-856
10. Michels NA (1942) The variational anatomy of the spleen and splenic artery. Am J Anat 70:21
11. Mebius RE, Kraal G (2005) Structure and function of the spleen. Nat Rev Immunol 5:606-16
12. Foster PN, Bolton RP, Cotter KL et al (1985) Defective activation of neutrophils after splenectomy. J Clin Pathol 38:1175–1178
13. Casaccia M, Torelli P, Pasa A, Sormani MP, Rossi E; IRLSS Centers (2010) Putative predictive parameters for the outcome of laparoscopic splenectomy: a multicenter analysis performed on the Italian Registry of Laparoscopic Surgery of the Spleen. Ann Surg 25:287-91
14. Park A, Targarona EM et al (2001) Laparoscopic surgery of the spleen: state of the art. Langenbecks Arch Surg 386:230-9
15. Weiss CA, Kavic SM, Adrales GL et al (2005) Laparoscopic splenectomy: What barriers remain? Surg Innov 12:23
16. Altaf AM, Ellsmere J, Jaap Bonjer H et al (2012) Morbidity of hand-assisted laparoscopic splenectomy compared to conventional laparoscopic splenectomy: a 6-year review. Can J Surg 55:227-32
17. Maartense S, Bemelman WA, Gerritsen van der Hoop A, Meijer DW, Gouma DJ (2004) Hand-assisted laparoscopic surgery (HALS): a report of 150 procedures. Surg Endosc 18:397-401
18. Lindgren PG, Hagberg H, Eriksson B, Glimelius B, Magnusson A, Sundström C (1985) Excision biopsy of the spleen by ultrasonic guidance. Br J Radiol 58:853–857
19. Tam A, Krishnamurthy S, Pillsbury EP et al (2008) Percutaneous image-guided splenic biopsy in the oncology patient: an audit of 156 consecutive cases. J Vasc Interv Radiol 19: 80 – 87
20. Gómez-Rubio M, López-Cano A, Rendón P, et al (2009) Safety and diagnostic accuracy of percutaneous ultrasound-guided biopsy of the spleen: a multicenter study. J Clin Ultrasound 37:445–450
21. McInnes MD, Kielar AZ, Macdonald DB (2011) Percutaneous image-guided biopsy of the spleen: systematic review and meta-analysis of the complication rate and diagnostic accuracy. Radiology 260:699-708
22. Wu Z, Zhou J, Pankaj P, Peng B (2012) Comparative treatment and literature review for laparoscopic splenectomy alone versus preoperative splenic artery embolization splenectomy. Surg Endosc 26:2758-66

23. Reso A, Brar MS, Church N, Mitchell P, Dixon E, Debru E (2010) Outcome of laparoscopic splenectomy with preoperative splenic artery embolization for massive splenomegaly. Surg Endosc 24:2008-12
24. Naoum JJ, Silberfein EJ, Zhou W et al (2007) Concomitant intraoperative splenic artery embolization and laparoscopic splenectomy versus laparoscopic splenectomy: Comparison of treatment outcome. Am J Surg 193:713
25. Madoff DC, Denys A, Wallace MJ et al (2005) Splenic arterial interventions: anatomy, indications, technical considerations, and potential complications. Radiographics 25 Suppl 1:S191-211
26. Baccarani U, Terrosu G, Donini A et al (1999) Splenectomy in hematology. Current practice and new perspectives. Haematologica 84:431-6
27. Katkhouda N, Hurwitz MG, Rivera RT et al (1998) Laparoscopic splenectomy: Outcome and efficacy in 103 consecutive patients. Ann Surg 228:1
28. Winslow GA, Nelson EW (1995) Thrombotic thrombocytopenic purpura: Indications for results of splenectomy. Am J Surg 170:558
29. Schwartz SI (1996) Role of splenectomy in hematologic disorders. World J Surg 20:1156
30. Casaccia M, Torelli P, Cavaliere D et al (2007) Laparoscopic lymph node biopsy in intra-abdominal lymphoma: High diagnostic accuracy achieved with a minimally invasive procedure. Surg Laparosc Endosc Percutan Tech 17:175
31. Taylor MA, Kaplan HS, Nelsen TS (1985) Staging laparotomy with splenectomy for Hodgkin's disease: The Stanford experience. World J Surg 9:449–460
32. Brodsky J, Abcar A, Styler M (1996) Splenectomy for non-Hodgkin's lymphoma. Am J Clin Oncol 19:558–561
33. Morel P, Dupriez B, Gosselin B, et al. (1993) Role of early splenectomy in malignant lymphomas with prominent splenic involvement (primary lymphomas of the spleen): A study of 59 cases. Cancer 71:207–215
34. http://www.nccn.org
35. Golomb HM, Vardiman JW (1983) Response to splenectomy in 65 patients with hairy cell leukemia: An evaluation of spleen weight and bone marrow involvement. Blood 61:349
36. Cusack JC Jr, Seymour JF, Lerner S et al (1997) Role of splenectomy in chronic lymphocytic leukemia. J Am Coll Surg 185:237–243
37. Mesa RA, Nagorney DS, Schwager S et al (2006) Palliative goals, patient selection, and perioperative platelet management: Outcomes and lessons from three decades of splenectomy for myelofibrosis with myeloid metaplasia at the Mayo Clinic. Cancer 107:361
38. Rupolo M, Berretta M, Buonadonna A, et al. (2001) Metastatic angiosarcoma of the spleen. A case report and treatment approach. Tumori 87:439-43
39. Hsu JT, Chen HM, Lin CY et al (2005) Primary angiosarcoma of the spleen. J Surg Oncol 92:312-6
40. Neuhauser TS, Derringer GA, Thompson LD et al (2000) Splenic angiosarcoma: a clinicopathologic and immunophenotypic study of 28 cases. Mod Pathol 13:978-87
41. Falk S, Krishnan J, Meis JM (1993) Primary angiosarcoma of the spleen. A clinicopathologic study of 40 cases. Am J Surg Pathol 17:959-70
42. Morgenstern L, Rosenberg J, Geller SA (1985) Tumors of the spleen. World J Surg 9:468-476
43. Schön CA, Görg C, Ramaswamy A, Barth PJ (2006) Splenic metastases in a large unselected autopsy series. Pathol Res Pract 202:351-6
44. Sauer J, Sobolewski K, Dommisch K (2009) Splenic metastases--not a frequent problem, but an underestimate location of metastases: epidemiology and course. J Cancer Res Clin Oncol 135:667-71
45. Harman JW, Dacorso P (1948) Spread of carcinoma to the spleen. Arch Pathol 45:179–186

What's New in Surgery for Kidney Cancer?

12

Marco Carini, Sergio Serni, Alberto Lapini and Andrea Minervini

12.1 Introduction

Based on the GLOBOCAN 2008 estimates published in 2011, >110.000 new cases of kidney cancer were expected in 2011, which account for ≈43.000 deaths among men from "developed" countries [1]. Due to increased utilization of diagnostic imaging for evaluation of patients with abdominal symptoms, incidentally discovered small renal masses (SRMs) are being diagnosed with greater frequency. Stage-T1 renal tumors (i.e., organ-confined and ≤7 cm in diameter) account for >60% of cases. Over the last three decades, stage migration has been observed, with an overall decreasing size at diagnosis of stage-1 renal cell carcinoma (RCC) [2].

12.2 Cytogenetics of Kidney Cancer

Understanding of RCC is evolving continuously, and cytogenetics promises to provide valuable tools for defining tumor biology to predict recurrence or response to therapy. Conventional renal cell carcinoma (ccRCC) carries a higher prevalence (75–80%) than other types, and occurs in sporadic and familial varieties (VHL syndrome).

It has been confirmed that sporadic and VHL-disease ccRCC tumors have similar molecular profiles, but sporadic tumors are more heterogenous and contain more events per tumor [3]. The biology of the VHL gene product (pVHL) and its regulation of the hypoxia-inducible factor (HIF) family (and consequently of some dynamically regulated transcription factors) are indelibly

M. Carini (✉) · S. Serni · A. Lapini · A. Minervini
Department of Oncology, Urology Clinic I
Careggi Hospital, Florence, Italy
e-mail: carini@unifi.it

A. Valeri et al. (eds.), *What's New in Surgical Oncology*,
DOI: 10.1007/978-88-470-5310-6_12, © Springer-Verlag Italia 2013

linked to ccRCC biology. In sporadic and familial forms, the molecular pathogenesis is due to mutations inactivating the tumor onco-suppressor gene VHL, which is responsible for the ubiquitination of HIF-1α and 2α. This process is sensitive to oxygen concentrations in tissues. In the presence of hypoxia or VHL-inactivating mutations, HIF-1α and 2α accumulate and dimerize with HIF-1β and 2β, and then bind to hypoxia-responsive elements (HREs) to regulate the survival, angiogenesis and metabolism of cells. If VHL is inactivated and HIF expression thereby stabilized, various other genes are transcriptionally upregulated: transforming growth factor α (TGF-α), vascular endothelial growth factor (VEGF), platelet-derived growth factor β (PDGF-β), stromal cell-derived factor (SDF-1), chemokine C-X-C motif ligand 12 (CXCL12), the chemokine receptor (CXCR4), and carbonic anhydrase IX and XII.

One HIF target, VEGF, has been found to be highly upregulated in kidney tumors [4]. This factor contributes to the highly vascular nature of this tumor, acting as a mitogen for endothelial cells. However, the effect on HIF deregulation is not uniform. Variant mutations in VHL may contribute to imbalances of the deregulation of HIF1α and HIF2α, leading to different effects on cell growth [5]. RCC can be characterized as H1H2 (expressing HIF1α and HIF2α) or H2 (expressing only HIF2α), with dramatically differing effects on the metabolism of tumor cells. Recent evidence suggests that H2 tumors may lose expression of HIF1α as a result of nonsense missense mutations in a subset of tumors [6]. This finding suggests a potentially selective pressure to lose the HIF1α gene during tumor progression.

Mammalian target of rapamycin (mTOR) is a serine/threonine protein kinase that regulates the growth, proliferation, motility, survival, protein synthesis, and transcription of cells. Its interaction with other proteins forms mTORC1 and 2 complexes, which are responsible for the production of HIF1-α and the control of protein synthesis. The mTOR signaling pathway is frequently overactive in RCC and an important prognostic factor.

With regard to ccRCC, the largest study on the prognostic role of molecular markers was recently reported at the University of California at Los Angeles. The authors tested the expression of 29 markers related mainly to the hypoxia-inducible and mTOR pathways in the surgical specimens of 170 patients with clinically localized RCC undergoing nephrectomy. The authors showed that expression of Ki-67, p53, endothelial VEGFR-1, epithelial VEGFR-1, and epithelial VEGFR-D were independent predictors of disease-free survival (DFS) once adjustment for the effects of standard clinical and pathologic variables (Eastern Cooperative Oncology Group (ECOG) performance status, pathologic stage of the primary tumor, and nuclear grade) was carried out. Interestingly, a nomogram that included molecular, clinical, and pathologic factors to predict DFS was generated; this nomogram yielded a prognostic accuracy of 90% [7]. It has been demonstrated that loss of 3p is significantly associated with increased DFS, whereas loss of 4p, 9p, and 14q are significantly associated with decreased DFS. Only loss of 9p is an independent predictor of survival upon adjustment for standard clinical and pathologic variables.

Papillary RCC (incidence among RCCs 10–15%) also occurs in sporadic or familial variety. In type 1, mutations activate the MET oncogene, whereas in type 2 mutations inactivate the tumor onco-suppressor fumarate hydratase (FH). Chromophobe RCC (incidence among RCCs, 4–6%) has a better prognosis. The molecular mechanisms involved are virtually unknown, but mutations of the Birt–Hogg–Dube tumor suppressor gene FLCN have been identified.

12.3 Nephron-sparing Surgery (NSS)

12.3.1 Functional and Oncological Results

The increased diagnosis of small intracapsular renal tumors has led to a concurrent rise in the rates of surgical intervention and to an augmented interest in the various methods of NSS. At the end of the twentieth century, NSS evolved from an uncommon procedure to the current standard of care for two main reasons [8].

Firstly, radical nephrectomy (RN) has been considered to be the standard for treatment of renal tumors for many decades, whereas NSS was limited to imperative indications. Since the mid-1990s, several studies compared the oncological result of open conservative surgery to those of RN for treating SRMs. They reported similar oncological results, and recent studies on large series confirmed the oncological equivalence of these two procedures [9–10]. Data on 3,480 patients from the Surveillance and Treatment Update on Renal Neoplasms (SATURN) database displayed no significant difference in cancer-specific survival (CSS) and recurrence-free survival between patients with clinical stage T1 RCC treated with NSS or RN, thereby strongly supporting NSS [10]. One drawback of NSS is the risk of positive surgical margins (PSMs) that have been reported in 0–7% of cases. However, whether or not PSM can influence recurrence-free and CSS is controversial, and indeed active surveillance is the recommended treatment for PSMs [8].

Secondly, in recent years, renal preservation has been progressively prioritized because ≈26% of patients have impaired renal function before undergoing NSS or RN. RN is a recognized independent risk factor in the development of chronic kidney disease postoperatively, cardiovascular events and overall mortality [11]. Weight et al. reviewed the data of patients with clinical T1b renal masses undergoing NSS (524 patients) or RN (480 patients). Those patients undergoing RN lost significantly more renal function than those undergoing NSS. The average excess loss of renal function observed with RN was associated with a 25% (95% confidence interval (CI), 3–73) increased risk of cardiac death and 17% (95% CI, 12–27) increased risk of death from any cause upon multivariate analyses [12].

Besides the advantages of NSS mentioned above, the surgical risk related with conservative surgery of the kidney as compared with RN should also be considered, in particular in terms of hemorrhage, as shown by the only randomized study comparing the two procedures [13].

For the purpose of improving haemostasis during NSS, several haemostatic agents (HAs) that can enhance physiologic coagulation mechanisms have been used. Even though such agents have been widely adopted in urology and seem to protect against postoperative bleeding [14], publications on their results during NSS are limited.

12.3.2 Warm Ischemia Time (WIT) and Renal Damage

In addition to oncologic and surgical outcome, postoperative renal function is a central issue in NSS. If ischemia is required, the tumor should be removed within the minimum possible duration. At which point does WIT cause permanent renal damage during partial nephrectomy? Several studies have attempted to establish the cutoff time point beyond which ischemia can lead to irreversible damage of the renal parenchyma: this value is 20–30 min [8]. In a recent single-center series on 362 patients with RCC in a solitary kidney evaluating short- and long-term renal effects, for each 1 min of increase in the WIT, there was a 5% increase in the risk of postoperative acute renal failure (ARF). Moreover, evaluating warm ischemia in 5-min increments, a cutoff of 25 min provided the best stratification of risk of developing ARF, or an acute glomerular filtration rate (GFR) <15 mL/min or new-onset stage-IV chronic kidney disease in the postoperative period [15]. Therefore, two key messages can be extrapolated from this study. Firstly, every minute is important and great effort should be mad to reduce the WIT as much as possible. Secondly, a cutoff value of 25 min seems to be the best stratification value to discriminate between the onset of acute and chronic renal damage and its avoidance.

12.3.3 Indications for NSS

The indications for NSS can be:

- Absolute/Imperative: anatomical or functional solitary kidney;
- Relative: the functioning opposite kidney is affected by a condition that might impair renal function in the future; relative indications include hereditary forms of RCC (which carry a high risk of developing a tumor in the contralateral kidney);
- Elective: localized unilateral RCC with a healthy contralateral kidney.

NSS is an attractive option for the elective treatment of SRMs. According to the most recent European guidelines on kidney cancer, NSS should be undertaken if technically feasible in the case of intracapsular RCC ≤7 cm in greatest diameter (T1a/b stage). Nevertheless, they are few consistent data concerning the oncologic outcomes of clinical T1b >5 cm treated with NSS, whereas the decision about the feasibility and oncologic safety of NSS in clinical T2a tumors is pending [8].

12.3.4 Open, Laparoscopic and Robotic NSS

Due to its wide use, open NSS remains the cornerstone of the management of SRMs. Nevertheless, due to its highly invasive nature, it is associated with postoperative pain, scarring, longer hospitalization and a slower return to ordinary activities. In the future, fewer NSS procedures will be approached in an open fashion.

First described by Winfield et al. in 1993, Laparoscopic nephron-sparing surgery (LNSS) duplicates the principles of open surgery and, with several technical variations, has been standardized [16]. LNSS is a viable treatment offering outcomes comparable with open surgery with reduced intraoperative and postoperative morbidity [17–18]. Proponents of LNSS cite the similar results to open surgery. Nevertheless, it continues to be carried out in a minority of centers due to its steep learning curve. It is technically demanding for the limited variation of the degree of incidence with the target structures in the extirpative and reconstructive steps of the procedure [17–19]. Indeed, LNSS can offer the advantages of reduced blood loss and shorter hospital stay with similar oncologic outcomes when compared with open NSS [18]. However, in some retrospective observational studies, LNSS has been associated with longer ischemia time, more postoperative complications (particularly urological) and an increased number of subsequent procedures [20].

First reported in 2004 by Gettman et al., [21], robot-assisted-NSS (also called robot-assisted partial nephrectomy (RAPN)) using the da Vinci Surgical System™ represents an alternative procedure to LNSS and open NSS for the treatment of intracapsular RCCs, and has steadily gained acceptance [22]. In recent years, several studies have compared the perioperative results of RAPN and LNSS, and evidence suggests that RAPN can reproduce the advantages of minimal invasiveness with a shorter learning curve because it entails excellent perioperative outcomes after about 30 cases [23]. Recent studies have also shown that RAPN can be utilized effectively for the treatment of larger renal tumors (>4 cm in diameter) and parahilar lesions [24]. Ideally, every surgical option for the conservative treatment of renal tumors should be compared with open NSS, i.e., matching the standard of treatment and robustness of data with respect to surgical and oncological results. Only one prospectively derived comparative study of perioperative outcomes of RAPN *vs* open NSS has been published: Simhan and colleagues showed that RAPN offered comparable perioperative and functional outcomes (including the WIT and change in estimated glomerular filtration rate (eGFR)) with decreased hospitalization [25].

12.3.5 Standard Partial Nephrectomy vs. Simple Enucleation (SE)

The treatment of SRMs represents an area of increasing interest and controversy that is also driven by the trend towards narrowing of the recommended surgical margins. Several studies have been published recently on the amount of normal tissue that should be excised with the tumor to avoid the risk of local recurrence. These studies concluded that, if the tumor is completely excised, the width of the resection margin is not relevant and not correlated with disease progression [26]. Guidelines set by the European Association of Urology (EAU) recommend a minimal tumor-free surgical margin of healthy renal tissue surrounding the resected tumor without specifying the exact minimum thickness of the healthy parenchyma to be removed [8].

NSS can be undertaken as standard partial nephrectomy defined as excision of the tumor and an additional margin of healthy peritumor renal parenchyma or as SE (i.e., a tumorectomy done by blunt dissection using the natural cleavage plane between the tumor and normal parenchyma without ablation of the tumor bed) [27]. In recent years, considerable data have emerged demonstrating the good oncological, functional and perioperative outcomes of SE [27–29] and some reports have shown a reduced incidence of PSM by adopting SE. This is probably because SE provides constant visual detection of the correct cleavage plane, whereas the sharp excision in the case of standard PN can mislead the surgeon (especially in the case of endophytic tumors). In the large multicenter series from the SATURN-LUNA project involving >1,500 patients, the prevalence of PSM was 3.4% and 0.2% after conventional PN and SE, respectively [27]. However, only prospective randomized studies will be able to shed light on this dualism.

12.3.6 Complications of NSS

The complication rates observed with NSS are slightly higher (but very tolerable) when compared with RN (level of evidence, 1b) [8, 13]. Results focusing on morbidity are extremely variable and the overall complication rate after NSS ranges between 4% and 37% [30].

Several predicting factors for postoperative complications have been reported in the literature, the most relevant are: imperative indication for NSS; tumor stage ≥T1b (maximal tumor dimension >4 cm); perihilar localization of the tumor; length of WIT (>20 minutes); endophytic tumor growth; and involvement of the collecting system [30]. Pasticier et al. retrospectively reported a prevalence of 30.7% (including 18.1% minor and 12.6% major adverse events) with a mean hospital stay of14.1 days [31]. However, the indications for surgery were imperative in 42% of patients, and this variable was the most relevant risk factor for complications. Other reseachers have reported a lower morbidity rate after standard NSS. Thompson et al. retrospectively reported an overall complication rate of 9.6% [30]. Among postoperative complications, bleeding, acute renal failure (ARF) and urinary fistulas are the most frequent, and deserve further discussion.

Acute or delayed postoperative hemorrhage occurs in ≈1.3–7.9% of patients, as described in different series [31]. Percutaneous super-selective embolization of the feeding arteries contributing to the bleeding site is preferred to open surgery, which often results in nephrectomy.

ARF has been reported in 1.3–12.7% of patients and is obviously increased in patients with imperative indications for surgery. The WIT and quantity of remnant healthy parenchyma are the only modifiable variables that can reduce the deterioration in renal function after NSS. To shorten the WIT, extracorporeal "on-demand" clamping and early unclamping as well as methods to facilitate the reconstructive phase (e.g., sliding clip renorrhaphy with Hem-O-Lok™ ligation clips) have been developed. Furthermore, super-selective clamping of the renal artery and clamp-less methods to have a zero-ischemia partial nephrectomy have been described, and are beginning to be the standard of treatment in several centers. However, although the WIT has been strongly associated with ARF, its correlation with chronic renal damage is controversial because other factors (e.g., width of healthy tissue removed with the tumor, the method of renorrhaphy or the hemostatic energy applied on the surgical bed) may play a part in its development. More detailed biomolecular and imaging tools are needed to assess the real renal damage after this type of surgery.

Urinary leakage is one of the most common early complications, occurring in 1.4–17.4% of patients [31]. Pasticier et al. reported urinary fistula in 10.1% of patients, Duque et al. in 9.1%, and Campbell et al. in 17.4% [31]. Not surprisingly, the factors most associated with urine leakage are tumor size, endophytic tumor growth, and tumor resection requiring repair of the collecting system [31]. Most of the urinary fistulas recover spontaneously after several days of drain manipulation but, sometimes, can require endoscopic procedures such as placement of a ureteric stent or percutaneous drainage if urinoma develops. Positioning a ureteral stent probably allows: (i) a pathway of least resistance for urine to drain, and (ii) the reconstructed collecting system to heal.

Recent advances in correct reporting of complications after the surgical treatment of kidney cancer include the Charlson and age-adjusted Charlson Comorbidity Index for precise and standardized comorbidity reports as well as grading of medical and surgical complications according to an established modification of the original Clavien system (a reliable and validated tool for the reporting of complications) [32, 33]. Moreover, two nephrometric scores have been validated: PADUA and RENAL nephrometric scores [34, 35].

The PADUA score is based on seven critical and reproducible anatomical features of solid renal masses. Of the seven components, six (i.e., longitudinal (polar) location; exophytic rate; renal rim; involvement of the renal sinus; involvement of the urinary collecting system; and tumor size (cm)) are scored on a one-, two- or three-point scale with the seventh feature indicating the anterior or posterior location of the mass relative to the coronal plane of the kidney.

The RENAL score is based on the five critical and reproducible anatomical features of solid renal masses. Of the five components, four are scored on a one-, two- or three-point scale (i.e., maximal diameter (cm); exophytic properties; proximity of the tumor to the collecting system or sinus (mm); and location relative to the polar lines) with the fifth feature indicating the anterior or posterior location of the mass relative to the coronal plane of the kidney.

These nephrometric scores have been used widely in recent studies with the aim to improve scientific accuracy. These scores are based on a simple anatomical system that can be used to predict the risk of surgical and medical perioperative complications in patients undergoing NSS. The use of an appropriate score can help clinicians stratify patients suitable for NSS into subgroups with different risks of complications. Moreover, they can help researchers evaluate the true comparability among patients undergoing NSS with different surgical approaches.

12.3.7 New Intraoperative Tools for NSS

Increasingly refined methods, instruments and probes are becoming available to help surgeons identify the correct margins during NSS. These include intraoperative ultrasound and near-infrared fluorescence (NIRF) of intravenously injected indocyanine green (ICG). Apart from the information obtained by preoperative imaging, intraoperative ultrasonography is the primary method for the identification of complex or intraparenchymal renal masses. Intraoperative ultrasonography with Doppler evaluation of vascular anatomy and the collecting system can be used to accurately locate the tumor and its burdens.

During RAPN, the ultrasound probe is controlled by the assistant rather than the surgeon. Use of a newly available robotic ultrasound probe that has a grooved ridge on its ventral aspect that fits robotic grasping instruments allows the surgeon to optimize tumor identification with maximal autonomy, and to benefit from the precision and articulation of the robotic instrument during this key step of partial nephrectomy [36].

Intraoperative imaging of ICG with NIRF is a new method that aims to accurately identify the renal vasculature and to differentiate renal tumors from surrounding normal parenchyma. ICG is a fluorescent tricarbocyanine dye that absorbs and emits light in the near-infrared region of the electromagnetic spectrum. If injected intravenously, ICG interacts with blood components, producing a large increase in the quantum efficiency of fluorescence. ICG binds to albumin and lipoproteins, so it remains predominantly intravascular until hepatobiliary excretion. NIRF imaging after ICG administration permits excellent definition of the vascular system, and has been used in several other surgical specialties as a method of fluorescent angiography.

12.4 Ablative Treatments

New minimally invasive ablative percutaneous procedures such as cryotherapy, radiofrequency ablation (RFA) and high-intensity focused ultrasound (HIFU) represent another area of research by many urological and radiological centers, and might be an alternative to surgery for selected patients and tumors [37].

According to the EAU 2010 guidelines, ablative therapies should be offered to elderly patients with small, incidentally found, renal cortical lesions. Due to the lack of adequate oncological follow-up and several drawbacks (e.g., accuracy of pre- and post-ablation biopsy, need for frequent imaging, and the high rate of benign disease in SRM), ablative methods are reserved for patients unfit for surgery [8].

Of the available ablative methods, RFA and cryoablation are the most intensively investigated approaches in terms of practicality, complication rate and oncological safety. In a recent study on computed tomography (CT)-guided RFA for single, biopsy-proven (T1a and T1b) RCC with follow-up of ≤10 years, RFA was shown to be highly efficient for managing T1a RCC. In this group, the authors reported 5- and 10-year recurrence-free survival as high as 96% and 93%, respectively [37]. The 5-year DFS and CSS were 91% and 100%, respectively [37]. The outcomes of RFA in T1b tumors was less spectacular, with 5-year DFS of 74%, suggesting that RFA in tumors >4 cm should be considered only in infirm patients [37]. Similar findings in T1a tumors were reported by Olweny et al. [38].

Data regarding cryoablation are not mature, but early results seem promising. Cryoablation seems to have a lower rate of re-ablation and local recurrence as well as good intermediate oncological outcomes in comparison with RFA [39].

Clearly, further prospective ideally, multi-institutional studies are needed to enable widespread use of these ablative procedures. Undoubtedly methods as well as devices should be standardized, and this is especially true for RFA. Moreover, better definitions of the success and failure of treatments are necessary because radiologic criteria vary between studies and might be inconsistent. Comparative studies should be done to assess if these approaches can be alternatives to partial nephrectomy.

12.5 Role of Surgical Treatment for Metastatic and Locally Advanced Kidney Cancer

Surgery represents a crucial therapeutic tool also for the treatment of metastatic kidney cancer. The role has evolved over time. It began with reports about the spontaneous regression of metastases after removal of the primary tumor, and continued with other experiences that led it to become the cornerstone of the current multidisciplinary approach.

Two randomized studies based on cytokine research and surgery (SWOG-8949 and EORTC-30947) compared the oncological outcomes of cytoreductive nephrectomy plus immunotherapy *vs* immunotherapy alone in patients with metastatic RCC: higher long-term survival was found in patients who underwent surgery [40, 41]. Today, even if matching comparative studies using molecular targeted therapies (TTs) are not available, cytoreductive nephrectomy remains the "gold standard" treatment in these settings [8]. Some authors suggest that, in metastatic RCC, TT is so much more effective than cytokines that the need for surgery could be questioned. The CARMENA trial is ongoing to evaluate the role of cytoreductive nephrectomy in the TT era, but the non-randomized studies completed so far have shown a limited effect of TT on the primary lesion [42] (Table 12.1).

Current studies are oriented more towards the potential role of the neoadjuvant effect of TTs (NCT01099423-SURTIME) because it could have potential benefits such as:

- Tumor downsizing to facilitate tumor removal;
- More rapid initiation of therapy that may translate into decreased cancer-related morbidity;
- Evaluation of tumor susceptibility to select only patients that respond to surgery [43].

Some aspects of neaoadjuvant therapy have been questioned, as discussed below.

12.5.1 Effect on Primary Tumor

Several studies have shown volume modifications of the primary lesion after TT (Table 12.2). After 8 weeks of therapy, Jonasch et al. reported a reduction of the size of primary lesions of between 10% and 30% using RECIST criteria in 23% of patients [44]. It is questionable whether RECIST criteria are suitably accurate for the evaluation of TT results because they consider only the dimensional reduction of the mass and not the increase of its necrotic component and other imaging signs of tissue modifications. Indeed, many lesions greatly increase the content of necrosis after TT, which does not always corre-

Table 12.1 Tumor measurements after initiating sunitinib treatment

Patient number	RECIST					PFS (months)	Survival (months)
	SLTS (%)	Primary (%)	Metastates (%)	Overall (%)	Overall		
1	-9	-9	4	-1	SD	10	18+
2	–	–	–	–	–	1	2
3	–18	–18	–56	–32	PR	10	15
4	–11	–11	–45	–32	PR	14	15+
5	46	10	77	41	PD	0.02	4
6	–20	–20	–100	–29	SD	10	14+
7	–16	7	–16	–10	SD	6	14
8	–12	–12	–28	–17	SD	15	22
9	11	11	50	18	SD	1	4
10	13	-1	11	4	SD	4	15+

Table 12.2 Volume modifications of primary lesions after targeted therapies reported in the literature

Author	Number of cases	Drug	Percentage of patients with downsizing of primary tumor	Mean reduction (range) of primary tumor
Amin et al. [45]	9	Suni/Sora	90	12% (1–54%)
van der Veldt et al. [48]	17	Sunitinib	76	12%
Cowey et al. [46]	30*	Sorafenib	82	13% (1–40%)
Thomas et al. [47]	19	Sunitinib	53	9% (0–24%)
Bex et al. [42]	10	Sunitinib	60	14%
Jonasch et al. [44]	50	Beva/Beva+ Erl	52	<10% (1–30%)

late with a reduction in volume of the tumor. Conversely, in many cases we observe increases in their volume.

Beyond tissue modifications, a minimal reduction in volume is not useful from a surgical perspective. Frequently, in metastatic RCC, the primary tumor is >10 cm and a reduction of 10% of the volume does not simplify the procedure significantly. Recently, Kroon et al. investigated the correlation between tumor size and downsizing after TT therapy. Median downsizing in tumors of diameter 7–10 cm, 5–7 cm, <5 cm were 14%, 11% and 34%, respectively. Hence, small primary lesions showed increased susceptibility to TT in terms of downsizing [45]. These results are in agreement with the potential application of TT before elective NSS, which aims to simplify the procedure and reduce complications, as suggested by Ficarra et al.

Sometimes, the clinical scenario in metastatic kidney cancer is characterized by minimal metastatic disease associated with retroperitoneal bulky disease due to a large primary tumor with extension to an adjacent organ and/or with an associated confluent nodal mass involving the great vessels [47]. In these cases, which are defined as "surgery-limiting tumor sites (SLTSs)", effective preoperative therapy can allow complete tumor removal with an acceptable risk of complications. Unfortunately, experiences with SLTSs shows good results at metastatic sites but poor results against primary complex tumors [42].

12.5.2 Effect on Caval Thrombus

A total of 4–10% of RCCs have thrombus in the inferior caval vein (IVC) and, in 1% of cases, the thrombus involves the right atrium. Up to 60% of these patients have also concurrent subclinical metastases [48]. Surgical patients N0M0 show a median overall survival of 51.7 months compared with 10.7 months for N+M0 and 6.9 months for NxM+ [49].

The risk of perioperative morbidity and mortality from RN and thrombectomy is related to the level of the thrombus. Whether the level of the thrombus (independent from pathologic stage) has an impact on survival is controversial. It is known, however, that higher-level tumor thrombi tend to be associated with a higher grade and a more advanced T stage.

Neoadjuvant systemic therapy can potentially decrease the burden of the tumor thrombus and thus improve the safety and feasibility of resection. Many case reports have been published stating this viewpoint with positive results. We also have positive experiences with preoperative TT in the presence of IVC thrombi, but large cohorts (>25 cases) are present in few publications. Cost et al. did not report exciting results: 1 patient (4%) had an increase in the thrombus level (level II to level III), 21 (84%) had stable thrombi and, in 3 (12%), the thrombus level was decreased. Hence, there was only 1 case (4%) in which the surgical approach was potentially affected by regression of the tumor thrombus (level IV to level III) [50].

12.5.3 Surgical Complications and Discontinuation of Drug Administration

Major and overall complications are not influenced by neaoadjuvant therapy; only surgical wound healing represents a real risk due to preoperative therapy [51]. To evaluate the most appropriate time for therapy discontinuation, we must consider the half-life of the drugs: temsirolimus, 17 h; sorafenib, 24–48 h; sunitinib, 60–110 h; bevacizumab, 14–21 days; and pazopanib, 30.9 h. To be sure, we advocate therapy discontinuation by a time ≥2/3-times the half life of the drug.

Before the conclusion of the SURTIME trial, we do not know whether the best initial therapeutic approach for metastatic RCC is surgery or molecular therapy. However, considering different aspects we can identify certain useful criteria to select patients for cytoreductive nephrectomy or for neoadjuvant therapy.

We consider the ideal candidates for surgery (as the first treatment) those patients with resectable primary tumor (no bulky disease or involvement of adjacent organs), no lung metastases and good performance status, and when surgery can remove >90% of tumor volume [52]. In the other cases, neoadjuvant treatment with TT is probably a more rational approach.

12.6 Conclusion

We are in a phase of rapid transition in which NSS is increasing its role over RN as experiences with conservative surgery and the efficacy of hemostatic agents increases and in which minimally invasive approaches such us laparoscopy, robotics and ablative procedures are advancing. In particular, RAPN represents a viable alternative to open NSS with the goal of decreasing postoperative pain and accelerating the return to normal activities. For the open procedure, extreme attention must be paid to limiting the WIT to 20–30 min.

Preoperative systemic therapy seems to be safe and feasible but the potential advantages must be tested rigorously. Until further data become available, caution should be exercised in applying this treatment for potentially curable and resectable disease.

References

1. Jemal A, Bray F, Center MM et al (2011) Global cancer statistics. CA Cancer J Clin 61:69-90
2. Cooperberg MR, Mallin K, Ritchey J et al (2008) Decreasing size at diagnosis of stage 1 renal cell carcinoma: analysis from the National Cancer Data Base, 1993 to 2004. J Urol 179:2131-2135
3. Beroukhim R, Brunet JP, Di Napoli A et al (2009) Patterns of gene expression and copy-number alterations in von-Hippel Lindau disease-associated and sporadic clear cell carcinoma of the kidney. Cancer Res 69:4674-4681
4. Edgren M, Lennernas B, Larsson A, Nilsson S (1999) Serum concentrations of VEGF and b-FGF in renal cell, prostate and urinary bladder carcinomas. Anticancer Res 19:869-873
5. Rathmell WK, Hickey MM, Bezman NA et al (2004) In vitro and in vivo models analyzing von Hippel-Lindau disease-specific mutations. Cancer Res 64:8595-8603
6. Dalgliesh GL, Furge K, Greenman C et al (2010) Systematic sequencing of renal carcinoma reveals inactivation of histone modifying genes. Nature 21 463:360-363
7. Klatte T, Seligson DB, LaRochelle J et al (2009) Molecular signatures of localized clear cell renal cell carcinoma to predict disease-free survival after nephrectomy. Cancer Epidemiol Biomarkers Prev 18:894–900
8. Ljungberg B, Cowan NC, Hanbury DC et al (2010) EAU guidelines on renal cell carcinoma: the 2010 update. Eur Urol 58:398–406
9. Patard JJ, Shvarts O, Lam JS et al (2004) Safety and efficacy of partial nephrectomy for all T1 tumors based on an international multicenter experience. J Urol 171:2181-2185
10. Antonelli A, Ficarra V, Bertini R et al (members of the SATURN Project – LUNA Foundation) (2012) Elective partial nephrectomy is equivalent to radical nephrectomy in patients with clinical T1 renal cell carcinoma: results of a retrospective, comparative, multi-institutional study. BJU Int 109:1013-1018
11. Huang WC, Levey AS, Serio AM et al (2006) Chronic kidney disease after nephrectomy in patients with renal cortical tumours: a retrospective cohort study. Lancet Oncol 7:735–740
12. Weight CJ, Larson BT, Fergany AF et al (2010) Nephrectomy induced chronic renal insufficiency is associated with increased risk of cardiovascular death and death from any cause in patients with localized cT1b renal masses. J Urol 183:1317-1323

13. Van Poppel H, Da Pozzo L, Albrecht W et al (2007) A prospective randimized EORTC intergroup phase 3 study comapring the complications of elective nephron-sparing surgery and radical nephrectomy for low-stage renal cell carcinoma. Eur Urol 51:1606-1615
14. Breda A, Stepanian SV, Lam JS et al (2007) Use of haemostatic agents and glues during laparoscopic partial nephrectomy: a multi-institutional survey from the United States and Europe of 1347 cases. Eur Urol 52:798-803
15. Thompson RH, Lane BR, Lohse CM et al (2010) Every minute counts when the renal hilum is clamped during partial nephrectomy. Eur Urol 58:340-345
16. Winfield HN, Donovan JF, Godet AS, Clayman RV (1993) Laparoscopic partial nephrectomy: initial case report for benign disease. J Endourol 7:521–526
17. Marszalek M, Meixl H, Polajnar M et al (2009) Laparoscopic and Open Partial Nephrectomy: A Matched-Pair Comparison of 200 Patients. Eur Urol 55:1171–1178
18. Porpiglia F, Volpe A, Billia M, Scarpa RM (2008) Laparoscopic versus open partial nephrectomy: analysis of the current literature. Eur Urol 53:732–743, discussion 742–743
19. Colli J, Sartor O, Grossman L, Lee BR (2012) Underutilization of partial nephrectomy for stage t1 renal cell carcinoma in the United States, trends from 2000 to 2008. A long way to go. Clin Genitourin Cancer 10:219-224
20. Gill IS, Kavoussi LR, Lane BR et al (2007) Comparison of 1,800 laparoscopic and open partial nephrectomies for single renal tumors. J Urol 178:41–46
21. Gettman MT, Blute ML, Chow GK et al (2004) Robotic-assisted laparoscopic partial nephrectomy: technique and initial clinical experience with DaVinci robotic system. Urology 64:914–918
22. Patel HD, Mullins JK, Pierorazio PM et al (2012) Trends in Renal Surgery: Robotic Technology Is Associated with Increased Use of Partial Nephrectomy. J Urol [Epub ahead of print] doi: 10.1016/j.juro.2012.10.024
23. Benway BM, Bhayani SB, Rogers C et al (2009) Robot assisted partial nephrectomy versus laparoscopic partial nephrectomy for renal tumors: a multi-institutional analysis of perioperative outcomes. J Urol 182:866-72
24. Patel MN, Krane LS, Bhandari A et al (2010) Robotic partial nephrectomy for renal tumors larger than 4 cm. Eur Urol 57:310–316
25. Simhan J, Smaldone MC, Tsai KJ et al (2012) Perioperative outcomes of robotic and open partial nephrectomy for moderately and highly complex renal lesions. J Urol 187:2000-2004
26. Castilla EA, Liou LS, Abrahams NA et al (2002) Prognostic importance of resection margin width after nephron-sparing surgery for renal cell carcinoma. Urology 60:993-997
27. Minervini A, Ficarra V, Rocco F et al (2011) Simple enucleation is equivalent to traditional partial nephrectomy for renal cell carcinoma: results of a nonrandomized, retrospective, comparative study. J Urol 185:1604-10
28. Laryngakis NA, Van Arsdalen KN, Guzzo TJ, Malkowicz SB (2011) Tumor enucleation: a safe treatment alternative for renal cell carcinoma. Expert Rev Anticancer Ther 11:893-9
29. Minervini A, Serni S, Tuccio A et al (2012) Simple enucleation versus radical nephrectomy in the treatment of pT1a and pT1b renal cell carcinoma. Ann Surg Oncol 19:694-700
30. Ficarra V, Porta C (2010) Il carcinoma renale. Basi per un moderno approccio multidisciplinare. Il Pensiero Scientifico Editore, Roma
31. Pomara G, Campo G, Francesca F (2009) Intraoperative and postoperative complications of nephron sparing surgery: Prevention and possible treatments. Arch Ital Urol Androl 81:93-98
32. Charlson M, Szatrowski TP, Peterson J, Gold J (1994) Validation of a combined comorbidity index. J Clin Epidemiol 47:1245-1251
33. Dindo D, Demartines N, Clavien PA (2004) Classification of surgical complications: a new proposal with evaluation in a cohort of 6336 patients and results of a survey. Ann Surg 240:205-13
34. Ficarra V, Novara G, Secco S, Macchi V (2009) Preoperative aspects and dimensions used for an anatomical (PADUA) classification of renal tumours in patients who are candidates for nephron-sparing surgery. Eur Urol; 56(5):786-93

35. Kutikov A and Uzzo RG (2009) The R.E.N.A.L. nephrometry score: a comprehensive standardized system for quantitating renal tumor size, location and depth. J Urol 182:844-853
36. Kaczmarek BF, Sukumar S, Petros F et al (2012) Robotic Ultrasound probe for tumor identification in robotic partial nephrectomy: Initials series and outcomes. Int J Urol [Epub ahead of print] doi: 10.1111/j.1442-2042.2012.03127.x
37. Psutka SP, Feldman AS, McDougal WS et al (2012) Long-Term Oncologic Outcomes After Radiofrequency Ablation for T1 Renal Cell Carcinoma. Eur Urol [Epub ahead of print] doi: 10.1016/j.eururo.2012.08.062
38. Olweny EO, Park SK, Tan YK et al (2012) Radiofrequency ablation versus partial nephrectomy in patients with solitary clinical T1a renal cell carcinoma: comparable oncologic outcomes at a minimum of 5 years of follow-up. Eur Urol 61:1156-61
39. Kunkle DA, Egleston BL, Uzzo RG (2008) Excise, ablate or observe: the small renal mass dilemma--a meta-analysis and review. J Urol 179:1227-33, discussion 1233-4
40. Flanigan RC, Salmon SE, Blumenstein BA et al (2001) Nephrectomy followed by interferon alfa-2b compared with interferon alfa-2b alone for metastatic renal-cell cancer. New Eng J Med 345:1655-9
41. Mickisch G H J, Garin A, Van Poppel H; de Prijck L; Sylvester R (2001) Radical nephrectomy plus interferon-alfa-based immunotherapy compared with interferon alfa alone in metastatic renal-cell carcinoma: a randomised trial. Lancet 358:966-70
42. Bex A, van der Veldt AA, Blank C et al (2009) Neoadjuvant sunitinib for surgically complex advanced renal cell cancer of doubtful resectability: initial experience with downsizing to reconsider cytoreductive surgery. World J Urol 27(4):533-9
43. Winquist E, Rodrigues G (2012) Open clinical uro-oncology trials in Canada. Can J Urol 19:6587-91
44. Jonasch E, Wood CG, Matin SF et al (2009) Phase II presurgical feasibility study of bevacizumab in untreated patients with metastatic renal cell carcinoma. J Clin Oncol 27:4076-81
45. Amin C, Wallen E, Pruthi RS et al (2008) Preoperative tyrosine kinase inhibition as an adjunct to debulking nephrectomy. Urology 72(4):864-8
46. Cowey CL, Fielding JR, Rathmell WK (2010) The loss of radiographic enhancement in primary renal cell carcinoma tumors following multitargeted receptor tyrosine kinase therapy is an additional indicator of response. Urology 75(5):1108-13
47. Thomas AA, Rini BI, Lane BR et al (2009) Response of the primary tumor to neoadjuvant sunitinib in patients with advanced renal cell carcinoma. J Urol 181(2):518-23; discussion 523
48. van der Veldt AA, Meijerink MR, van den Eertwegh AJ et al (2008) Sunitinib for treatment of advanced renal cell cancer: primary tumor response. Clin Cancer Res 14(8):2431-6
49. Kroon BK, De Bruin R, Prevoo W et al (2012) Primary tumor downsizing in renal cell carcinoma is more prominent in smaller tumors and may enable nephron sparing strategies Eur Urol Suppl 11:abs 78
50. Ficarra V, Novara G (2010) Kidney cancer: neoadjuvant targeted therapies in renal cell carcinoma. Nat Rev Urol 7:63-4
51. Bromwich E, Hendry D, Aitchison M (2002) Cytoreductive nephrectomy: is it a realistic option in patients with renal cancer? BJU Int 89(6):523-5
52. Klatte T, Pantuck AJ, Riggs SB et al (2007) Prognostic factors for renal cell carcinoma with tumor thrombus extension. J Urol 178:1189-95
53. Haferkamp A, Bastian PJ, Jakobi H et al (2007) Renal cell carcinoma with tumor thrombus extension into the vena cava:prospective long-term followup. J Urol 177:1703-8
54. Cost NG, Delacroix SE Jr, Sleeper JP et al (2011) The impact of targeted molecular therapies on the level of renal cell carcinoma vena caval tumor thrombus. Eur Urol 59:912-8
55. Margulis V, Matin SF, Tannir N et al (2008) Surgical morbidity associated with administration of targeted molecular therapies before cytoreductive nephrectomy or resection of locally recurrent renal cell carcinoma. J Urol 180:94-8
56. Pierorazio PM, McKiernan JM, McCann TR et al (2007) Outcome after cytoreductive nephrectomy for metastatic renal cell carcinoma is predicted by fractional percentage of tumour volume removed. BJU Int 100:755-9

Well-Differentiated Carcinomas of the Thyroid Gland and Neoplasms of the Parathyroid Glands

13

Micaela Piccoli, Casimiro Nigro, Barbara Mullineris, Roberto Panconesi and Gianluigi Melotti

13.1 Well-differentiated Carcinoma (WDCs) of the Thyroid Gland

Papillary carcinoma and follicular thyroid carcinoma, called well-differentiated carcinomas (WDCs) of the thyroid gland, account for ≈1% of human cancers, with an incidence between 0.5 and 10 per 100,000 per year, and increasing steadily. The increasing incidence is probably due to the early diagnosis of the subclinical disease (i.e., of papillary microcarcinomas) even though the SEER analysis conducted in 2009 by the National Cancer Institute showed an increase in well-differentiated tumors of the thyroid gland irrespective of size, including tumors > 4 cm in diameter [1]. Despite the steady increase in prevalence observed in the last few decades, the mortality from thyroid carcinoma is gradually decreasing. Survival data at 30 years after diagnosis indicate that the overwhelming majority of patients with papillary or follicular carcinoma are alive as a result of early diagnosis and multidisciplinary treatment programs.

The parallel increase in the rates of obesity and thyroid cancer is intriguing but, without a much larger population study, it is not possible to determine if obesity causes thyroid cancer. A higher body mass index (BMI) seems to be associated with a later stage of thyroid cancer. One explanation could be that the

M. Piccoli (✉) · Barbara Mullineris · Gianluigi Melotti
Department of Surgery, Endocrine Surgery Unit
Nuovo Ospedale Civile Sant'Agostino Estense, Modena, Italy
e-mail: m.piccoli@ausl.mo.it

R. Panconesi
General, Emergency and Minimally Invasive Surgery
Careggi Hospital, Florence, Italy

C. Nigro
General Surgery, Tor Vergata Hospital, Rome, Italy

A. Valeri et al. (eds.), *What's New in Surgical Oncology*,
DOI: 10.1007/978-88-470-5310-6_13, © Springer-Verlag Italia 2013

biology of obesity increases the risk and severity of cancer (as is the case for patients with breast cancer). The possible role of leptin and insulin-like growth factor in the obesity–cancer relationship has also been mentioned recently [2].

13.1.1 Pathogenesis

13.1.1.1 Oncogenes

Thyroid carcinoma has a monoclonal origin. Major gene mutations lead to the activation of oncogenes and inactivation of tumor suppressor genes. The genes involved are: Ras, Gαs TSH-R, RET and TRK. In particular, oncogenes RET/PTC, TRK and BRAFV600E, due to their selective expression and high prevalence, are excellent markers of papillary thyroid carcinoma (PTC) [3].

The forms with the highest prevalence in PTC are RET/PTC1, RET/PTC2 and RET/PTC3. In particular, the RET/PTC rearrangement is very frequent in papillary carcinomas in children with a history of exposure to ionizing radiation, especially after the Chernobyl accident in Russia. This type of gene alteration has a role chiefly in the early stages of thyroid carcinogenesis because it is most frequent in papillary microcarcinomas [3].

It has been reported that the mutation of the BRAF gene is present in 44% of cases of PTC: BRAF V600E, the most frequent mutation, was associated with tumors featuring more invasive behavior and with the follicular variant of papillary carcinoma [4].

BRAF mutations have been detected in blood samples from patients with PTC. They are not found in benign nodules and in follicular thyroid carcinomas, so their identification can be helpful in the diagnosis and management of PTC. Searching for BRAF mutations during fine-needle aspiration (FNA) can be useful for the evaluation of follicular lesions. BRAF positivity during the follow-up of PTC patients is correlated with residual or metastatic disease [5].

13.1.1.2 Ionizing Radiation

There is a clear relationship between thyroid carcinoma and ionizing radiation: 70–97% of radio-induced thyroid tumors are papillary tumors. These are tumors with a good prognosis [6]. For the carcinogenesis to be triggered, the radiation dose should be <15–20 Gy, otherwise cell-death effects override the tumorigenic action.

13.1.1.3 Other Factors

Important risk factors for WDC of the thyroid gland are family history, a diet low in iodine, hormonal factors, and previous thyroid disease. Patients with Gardner's syndrome, a family history of adenomatous polyposis of the colon, and patients with Cowden syndrome are likely to experience the onset of PTC [7].

PTC is associated with family history in 3% of cases. Before menopause and after menopause, the female:male ratio is 1. During childbearing age, it reaches 2–4. Furthermore, goiter and thyroid nodules are often detected during pregnancy. Infertility is associated with a high risk of onset of thyroid carcinoma [8].

13.1.2 Histology

13.1.2.1 Papillary Carcinoma

Papillary carcinoma represents ≈80% of WTCs, and is the most widespread thyroid tumor. Depending on their extent and size, carcinomas are classified as: microcarcinomas, intrathyroid carcinomas or extrathyroid carcinomas.

The overwhelming majority of papillary carcinomas are confined to the thyroid gland. Metastases tend to follow the lymphatic pathway, and are found mainly in the cervical and upper mediastinic lymph nodes. Blood metastases occur less frequently and, if present, tend to involve the lungs and, more rarely, the bones.

The classic form is multifocal in 35% of cases, with bilateral involvement in 24% of cases. Multifocality has been shown to be the expression of a neoplastic growth which is synchronous and independent, unrelated to the dissemination of the primary tumor. Papillary tumors are slow-growing with a very good prognosis.

However, these tumors may become more aggressive over the years, characterized by greater local invasion and distant spread, and turn into anaplastic forms.

Microscopically, the typical structures of papillary carcinomas can be appreciated. That is, psammoma bodies characterized by calcium deposits in the stroma and by "ground glass" cells (cells with pale nuclei). Papillary carcinomas include several histotypes:

- The follicular variant, characterized by follicles filled with colloid, composed by cells morphologically similar to normal ones. It is a grossly encapsulated tumor. Psammoma bodies are often present; the lymphocyte infiltrate is also a frequent finding;
- The diffuse sclerosing variant, typically multifocal with malpighian metaplasia and fibrosis. It is a rare variant, which is present only in children. It is frequently characterized by lymph-node and blood metastases;
- The tall cell variant, typical in the elderly: these large tumors infiltrate the perithyroid muscles. Squamous metaplasia and tall cells are often detected; the prognosis is more severe than in the classic forms;
- The encapsulated variant: the capsule of this tumor is often invaded. The microscopic pattern shows the same features as the classic papillary carcinoma. The prognosis is favorable.

13.1.2.2 Follicular Carcinoma

Follicular carcinomas are characterized by follicular differentiation but without the nuclear inclusions typical of papillary carcinomas. Follicular carcinomas are more aggressive and less frequent than papillary carcinomas. They are most frequently diagnosed in subjects aged >40 years, and account for 10% of thyroid tumors. They may appear as solitary thyroid nodules, encapsulated or unencapsulated. They are slow-growing tumors with a relatively favorable prognosis, but are more aggressive than papillary carcinomas.

The World Health Organization (WHO) recognizes two forms of follicular carcinoma: the minimally invasive form and the highly invasive form. This distinction is based on vascular and capsular invasion and has remarkable prognostic value. Invasion, if limited to the tumor capsule, does not seem to be of relevance from a prognostic viewpoint, whereas vascular involvement is invariably an unfavorable prognostic sign.

Minimally invasive follicular carcinomas account for more than half of all follicular carcinomas. Cytology by means of thin-needle aspiration does not allow a clear differentiation compared with follicular adenomas because both share the same cytological characteristics. Only histology after excision of the nodule allows differentiation of carcinomas and follicular adenomas with certainty: capsular infiltration determines the diagnosis of carcinoma. In 85% of cases, the lesion is an adenoma.

Highly invasive follicular carcinomas are characterized by obvious vascular invasion; they may or may not be encapsulated. The degree of differentiation varies between tumors. There may be well differentiated tumors with follicles of varying sizes containing colloid, or poorly differentiated tumors formed by micro-follicles with solid or trabecular structures lacking colloid. The latter are usually associated with a worse prognosis and with a greater chance of metastases. Metastases from follicular carcinoma spread mainly through the bloodstream, involving especially the lungs, bones and brain.
There are three histotypes of follicular carcinoma:

- Clear cell carcinomas: a rare type characterized by the accumulation of fat or glycogen cells in the cytoplasm. Thyroglobulin immunohistochemical analyses should be used to differentiate these carcinomas from intrathyroid metastases of a kidney carcinoma or of a parathyroid carcinoma (PCa);
- Hurthle (or oxyphilic cell) carcinomas feature partially or totally encapsulated thyroid nodules. They cause locoregional recurrences in most cases. In some case series, the prognosis has been reported to be less favorable than for other carcinomas;
- Insular carcinomas are highly invasive, poorly differentiated tumors. They consist of monomorphic cells of smaller size than the other follicular carcinomas. They tend to metastasize very often through the lymphatic and the bloodstream pathways. The prognosis is unfavorable.

13.1.2.3 FNAC Diagnosis of Thyroid Cancer

The propagation of ultrasound technology and its increasing high-resolution power has resulted in an increased ability to detect nodular thyroid disease. Thus, the prevalence of subjects found to have nodular thyroid disease has increased to a staggering prevalence of 50% in Italy. This has imposed the need for screening to recognize the nodules which may develop malignancies.

The most important ultrasound features of a thyroid nodule that may suggest a malignant tumor are irregular margins, hypoechogenicity, and intranodular vascularization. However, none of these characteristics are completely diagnostic. Thus, if ultrasound reveals a nodule with these peculiarities, a fine-needle aspiration biopsy (FNAB) is essential. After a period when all nodules were considered FNAB candidates, the indications for this procedure have been restricted to exclude hyperfunctioning nodules (which are always benign) and those with a completely cystic aspect. If the nodule size is between 1 cm and 2 cm, the sensitivity of FNAB is the highest possible. If the nodule is <1 cm, this method must be very prescribed selectively and limited to cases with a highly suspicious ultrasound pattern. If focal lesions are >2 cm, FNAB sensitivity decreases in an inversely proportional manner.

The cytology sample is harvested with a fine needle (23 G). No aspiration maneuver is usually necessary, only a gentle movement of the needle in various directions (thereby applying the capillary method) until the sample appears in the cone of the needle. This maneuver must be completed with ultrasound guidance to check the correct origin of the sample. The cytological description may be as follows:

- Thy 1: not evaluable due to the absence of a sufficient number of thyrocytes;
- Thy 2: definitely benign;
- Thy 3: indeterminate/follicular proliferation;
- Thy 4: suspicion of malignancy;
- Thy 5: definitely malignant.

The subsequent therapeutic strategy (surgical or otherwise) should be determined based on the cytological result. In case of Thy 1, the examination must be repeated if the lesion is not cystic. If the result is Thy 2, further treatments are excluded. If Thy 3 is the cytological response, patients should undergo surgery because the chance of a malignant lesion may be ≤25–30% and the only way to obtain a definitve diagnosis is to examine the entire sample. The number of Thy 3 false-positives for malignancy is very high, so researchers have recently focused their attention on molecular biology to avoid surgical overtreatment. However, the results have still to be clarified. For Thy 4 and Thy 5, a surgical approach is essential. Furthermore, in each patient with nodular disease, the calcitonin level should be measured to diagnose a medullary cancer.

In all nodules, in particular for a focal lesion >2 cm, clinical examination is absolutely essential because it is likely to lead to the correct diagnosis. Indeed, if a "hardwood" mass is revealed at palpation, surgery is absolutely essential [9].

13.1.3 Treatment

13.1.3.1 Surgery

Total extracapsular thyroidectomy (TT) is the most suitable approach in the therapy of thyroid carcinoma. This view is supported by the following arguments:

- Papillary carcinoma foci may be present in both thyroid lobes in 36–85% of cases;
- Recurrences occur in the contralateral lobe in 5–10% of cases;
- TT improves the follow-up;
- The specificity of the value of serum thyroglobulin as a tumor marker is facilitated by total removal of normal thyroid tissue;
- Retrospective studies suggest that the risk of recurrence and mortality is dramatically reduced by TT if the tumor diameter is ≤1 cm.

However, guidelines by the American Thyroid Association (ATA) issued in 2009 [9] maintain that: "TT is recommended if the primary tumor is 1 cm in diameter or larger, if the tumor extends into the extrathyroid region, or if metastases are present. TT is mandatory in all thyroid carcinoma patients with a history of head and neck exposure to ionizing radiation due to the high recurrence rate of the tumor. Unilateral lobectomy and isthmectomy may be considered if the tumor is less than 1 cm in diameter and confined to one lobe of the gland." Some experts support this view, especially in 15–45-year-old patients and if the WDC is diagnosed after surgery. However, if the diagnosis of papillary cancer is reached preoperatively, the surgeon should strongly consider total thyroidectomy even in microcarcinomas because ≤20% may be multifocal [10].

Lymphadenectomy (LY) should be done if there is clinical and ultrasound evidence of metastatic lymph nodes. However, there is some debate as to which is the correct choice concerning LY. Some authors suggest that the procedure should be limited to the central compartment (VI) even in case of the absence of evident metastatic disease. Other researchers believe that LY should be reserved for cases in which it is really necessary, whereas other authors maintain that it should be undertaken only on the side of the neoplasm if the tumor is very aggressive [11]. Furthermore, some authors carry out the laterocervical LY only in case of positive, monolateral lymph nodes on the side of the tumor, whereas others undertake the ipsilateral LY in any case of thyroid cancer [12]. In conclusion, the most rational choice is probably to execute a TT with homolateral laterocervical or central-compartment LY only if it is absolutely necessary due to aggressive or metastatic disease in the lymph nodes. Even in the latter case, however, the rate of surgical complications (hypoparathyroidism, palsy in the inferior laryngeal nerve) is too high, and therefore LY should be considered too dangerous to be done in a disease with a substantially good prognosis [9]. One potential solution that has been used in many other domains of oncological surgery is sentinel lymph node (SLN) biopsy. However, the value of this method in WDC of the thyroid remains ambiguous [13].

13.1.3.2 Radioiodine Treatment

Radioiodine ablation enables the destruction of the residual thyroid tissue left after surgery. The iodine isotope used is ^{131}I. Ablation reduces the risk of recurrence and mortality [9]. Radioablation by ^{131}I entails:

- destruction of the residual normal thyroid tissue;
- destruction of the microscopic foci of residual disease;
- reduction of tumor recurrences in high-risk patients (history of head and neck irradiation or patients with genetic syndromes);
- improved reliability of thyroglobulin value as a tumor marker;
- improved specificity of ^{131}I scintigraphy.

Several prospective studies and one meta-analysis [14] have suggested that ablation by ^{131}I is associated with a reduction in the 10-year risk of recurrence by ≈50% and a reduction in the mortality rate of 3%. However, the cases considered were carcinomas of 1–1.5 cm in diameter, multifocal, with laterocervical lymph node metastases or with soft-tissue involvement at the time of diagnosis.

According to the 2009 ATA guidelines [9], radioiodine treatment is indicated:

- in all patients with distant metastases and extra-thyroid extension, regardless of tumor size;
- in all patients with tumor size >4 cm even in the absence of other high-risk characteristics;
- in all patients with lymph-node metastases;
- in patients whose risk is considered high (vascular invasion, more aggressive histological subtypes such as tall cell, columnar, insular, or poorly differentiated histology).

ATA also recognize the importance of clinical judgment and of a personalized approach to treatment.

Therapy with ^{131}I is not routinely recommended in unifocal carcinomas of diameter <1 cm in the absence of other risk factors (distant metastasis, vascular invasion, extrathyroid extension or aggressive histotypes) or in multifocal carcinomas in which all foci are <1 cm in the absence of other high-risk conditions. Pregnancy and lactation are absolute contraindications to therapy with ^{131}I. Fetal thyroid tissue is functional from the 10th to 12th week and could be destroyed by ^{131}I, resulting in cretinism. An absolute precondition for the administration of ^{131}I to women of childbearing age is a negative pregnancy test administered 72 h before treatment.

The absorption of ^{131}I by thyroid tissue is stimulated by thyroid-stimulating hormone (TSH). The values of TSH should therefore be higher than 25–30 μU/mL at the time of the ablative treatment. Thus, treatment is carried out after discontinuing hormone therapy for 4–6 weeks. Approximately 6–12 months after ablative therapy, the patient is assessed again by measuring thyroglobulin and by total body scintigraphy if necessary.

13.1.3.3 Hormone Therapy: TSH Suppressive Treatment with Levothyroxine (LT4)

TSH is an important growth factor for thyroid cells. TSH suppression with exogenous thyroid hormones reduces tumor progression and metastases, decreasing the prevalence of recurrence and cancer-specific mortality. Along with surgery and radioiodine therapy, TSH is a mainstay of the treatment of connective tissue diseases (CTDs) and is aimed at preventing or slowing down the growth of neoplastic foci and reducing the risk of disease recurrence.

To achieve TSH suppression, the LT4 dose is adjusted for each patient depending on the body weight and age. As a general rule, treatment (in μg/kg/day) is started with 2.5 in young patients, 1.5–2.5 in adults and 1.2–1.8 in the elderly. To assess TSH suppression, doses of TSH and of free triiodothyronine (FT3) and free thyroxine (FT4) are assessed 2 months after the beginning of treatment. Therapy is aimed at achieving a TSH value <0.1 μUI/mL, with normal values of FT3 and FT4 in the upper half of the normal range, using the minimum dose needed to inhibit TSH and preventing possible damage due to iatrogenic hyperthyroidism (especially as far as the heart and bones are concerned). Once the optimal dose in the individual is obtained, hormonal status must be assessed at 6- or 12-month intervals.

In the cases where complete remission of the disease seems to have been achieved (persistently undetectable thyroglobulin and negative post-therapy total body scintigraphy), the follow-up envisages semi-suppressive therapy, maintaining the level of serum TSH at ≈0.4 μUI/mL.

13.1.3.4 Radiotherapy

Radiotherapy is the adjuvant treatment of choice in patients with locally advanced disease whose tumors do not concentrate radioactive iodine or who cannot tolerate salvage surgery [15]. Typically, this indication is for known macroscopic tumors that remain after primary surgery, radioiodine remnant ablation (RRA), and/or revision surgery, as well as tumors that are unresectable without undue morbidity. It is not indicated for the final treatment of non-operated thyroid cancer except in palliative situations.

13.1.3.5 Chemotherapy

Conventional chemotherapy has been studied for metastatic WDC of the thyroid gland but success rates have been low. Chemotherapy is not indicated for the definitive treatment of locoregional WDC except in the case of refractory recurrent or metastatic disease. The cytotoxic chemotherapeutic agent doxorubicin is approved by the US Food and Drug Administration (FDA) for use in these cases. However, due to the lack of evidence on response, its use is not common [15].

13.1.3.6 Other

The most recent advances in the pharmacotherapy for PTC have been the advent of targeted therapies designed to affect biologic pathways such as BRAF and RET. Tyrosine kinase inhibitors are the targeted agents that have been studied to the greatest extent, but recent evidence has also shown encouraging pre-clinical results with other targeted agents. These agents may play a larger part in the treatment of WDC in the future, but they have no role in the primary treatment of well-differentiated PTC at the moment. Radiofrequency ablation (RFA) using percutaneous ethanol in the treatment of recurrent WDC has been reported but long-term results in a large series of patients have not [16].

13.1.4 Staging

The International Union Against Cancer (UICC) and the American Joint Committee on Cancer (AJCC) have developed a staging system for thyroid cancer based on the TNM system. The TNM staging system is based on three components: size and extent of the primary tumor (T), presence or absence of metastases involving regional lymph nodes (N) and presence or absence of distant metastases (M). These categories are further divided numerically to identify the progression of cancer (Tables 13.1-13.3).

Table 13.1 TNM staging (7th edition, 2010)

Papillary and follicular thyroid carcinoma	
Tx	Primary tumor cannot be assessed
T0	No evidence of primary tumor
T1	Tumor size ≤2 cm and limited to the thyroid gland
T1a: Tumor ≤1 cm in greatest dimension, limited to the thyroid gland	
T1b: Tumor with greatest dimension between 1 cm and 2 cm, limited to the thyroid gland	
T2	Tumor size >2 cm but ≤4 cm, limited to the thyroid gland
T3	Tumor size >4 cm, limited to the thyroid gland or any tumor with minimal extrathyroid extension (e.g., extension to the sternocleidomastoid muscle or perithyroid soft tissues)
T4a	Tumor of any size extending beyond the thyroid capsule to invade subcutaneous soft tissues, larynx, trachea, esophagus, or recurrent laryngeal nerve
T4b	Tumor invading the prevertebral fascia or encasing the carotid artery or mediastinal vessels
Categories T1, T2 and T3 must be divided into (s) single tumor and (m) multifocal tumor. The largest lesion determines the T classification. All anaplastic carcinomas are considered stage T4.	

Table 13.2 Regional lymph nodes

Nx	Regional lymph nodes cannot be assessed
N0	Absence of lymph node metastases
N1	Metastases in regional lymph nodes
N1a	Metastases to level VI (pretracheal, paratracheal, and prelaryngeal/Delphian lymph nodes)
N1b	Metastases to unilateral, bilateral, or contralateral cervical (levels I, II, III, IV, or V) or retropharyngeal or superior mediastinal lymph nodes (level VII).
Regional lymph nodes are formed by the central compartment (VI), lateral cervical (IV, III an II), and upper mediastinal (VII) lymph nodes.	

Table 13.3 Distant metastases

Mx	Distant metastases cannot be assessed
M0	Absence of distant metastases
M1	Presence of distant metastases

Table 13.4 Conditions associated with an increased risk of recurrence and mortality in individuals with well-differentiated cancers

Age	<16 years and >45 years
Histological subtype	Tall cell carcinoma Papillary carcinomas Columnar cell carcinoma Diffuse sclerosing carcinoma
Follicular carcinomas	Widely invasive carcinoma Poorly differentiated carcinoma Hurthle cell or oxyphilic carcinoma
Tumor size	Tumors >4 cm or extending beyond the thyroid capsule
Lymph-node involvement	

13.1.4 Classes of Risk

There have been many attempts to classify the risk of recurrence and mortality in patients with WDC. These include the scoring systems created by the European Organization for Research and Treatment of Cancer (EORTC), AMES, AGES, Mayo Clinic (i.e., the metastases, age, completeness, invasion and size (MACE) system) as well as the OHIO classification. Several conditions are associated with an increased risk of recurrence, as shown in Table 13.4.

A recent Consensus Conference held in 2010 [17] divided patients into three risk groups:

- Low: patients with unifocal microcarcinoma without extension beyond the thyroid capsule, without vascular invasion, and without lymph-node metastasis. Absence of aggressive histotype (such as insular, tall cell, columnar cell, Hurthle cell, and follicular carcinomas). In these patients, radionuclide therapy with ^{131}I is not indicated;
- Intermediate: patients with evidence of microscopic invasion in perithyroid tissue. Metastases in lymph nodes or total-body scintigraphy findings of cervical uptake outside the thyroid bed at the time of radioiodine therapy (which is indicated). Patients with aggressive histology (insular, tall cell, columnar cell, Hurthle cell, and follicular carcinomas).
- High: patients with persistent disease already documented or at high risk of persistent or recurrent disease as well as distant metastases. Administration of ^{131}I reduces the chance of recurrence and improves survival.

13.1.5 Follow-up

The methods for monitoring WDC patients after initial treatment are doses of TSH, thyroid hormones, circulating thyroglobulin and anti-thyroglobulin antibodies; neck ultrasound and diagnostic whole-body imaging (CT, magnetic resonance imaging (MRI) and positron emission tomography (PET) supplement follow-up; radiography is a second-choice test). In the past, all patients were monitored postoperatively with serum calcium measurements to detect downward levels, indicating hypoparathyroidism. However, the advent of rapid parathyroid hormone (PTH) detection has improved the ability to predict postoperative hypoparathyroidism. A study at the University of Cincinnati proposed an algorithm for management after TT. Patients with postoperative PTH levels (in nmol/L) >30 were eligible for hospital discharge without supplementation, those with 10–20 were discharged home on calcium supplementation, and those with <10 were started on supplementation with calcium and vitamin D and observed overnight [18]. The follow-up protocols for WDC patients submitted to initial treatment with thyroidectomy and ^{131}I ablation have changed over the years. The follow-up strategies involve four stages:

- Assessment of the thyroid remnant at the time of ablation by 131I followed by LTH suppression therapy;
- Follow-up after 3 months of treatment with LT4 to assess correct hormone dosage by TSH and measurement of serum thyroglobulin and free thyroid hormones;
- Follow-up after 6–12 months with serum thyroglobulin measurement after stimulation with recombinant human thyroid-stimulating hormone (rhTSH) or in hypothyroidism;
- Long-term follow-up.

13.1.5.1 Clinical and Ultrasound Examination

Palpation of the thyroid and of locoregional lymph nodes is a routine procedure but is not sensitive enough for assessing persistent or recurrent disease.

Ultrasound imaging supplements the clinical examination and is an operator-dependent method. It allows the identification of locoregional recurrences as small as 2–3 mm in diameter, and lymph nodes with abnormal morphology suggestive of malignancy, thereby making it possible to distinguish reactive and metastatic lymph nodes. Suspicious lymph nodes can be subjected to fine needle aspiration cytology (FNAC) under ultrasound guidance coupled with the measurement of thyroglobulin in lavage fluid [9]. This method allows detection of lymph-node metastases of the neck in almost all cases. Ultrasound monitoring at regular intervals are required for each lymph node >5 mm in diameter.

Radiography: Patients with unmeasurable thyroglobulin values are not subjected to chest radiography [9]. Radiography does not allow evaluation of lung metastases <1 cm in diameter which, conversely, can be visualized using ^{131}I total-body scintigraphy. Micronodular metastases, however, are best viewed with non-contrast CT or MRI. Radiography shows bone metastases from thyroid carcinomas as osteolytic lesions. Scintigraphic imaging detects them as hypocaptating or moderately hypercaptating foci [9].

Fluorodeoxyglucose positron emission tomography FDG-PET: In patients with evidence of distant metastases, FDG PET scintigraphy provides information about the prognosis. In fact, in a study of 125 patients who underwent FDG-PET, FDG uptake over a larger volume of tissue correlated with shorter survival [9].

Determination of thyroglobulin: Thyroglobulin is an extremely useful tumor marker in the follow-up of CTD patients. It is a high-molecular-weight (660 kDa) glycoprotein from which thyroid hormones are derived. It is produced by follicular cells (normal and neoplastic).
Thyroglobulin production is controlled by TSH, which stimulates the transcription genes of the protein and its release into the bloodstream. Therefore, it is essential that, whenever thyroglobulin is determined, TSH is also measured. During the follow-up of WDCs of the thyroid, determination of the thyroglobulin level when TSH levels are high (thanks to discontinuation of LT4 or administration of rhTHS) allows more sensitive results than during LT4 suppressive therapy.

After surgery and after radioablation, serum levels of thyroglobulin remain relatively high for a few months. Therefore thyroglobulin should not be measured until after 3 months, at which point in time it should be undetectable. Increased thyroglobulin values during hormone suppressive therapy are associated with distant metastases in the overwhelming majority of cases [20]. Thyroglobulin levels are directly correlated with the extension and severity of the tumor [21]. However, only 60% of patients with thyroid cancer forming local or distant metastasis during therapy with LT4 have detectable serum thyroglobulin levels [20]. In 20% of patients with isolated lymph-node metastases and in 5% of patients with small lung metastases not visible on radiography, thyroglobulin levels are undetectable: these are false-negatives. Other important causes of false-negative results may be methodological problems, structural abnormalities of thyroglobulin or presence of monoclonal antibodies that make the protein unrecognizable by standard measurement methods [20]. Patients with undetectable thyroglobulin levels while hypothyroid are free from disease 20 years after the diagnosis, whereas those with detectable circulating thyroglobulin (>10 ng/mL) develop neck or distant metastases in 60–80% of cases.

In low-risk patients not undergoing radioiodine ablation, the risk of tumor recurrence is very low, and TSH stimulation by discontinuation of LT4 or administration of rhTSH is not recommended. These patients can be cared for by measuring thyroglobulin during LT4 treatment and ultrasound of the neck. A total of 93% of low-risk individuals during hormone replacement therapy have undetectable thyroglobulin levels and, in the remaining 7%, thyroglobulin is detectable with levels <5 ng/mL. Thyroglobulin serum levels in low-risk patients after lobectomy are undetectable in 2/3 of patients on suppression therapy.

Thyroglobulin is a protein with many antigenic epitopes. In general, thyroglobulin antibodies are markers of autoimmune thyroid diseases. In patients with thyroid cancer, thyroglobulin antibodies are present in 20% of cases. The reasons for the increase in antibodies are not well understood. Their disappearance is associated with a reduction of the tumor and its severity (most likely linked to a lower antigenic stimulus [21]). Their presence interferes with the measurement of thyroglobulin serum levels, so patients with positive levels of thyroglobulin antibodies and with undetectable serum thyroglobulin cannot be considered in remission of disease. They should be monitored periodically with diagnostic whole-body imaging and ultrasound of the neck. The disappearance of thyroglobulin antibodies in the follow-up could be considered clear evidence of remission.

The importance and role of serum thyroglobulin in the follow-up of WDCs is well established. The option of avoiding the diagnostic examination with ^{131} I, with the consequent advantages that derive from this, have allowed rhTSH and the induction of hypothyroidism through LT4 discontinuation to play a crucial part in monitoring the possible recurrence of cancer.

Some studies have concluded that the diagnostic accuracy of thyroglobulin in patients negative for thyroglobulin antibodies is sufficient to decide if treatment is necessary because the test with ^{131}I adds very little information compared with thyroglobulin alone. It is however, recognized, that serum thyroglobulin concentration after discontinuation resulting in increased stimulation by TSH plays an important part in follow-up [9].

13.1.6 Outline of Surgical Methods

The specific decription of thyroidectomy is beyond the scope of this chapter. The surgeon should be proactive with regard to the removal of all thyroid tissue, but great care should be taken to identify and protect the recurrent laryngeal nerve, superior laryngeal nerve and parathyroid glands as well as their vascular supplies. Re-implantation of parathyroid glands should be considered if they must be removed. The past decade has seen numerous technological advances in thyroid surgery. Many of these include changes in instrumentation or the introduction of new instruments, but others concern minimally invasive surgical procedures (e.g., endoscopes, three-dimensional intraoperative viewing, and robotic surgery).

13.1.6.1 Changes in Instrumentation or the Introduction of New Instruments

In the early 2000s, the US FDA and the European Medical Device Directive approved the use of ultrasonic coagulating-dissecting and electrothermal bipolar vessel sealing systems to seal thyroid gland vessels and parenchyma [22].

Due to the vascularization of the thyroid gland, many surgeons utilize these instruments rather than bipolar cautery, ties, or clips. Some studies comparing these instruments with other haemostatic methods showed a decrease in operating time and intraoperative blood loss with no increase in complications [23–29].

Surgeon preferences may also include the use of intraoperative nerve monitoring with an electrode attached to an endotracheal tube to allow detection of stimulation of the recurrent laryngeal nerve. This may be helpful in the identification of the recurrent and superior laryngeal nerves (even though studies have not identified a significant decrease in the rate of vocal-cord paralysis with this technology [30]). Common indications for the use of this technology are thyroid revision surgery or tumors with extrathyroid extension when identification of the nerve is more difficult.

Although drains are used for major surgical procedures of the head and neck, their use for routine thyroidectomy has been questioned. A Cochrane review of studies on drain use did not show a decrease in complications for patients undergoing goiter surgery without substernal extension, lateral neck dissection, or coagulation abnormalities, but it did find an increase in the duration of hospital stay [31]. However, the decision to use drains should be guided by the surgeon's experience and intraoperative findings.

13.1.6.2 Minimally Invasive Surgical Procedures

WDCs of the thyroid are more prevalent in young women, and usually show favorable biological behavior and better prognosis than other cancers of the head and neck. Furthermore, the evolution of minimally invasive methods for the treatment of thyroid cancer has been driven by cosmetic results [32].

Video-assisted thyroidectomy (VAT), first described by Miccoli et al. in 1999, [33] is an entirely gasless method. It involves a 1.5–2.5-cm incision directly over the thyroid and reproduces the same steps used in conventional surgery with the technical support of a camera and a set of dedicated instruments [34–38].

A problem which remains partially unsolved is the treatment of malignant thyroid disease. However, several authors, after developing, evaluating, validating and standardizing the procedure, have proposed that VAT can also be used in the treatment of in low-risk, small size PTCs (T1) [39, 40].

Concerns regarding the adequacy of resection were addressed by Miccoli et al. in a prospective randomized trial for papillary cancer. Postoperative thyroglobulin, levels of uptake of radioactive iodine, and complication rates were found to be equivalent to those of patients treated with conventional open thyroidectomy or minimally invasive video-assisted thyroidectomy (MIVAT). This method was described initially with some contraindications, including large nodules (>2.5 cm to 3.0 cm), thyroiditis, an enlarged thyroid gland (>20 cm^3), previous neck surgery, central compartment neck metastases, and large malignant tumors with extrathyroid extension. Recently, some authors explored several cases using expanded indications for MIVAT, and demonstrated oncologic completeness by evaluating postoperative uptake of radioiodine [41, 42].

The only universally recognized indication to the radical ablation of central compartment lymph nodes is preoperative or intraoperative evidence of macroscopic metastatic involvement of these same lymph nodes [43], this, therefore, being a condition in which lymphadenectomy is undertaken with intent to treat.

13.1.6.3 Robotic Transaxillary Thyroidectomy (RAT)

RAT has gained popularity due to the avoidance of a neck incision. This procedure was popularized by Chung et al. in Korea and the method provides excellent optics with three-dimensional visualization, elimination of tremor, and the ability to work with precision through a longer approach. Initial cases were limited to WDCs of the thyroid gland with a tumor size of 2 cm without definite extrathyroid tumor invasion (T1 lesions) or to follicular neoplasms with a tumor size of 5 cm. After demonstrating the safety, feasibility, and functional benefits of robotic thyroidectomy, some comparative studies were conducted *vs* conventional methods and multicenter trial studies to determine its technical reproducibility. As robotic experience accumulated, it made possible the successful management of unexpectedly encountered advanced cases, such as cases with definite invasion of adjacent muscles or multiple nodal metastases, in which the procedure was completed without open conversion. Thus, over time, the indications for robotic bilateral total thyroidectomy were extended and more advanced cases were included. The indications for robotic thyroidectomy have been expanded to include patients with T3 or larger size lesions (<4 cm) and N1a or N1b (limited metastasis to the lateral neck compartment) [32].

Axillo-breast robotic thyroidectomy has also been shown to be feasible. Preliminary studies have been conducted on facelift incision robotic surgery and transoral robotic thyroidectomy, which may prove to be applicable in the future [44–47].

13.2 Neoplasms of the Parathyroid Glands

Parathyroid carcinoma (PCa) is a rare neoplasm. In patients with primary hyperparathyroidism (PHPT) the prevalence is <1%. The incidence of parathyroid carcinoma, however, appears to be increasing [48–49]. The Surveillance, Epidemiology, and End Results Cancer Registry showed a 60% increase in incidence from 1988 to 2003. PCa affects both sexes equally. The peak age of diagnosis in the fifth decade is only slightly younger than that for patients with benign hyperparathyroidism (BHPT) [50].

13.2.1 Presentation

The histopathological features of PCa cannot always be clearly defined or differentiated from the more common adenoma. The definitive diagnosis of PCa is made only if recurrence or metastasis occurs. Every case that involves the rapid-onset symptoms of HPT should be considered suspicious for carcinoma, but it usually cannot be confirmed preoperatively. This complicates the treatment strategy. In some patients, the pathologic diagnosis of PCa begins during surgery due to the finding of an indurate mass (5%) invading surrounding structures (which may include the strap musculature, ipsilateral thyroid lobe, muscularis of the esophagus, trachea, and/or recurrent laryngeal nerve) [51]. Marked hyperkalcemia, low serum phosphorus (if renal function is not impaired), and substantial elevation of serum PTH are common findings. An initial *en bloc* resection is recommended if the diagnosis is suspected at the beginning of the procedure. A right surgical procedure reduces metastases and increases recurrence-free survival. Fifty percent of the procedure could be considered to be curative but only a long follow-up shows the complications of the recurrences that lead to death. Patients with PCa commonly die from metabolic complications and due to the infiltration of vital organs by tumor [52]. More than 50% of patients with PCa treated by surgery have signs and symptoms involving the skeleton (40% to 70%), the kidneys (30% to 60%) and the digestive system (stomach–duodenum, pancreas; 15%). Non-functioning PCa, with a normal serum level of PTH, occurs but only in 5% of all PCa [50].

13.2.2 Localization

Normally, PCa tends to be larger in diameter (>2 cm) [53]. The localization studies are: ultrasonography (offering the advantage of intraoperative use), CT, MRI and scintigraphy with thallium or sestamibi. Scintigraphy can also be used to detect ectopic parathyroid glands but yields less information about the dimension and morphological features of the parathyroid glands. In general, FNAC of PCa is not necessary and should be avoided in resectable cases because disruption of the tumor capsule increases the possibility of tumor implantation [54].

13.2.3 Biologic Markers

The histological features of PCa have been described by Shantz and Castelman: (i) uniform sheets of cells arranged in a lobulated fashion with intervening fibrous trabeculae; (ii) capsular and/or vascular invasion; and (iii) mitotic figures, which should be clearly differentiated from those observed in endothelial cells [48]. Several oncogenes and tumor suppressor genes have been linked to PCa. Altered DNA content is overexpressed frequently in PCa (somatic or germline mutations in HRPT2; loss of a region on chromosome 13); the cyclin D1 or parathyroid adenoma 1 (PRAD1) oncogene is frequently overexpressed in PCa and it also has been suggested that *PRAD*1 plays an important part in the malignant transformation of PCa [55] .

13.2.4 Treatment

The treatment of PCa is *en bloc* excision of the tumor with the contiguous ipsilateral thyroid lobe and isthmus. If there is an evidence of soft-tissue extension a wider excision must be done. Efforts must be made not to violate or rupture the parathyroid capsule, which often leads to tumor spillage and eventual disease recurrence. Prophylactic neck dissection does not improve the prognosis [56]. Any sacrifice of a normally functioning recurrent laryngeal nerve is not required unless it is involved circumferentially by malignancy and has been shown to be dysfunctional preoperatively. Intraoperative PTH (IPTH) measurement is a method for optimizing tumor removal while minimizing the invasiveness of parathyroid surgery. Multiple studies have investigated its use in the surgical management of PHPT but its role in the management of PCa remains unclear. It can be postulated that IPTH measurement may be of limited application to PCa if metastases are present. The most common site for implants and local metastatic disease is the cervical region, followed by the lungs, liver and skeleton. Because external beam radiation and chemotherapy are generally ineffective for the treatment of persistent or recurrent PCa, re-operation is often recommended to: relieve symptoms; eradicate residual disease; remove metastases. PTH secretion and hypercalcemia are the true causes of mortality and morbidity rather than tumor dimension and local compression/infiltration. Treatment modalities for hypercalcemia (if possible) are an aggressive cervical surgical approach and surgical exicision of distant metastases (such as wedge lung resection). In patients with unresectable disease, the aim is to ameliorate the symptoms of hypercalcemia. Conventional treatment with intravenous fluids, diuretics, and anti-resorptive agents (such as bisphosphonates, gallium, or mithramycin) and calcimimetic agents are usually employed to reach this goal [55].

13.2.5 Staging

Because of the low incidence of PCa, an AJCC staging system has not yet been formulated and thus is not applicable for this malignancy. Neither tumor size nor lymph-node status appear to be important prognostic markers for this malignancy. Patients are considered to have localized or metastatic disease. For localized PCa the disease involves the parathyroid gland with or without invasion of adjacent tissues. For metastatic PCa, the disease spreads beyond the tissues adjacent to the involved parathyroid gland(s). PCa most frequently metastasizes to regional lymph nodes and lungs, and it may involve the liver, bone, pleura, pericardium, and pancreas.

13.2.6 Prognosis

Patients with PCa represent a heterogeneous group. PCa is often indolent but with a progressive course. Some patients are cured for as long as a decade or more, whereas some with aggressive tumors experience early recurrence with local and distant spread. The 5-year survival rate is of 40–50%.

References

1. Chen AY, Jemal A, Ward EM. (2009). Increasing incidence of differentiated thyroid cancer in the United States, 1988-2005. Cancer Aug 15; 115 (16):3801-7.
2. Duh QY (2012). Thyroid cancer operations for obese patients: the bad news and the good news. Arch Surg 147(9):811-2. doi: 10.1001/archsurg.2012.911
3. Suarez H.G. (1998). Genetic alterations in human epithelial tumors. Clin Endocrinol, May 48 (5): 531-546.
4. Lupi C, Giannini R, Ugolini C et al. (2007). Association of BRAF V600 E mutation with poor clinicopathological outcomes in 500 consecutive cases of papillary thyroid carcinoma. J Clin Endocrinol Metab 92(11):4085-90)
5. Cradic KW, Milosevic D, Rosenberg AM et al (2009). Mutant BRAF(T1799A) can be detected in the blood of papillary thyroid carcinoma patients and correlates with disease status. J Clin Endocrinol Metab; 94(12):5001-9.
6. Schneider AB., Recant W., Pinsky SM (1986). Radiation-induced thyroid carcinoma. Clinical course and results of therapy in 296 patients. Ann. Intern. Med; 105 (3), 405-412
7. Franceschi S., Boyle P., Maisonneuve P et al (1993). The epidemiology of thyroid carcinoma. Critical Review in Oncogenesis 4(1): 25-52
8. Ron E, Lunenfeld B, Menczer J et al (1987). Cancer incidence in a cohort of infertile women. Am J Epidemiol May;125(5): 780-790
9. Cooper DS, Doherty GM, Haugen BR et al (2009). Revised American Thyroid Association management guidelines for patients with thyroid nodules and differentiated thyroid cancer..American Thyroid Association (ATA) Guidelines Taskforce on Thyroid Nodules and Differentiated Thyroid Cancer. Thyroid; 19(11):1167-214.
10. Baudin E, Travagli JP, Ropers J et al (1998). Microcarcinoma of the thyroid gland: the Gustave-Roussy Institute experience. Cancer83(3):553–9;
11. Dralle H, Machens A (2012). Surgical management of the lateral neck compartment for metastatic thyroid cancer. Curr Opin Oncol Oct 17
12. Yu WB, Tao SY, Zhang NS (2012). Is Level V Dissection Necessary for Low-risk Patients with Papillary Thyroid Cancer Metastasis in Lateral Neck Levels II, III, and IV. Asian Pac J Cancer Prev;13(9):4619-22
13. Amir A, Payne R, Richardson K et al. (2011) Sentinel lymph node biopsy in thyroid cancer: it can work but there are pitfalls. Otolaryngol Head Neck Surg Nov;145(5):723-6.
14. Sawka AM, Thephamongkhol K, Brouwers M, et al (2004). Clinical review 170: A systematic review and metanalysis of the effectiveness of radioactive iodine remnant ablation for well-differentiated thyroid cancer. J Clin Endocrinol Metab 89(8):3668-76
15. Byrd JK, Yawn RJ, Wilhoit CS et al (2012). Well Differentiated Thyroid Carcinoma: current treatment. Curr Treat Options Oncol 13(1):47–57
16. Monchik JM, Donatini G, Iannuccilli J et al. (2006). Radiofrequency ablation and percuta-

neous ethanol injection treatment for recurrent local and distant well-differentiated thyroid carcinoma. Ann Surg 244(2):296–304.
17. Tuttle RM, Tala H, Shah J et al (2010). Estimating risk of recurrence in differentiated thyroid cancer after total thyroidectomy and radioactive iodine remnant ablation: using response to therapy variables to modify the initial risk estimates predicted by the new American Thyroid Association staging system. Thyroid 20(12):1341-9.
18. Sabour S, Manders E, Steward DL (2009). The role of rapid PACU parathyroid hormone in reducing post-thyroidectomy hypocalcemia. Otolaryngol Head Neck Surg 141(6):727–9
19. Robbins RJ, Wan Q, Grewal RK, et al. (2006). Real-time prognosis for metastatic thyroid carcinoma based on 2-[18F]fluoro-2-deoxy-D-glucose-positron emission tomography scanning. J Clin Endocrinol Metab 91(2):498-505.
20. Ringel MD., Ldenson P W (2004). Controversies in the follow-up and management of well-differentiated thyroid cancer. Endocr Relat Cancer, 11(1): 97-116.
21. Schlumberger M (1992). Can iodine-131 whole body scan be replaced by thyreoglobulin measurement in the post surgical follow-up of differentiated thyroid carcinoma. J Nucl Med; 33(1): 172-173
22. Dionigi G, Van Slycke S, Rausei S et al (2012). Parathyroid function after open thyroidectomy: A prospective randomized study for ligasure precise versus harmonic FOCUS. Head Neck. 2012 Jun 19 (doi: 10.1002/head 23005).
23. Ecker T, Carvalho AL, Choe JH et al (2010). Hemostasis in thyroid surgery: harmonic scalpel versus other techniques–a meta-analysis. Otolaryngol Head Neck Surg;143(1):17–25.
24. Chang J. O'Neill C, Suliburk J et al (2011). Sutureless total thyroidectomy: a safe and cost effective alternative. ANZ J Surg Jul-Aug;81(7-8):510-4
25. Lepner U, Vaasna T (2007). Ligasure vessel sealing system versus conventional vessel ligation in thyroidectomy. Scand J Surg ;96(1):31–34.;
26. Manouras A, Markogiannakis H, Koutras AS et al (2008). Thyroid surgery: comparison between the electrothermal bipolar vessel sealing system, harmonic scalpel, and classic suture ligation. The American Journal of Surgery 195(1):48–52
27. Shen WT, Baumbusch MA, Kebebew E et al (2005). Use of the electrothermal vessel sealing system versus standard vessel ligation in thyroidectomy. Asian J Surg ;28(2):86–89
28. Lombardi CP, Raffaelli M, Cicchetti A et al (2008). The use of 'harmonic scalpel' versus 'knot tying' for conventional 'open' thyroidectomy: results of a prospective randomized study. Langenbecks Arch Surg 393 (5):627–631;
29. Saint Marc O, Cogliandolo A, Piquard A et al (2007). LigaSure vs clamp-and-tie technique to achieve hemostasis in total thyroidectomy for benign multinodular goiter. A prospective randomized study. Arch Surg 142(2):150–6
30. Higgins TS, Gupta R, Ketcham AS et al (2011). Recurrent laryngeal nerve monitoring versus identification alone on post-thyroidectomy true vocal fold palsy: a meta-analysis. Laryngoscope; 121(5):1009–17
31. [Samraj K, Gurusamy KS (2007). Wound drains following thyroid surgery. Cochrane Database Syst Rev 17(4): CD006099
32. Kang SW, Park JH, Jeong JS et al (2011). Prospects of robotic thyroidectomy using a gasless, transaxillary approach for the management of thyroid carcinoma. Surg Laparosc Endosc Percutan Tech 21(4):223–229
33. Miccoli P, Berti P, Conte M et al (1999). Minimally invasive surgery for thyroid small nodules: Preliminary report. J Endocrinol Invest. 22(11):849–51
34. Bellantone R, Lombardi CP, Raffaelli M, et al (1999). Minimally invasive, totally gasless video-assisted thyroid lobectomy. Am J Surg 177(4): 342-3
35. Miccoli P, Berti P, Bendinelli C et al (2000). Minimally invasive video-assisted surgery of the thyroid: a preliminary report. Langenbecks Arch Surg; 385(4): 261-4
36. Mourad M, Saab N, Malaise J et al (2001). Minimally invasive video-assisted approach for partial and total thyroidectomy: initial experience. Surg Endosc 2001 15(10): 1108-11
37. Bellantone R, Lombardi CP, Raffaelli M et al (2002). Video-assisted thyroidectomy. J Am Coll Surg 194(5): 610-4

38. Miccoli P, Berti P, Raffaelli M et al (2001). Minimally invasive video-assisted thyroidectomy. Am J Surg 181(6): 567-70
39. Bellantone R, Lombardi CP, Raffaelli M et al (2003). Video-assisted thyroidectomy for papillary thyroid carcinoma Surg Endosc 17(10): 1604-8
40. Miccoli P, Elisei R, Materazzi G et al (2002). Minimally invasive video-assisted thyroidectomy for papillary carcinoma: a prospective study of its completeness. Surgery; 132(6):1070-4
41. Lai SY, Walvekar RR, Ferris RL (2008). Minimally invasive videoassisted thyroidectomy: expanded indications and oncologic completeness. Head Neck 30(11):1403–7;
42. Kim AJ, Liu JC, Ganly I et al (2011). Minimally invasive video-assisted thyroidectomy 2.0: expanded indications in a tertiary care cancer center. Head Neck 33(11): 1557-60 doi: 10.1002/hed 21633
43. Bellantone R, Lombardi CP, Boscherini M et al (1998). Prognostic factors in differentiated thyroid carcinoma: a multivariate analysis of 234 consecutive patients. J Surg Oncol 68(4): 237-241
44. Kuppersmith RB, Holsinger FC (2011). Robotic thyroid surgery: an initial experience with North American patients. Laryngoscope 121(3):521–6.
45. Tae K, Ji YB, Cho SH et al (2012). Early surgical outcomes of robotic thyroidectomy by a gasless unilateral axillo-breast or axillary approach for papillary thyroid carcinoma: 2 years' experience. Head Neck, 34(5):617-25
46. Terris DJ, Singer MC, Seybt MW (2011). Robotic facelift thyroidectomy: patient selection and technical considerations. Surg Laparosc Endosc Percutan Tech 21(4):237–42.
47. Wilhelm T, Metzig A (2011). Endoscopic minimally invasive thyroidectomy (eMIT): a prospective proof-of-concept study in humans. World J Surg 35(3):543–51
48. Shantz A, Castelman B (1973). Parathyroid carcinoma. A study of 70 cases. Cancer. 31:600–605.
49. Shane E (2001). Parathyroid carcinoma. J Clin Endocrinol Metab 86:485–493.
50. Clark-Duh-Kebebew (2005). Text Book of Endocrine Surgery 549-554 ISBN 0721601391
51. Koea JB, Shaw JH (1999). Parathyroid cancer: biology and management. Surg Oncol. 8:155–165.
52. Obara T, Fujimoto Y (1991). Diagnosis and treatment of patients with parathyroid carcinoma:an update and review. World J Surg 15:738-744.
53. Rosato L (2000) La patologia chirurgica della tiroide e delle paratiroidi 266-269. Grafica Santhiatese Editrice ISBN 8887374511
54. Shen W, Düren M, Morita E, et al (1996). Reoperation for persistent or recurrent hyperparathyroidism. Arch Surg 131: 861 – 869
55. Gary L. Clayman (2004). Parathyroid Carcinoma: Evaluation and Interdisciplinary Management. Cancer 5:900-905
56. Vetto JT, Brennan MF, Woodruf J, et al (1993). Parathyroid Carcinoma: diagnosis and clinical history. Surgery 114 (5):882-92

Non-invasive and Invasive Breast Cancer 14

Carlo Mariotti and Luis J. Sánchez

14.1 Introduction

There are 1 million cases of breast cancer (BC) worldwide. This statistic explains the extent to which the health sector and health policies are involved in dictating and supporting guidelines on behavior. The extent of BC results in several problems:

- Social: BC has an impact on the family and workplace, the organization of an adequate network of centers and hospital services, as well as staff training and related costs;
- Diagnosis: an early diagnosis is required in a large proportion of the female population;
- Therapeutic: due to the complexity and variety of treatment;
- Psychological: due to the overpowering impact on the female population;
- Rehabilitation for the family and social recovery of patients;
- Scientific: due to the possibility of carrying out research and the biological complexity of this tumor (which has already been well studied) so that research on BC can be a model for other types of cancer.

The upshot of these problems is national and international screening campaigns, social/health protection movements, as well as the pursuit of greater efficiency of detection (breast units, breast clinics). The latter is an issue of interest not only for major health organizations but also for politicians (European Parliament, Resolution 2002/2279). Non-invasive and invasive BC are different clinical entities and are described separately.

C. Mariotti (✉)
Azienda Ospedaliero-Universitaria "Ospedali Riuniti", Breast Surgery Unit
Ancona, Italy
e-mail: mariotticarlo@alice.it

L.J. Sánchez
Oncology, Breast Surgery Unit, Careggi Hospital, Florence, Italy

A. Valeri et al. (eds.), *What's New in Surgical Oncology*,
DOI: 10.1007/978-88-470-5310-6_14, © Springer-Verlag Italia 2013

14.2 Non-invasive Breast Cancer

According to the seventh edition of the cancer staging manual of the American Joint Committee on Cancer (AJCC), [1] three categories can be identified among non-invasive forms of BC or *in situ* types of BC (pTis). That is: ductal carcinoma *in situ* (DCIS); lobular carcinoma *in situ* (LCIS); and Paget's disease (PD), nipple areola *in situ* (without an associated intramammary DCIS or intramammary invasive BC).

14.2.1 Ductal Carcinoma in Situ (DCIS)

14.2.1.1 Epidemiology

The incidence of BC in Italy is 139/100.000 per year, and the incidence of mortality is 32/100.000 per year [2]. These values differ by ≤40% from northern to southern Italy. A national increase in incidence ranging from 2% to 17% has been recorded, but mortality has been declining from the 1990s in Italy (as in most developed countries). The incidence of DCIS (in particular and DCIS/invasive BC ratio) has been increasing. This is significantly related to the introduction of the screening programs which have been introduced in Italy and most of Europe. The results of IMPATTO project in Italy show this trend and that DCIS comprise 10–15% of all BC cases in Italy. This trend in the increasing number of DCIS diagnoses has been shifted to younger women not involved in screening programs, such as women aged <50 years [3]. This finding could be the effect of greater sensitivity of mammography and of spontaneous screening among different age cohorts. Such an increase has also been recorded in the USA, where screening programs are spontaneous. There is, however, a significant difference in percentages of DCIS and DCIS/invasive BC between Europe and the USA. Another difference is in grading and size of DCIS. This could be explained by differences in the approaches and standardization of diagnoses, though such differences have not been investigated.

Another issue is over-diagnosis. Would all the DCIS discovered by screening have developed into invasive BC and resulted in death, or could many of them have remained occult until the death of patients from different causes? Some cancers have a very slow rate of growth and favorable biology, so continuing research in this area might answer the question of over-diagnosis.

Although the introduction of screening programs correlates with higher rates of DCIS, there could be additional causes from different factors involved in BC pathogenesis.

14.2.1.2 Pathology

DCIS can be defined as a proliferation of malignant epithelial cells within mammary glandular structures without stromal invasion and breakdown of the basement membrane. According to Tavassoli et al., [4] DCIS can be classified within ductal intraepithelial neoplasia (DIN):

- DIN 1a: flat lesion with atypia;
- DIN 1b: atypical intraductal hyperplasia;
- DIN 1c: extended atypical intraductal hyperplasia: low grade DCIS;
- DIN 2: intermediate-grade DCIS;
- DIN 3: high-grade DCIS.

DCIS is a very diverse entity in terms of presentation, morphology, histology, biology and risk of progression towards invasive BC. The histologic classification of DCIS is based on three main features: type, grade, necrosis. The histotypes can be:

- Papillary/micropapillary;
- Cribriform;
- Solid;
- Comedo;
- Pleomorphic clinging type;
- Signet ring;
- Apocrine;
- Intracystic papillary;
- Cystic hypersecretory;
- Clear cell;
- Neuroendocrine;
- Spindle cell.

Necrosis can be central ("comedo") or focal ("punctuate").

Grading is very important because low-grade G1 DCIS and high-grade G3 DCIS are considered to be two distinct classes of BC due to their very different biomolecular characteristics. In a study conducted on the biological subtypes of DCIS, [5] it appears that basal-like subtypes are G3 in 84% of cases and G1–2 in only 16%. Luminal-A DCIS are G3 in 28% and G1–2 in 72% of cases. Luminal-B are G3 in 61% and G1–2 in 39%. Human epidermal growth factor receptor (HER)2+/estrogen receptor (ER)-DCIS are high grade in 92% of cases and low–intermediate in 8%. Thus, grading is a very important predicting factor for favorable/unfavorable biology. A pathology report for DCIS should always deatil: dimensions, margin status, histotype, grading, necrosis, and status of hormone receptors.

Microinvasive Breast Cancer (MIBC)

Although not part of non-invasive BC, MIBC should be dealt with as a part of DCIS because MIBC is often diagnosed after a preoperative diagnosis of DCIS (very rarely in LCIS cases).

Lagios et al. first introduced this term in 1982 to define DCIS with microscopic invasion <1 mm. Since then, many definitions have been reported, from differentiation between single-cell invasion and clusters or tubules of cells, to expression of the percentage (≤10%) of invasion seen among all the section examined. Other definitions have been stated even without defining the maximum extent of invasion.

In the seventh edition of the AJCC cancer staging manual (2010), as in previous editions, MIBC has a specific pT category: pT1mi. It is defined as invasive BC with a single focus <1mm or multiple foci with none of them measuring >1 mm in greatest dimension (without adding together all the different foci). In case of difficulties in reporting the number of foci, an estimate of such a number should be provided.

MIBC comprises 0.7–2.4% of all BC cases [6]. It is nearly always encountered in the setting of DCIS, less often in LCIS: this is why it is also referred to as "DCIS with microinvasion" (DCISM). Rare cases are encountered in the absence of non-invasive disease.

From a strict pathological perspective, the diagnosis of MIBC might be very challenging. Several artifacts may imitate such a condition. Therefore, immunohistochemistry is essential to clarify this situation, and several markers have been proposed. Myoepithelial cell markers (in particular, smooth muscle myosin heavy chain (SMM-HC), calponin and p63) are considered the most reliable.

The prognosis of MIBC is deemed to be intermediate between pure DCIS and early-stage BC. MIBC is an invasive BC and, as such, axillary staging is warranted, as well as taking into consideration adjuvant systemic therapy. Different definitions of MIBC, few cases, and short follow-ups hinder reliable clinical appraisal of MIBC. Two recent studies regarding axillary staging and clinical outcomes [7, 8] with a consistent number of cases and follow-up found axillary involvement after sentinel lymph-node biopsy (SLNB) in 12% and 10% of cases, respectively. In one of these studies, among the 14 cases deemed positive, out of 112 patients with DCISM who had SLNB, 6 were isolated tumor cells (ITCs), 5 were micrometastases and 3 were macrometastases. In the other study, among 68 cases of SLNB in MIBC, 3 patients had micrometastases and 4 had ITCs. Most authors recommend SLNB after a diagnosis of MIBC even though node involvement is quite rare and mostly micrometastatic. Furthermore, one could argue whether these micrometastases are prognostically important. Axillary involvement was not a prognostic risk factor for recurrences in these studies, but positive SLNB received chemotherapy and some of them had completion axillary lymph-node dissection (ALND), mostly with no further positive nodes. Completion ALND topic has been highlighted recently by the ACOSOG Z0011 trial for T1-2 BC. The results from this trial can also change the strategy for axilla management for MIBC. Further studies with larger cohorts and longer follow-up are necessary to draw conclusions about the routine use of SLNB in MIBC. In terms of immunophenotypes, ER, progesterone receptor (PR) and HER-2/neu status does not seem to be associated with recurrence [8].

14.2.1.3 Diagnosis

The first step in the diagnostic workup of DCIS is usually a mammographic X-ray (MXR). The signs of DCIS are most often microcalcifications (60% of cases). A nodule image is definitely less frequent (20%), along with architectural distortions and focal asymmetry (10% each).

In the case of microcalcifications in a MXR, diagnostic management is mainly based upon the BI-RADS classification set by the American College of Radiology (ACR). Grade 1 to grade 2 is benign and a further approach is not needed. Grade 3 warrants close follow-up at 6 months. For grades 4 and 5, immediate further investigations are necessary, such as fine-needle aspiration cytology (FNAC) or percutaneous biopsy.

A diagnosis of DCIS is possible only by biopsy because cytology cannot distinguish between a breakdown of the basement membrane of a cell or not. Nodules, unless clearly benign, should also be biopsied. When a diagnosis of DCIS has been reached (i.e., after the initial workup, physical examination, MXR and breast ultrasound), the need for MRI of the breast should be taken into account due to the multicentric nature of DCIS and its propensity to spread within the ductal tree. Breast MRI can give a better "map" of DCIS extension within the gland, showing areas of neoangiogenesis which have not developed microcalcifications and therefore did not appear at MXR. There is little accordance in the literature about this topic; a study published in *The Lancet* in 2007 [9] showed very good sensitivity for breast MRI in the diagnosis of DCIS (especially for high-grade tumors). A true and clear awareness of DCIS spread is essential to plan correct surgical interventions and achieve negative margins. The drawback of this imaging method is low specificity that mandates continuous comparison with conventional mammography and ultrasound.

14.2.1.4 Surgery

Surgery is the first therapeutic step after a DCIS diagnosis. Several surgical approaches can be chosen to treat DCIS: lumpectomy (if there is a palpable nodule), wide excision, quadrantectomy or mastectomy (usually skin- or nipple-sparing). These very diverse approaches are due to the difficult nature of DCIS, which can have intraductal spread throughout an entire ductal tree. In addition, DCIS can also exhibit peritumoral spread in a discontinuous fashion (Fig. 14.1).

These issues warrant thorough preoperative assessment (usually breast MRI). Most DCIS are non-palpable lesions (mostly microcalcifications) so careful preoperative localization of the index lesion is essential to guide the surgeon and avoid wider or incorrect excisions (unless mastectomy is the scheduled treatment). Such localization must be programmed preoperatively and undertaken by a radiologist using permanent dye, a radioisotope (radioguided occult lesion localization (ROLL)), a metal wire, or a gel-mark for the rare lesions seen only upon ultrasound.

Stereo-guided mammography is a technical method for localizing a non-palpable DCIS. Moreover, a clip must be left within the breast gland by the radiologist once carrying out percutaneous stereo-guided biopsy. This is because microcalcifications can be removed completely by the biopsy and because a clip can be used as a label by the surgeon after the excision. For non-palpable lesions treated by conservative procedures, the surgeon, in addition to the use of preoperative guides, ought to confirm the correctness of the excision

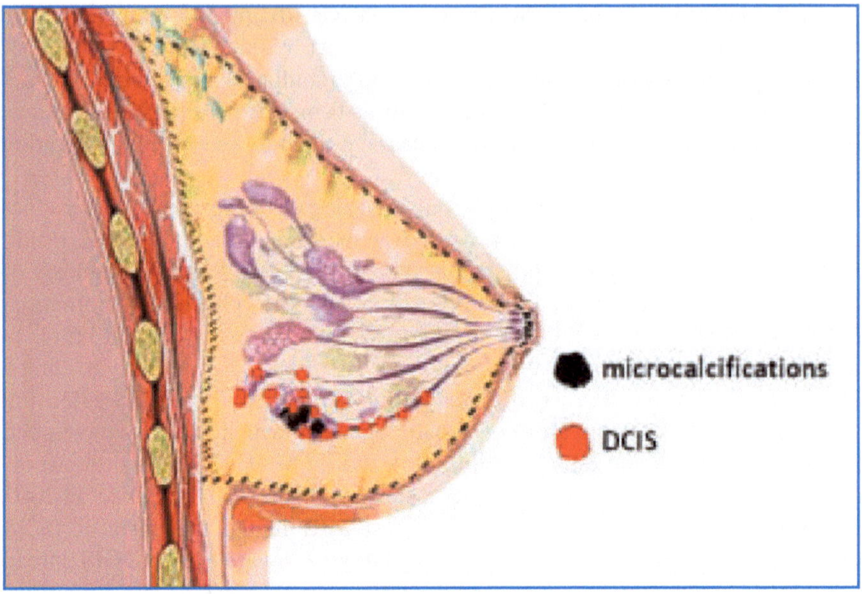

Fig. 14.1 Possible intraductal and discontinuous peritumoral spread of DCIS

through an intraoperative radiograph of the removed breast tissue. The radiograph can demonstrate the radiologic clip or the index microcalcifications, and give an idea of resection margins. Rarely, an ultrasound has to be carried out to confirm the lesion (or a gel-mark) in removed tissue if the tumor is not seen by mammography.

As mentioned above, mastectomy is sometimes necessary for DCIS. Three conditions mandate a mastectomy [10]: high tumor extension/breast volume ratio; multicentric tumors; postoperative radiotherapy (RT) is not possible.

If a conservative procedure is chosen, which minimum value of the margin value can be considered to be sufficient? This is definitively a controversial topic in the surgical treatment of DCIS. At the Philadelphia 1999 consensus conference [10] a 10-mm margin was deemed necessary. However, at the St. Gallen consensus conference in 2009, a 2-mm margin was considered acceptable. At the same consensus conference, for margins <2 mm, 48% of experts considered re-excision not to be necessary, whereas it was debatable for 9%, and absolutely necessary only for 43% of those present. RT is usually carried out after DCIS surgery, several authors from North America consider a margin to be negative if the tumor does not extend to the surface of the inked specimen.

In summary, because DCIS is, by definition, a local disease, appropriate local treatment with complete tumor removal is the primary goal of DCIS therapy. A failure in DCIS treatment is represented by local recurrence. Recurrences are invasive in 50% of cases and even more for young patients with G3, comedo-necrosis tumors.

Table 14.1 Van Nuys Prognostic Index

Score	Dimension (mm)	Margin Status (mm)	Histology	Age (years)
1	<15	>10	Non-high grade No necrosis Nuclear grade 1–2	>61
2	16–40	1–10	Non-high grade Necrosis Nuclear grade 1–2	40–60
3	>40	<1	High grade Nuclear grade 3	<39

A practical guide to local treatment is the validated van Nuys Prognostic Index (VNPI) score (Table 14.1). If the score ranges from 4 to 6, lumpectomy alone is sufficient; a score of 7 to 9 mandates radiotherapy; and a score of 10 to 12 necessitates mastectomy.

Axillary Surgery

Infiltration of lymphatic vessels and lymph-node involvement are, by definition, not possible for DCIS, because the basement membrane is not broken by tumor cells. Notwithstanding this principle, SLNB has a role in DCIS surgery. From 5% to 44% (mean, 20%) [11] of preoperative diagnoses of DCIS are micro-invasive or invasive cancers at definitive pathology report. Thus, a second intervention for axillary staging is necessary in such cases.

Another issue is positive SLNB at definitive pathology report, even in confirmed cases of DCIS (which has been estimated to be 3.7% in a recent study [12]). This could be interpreted as a pathology sampling failure and therefore a sign of infiltration or a sign of cell dislocation during diagnostic and surgical procedures.

No randomized trials have shed light on this topic. The choice to carry out SLNB in the case of a preoperative diagnosis of DCIS is based mainly on the *rationale* of avoiding further interventions. Several risk factors were identified in one study [13]. Four conditions can be identified as risk factors of invasion after a core biopsy diagnosis of DCIS:

- Palpable lump;
- Mass on mammography;
- Intermediate or poor tumor grade;
- Microcalcification area wider than 2.5 cm.

In the case of mastectomy, SLNB should always be done because this surgical procedure hinders the future possibility of undertaking SLNB. Some authors advocate that this policy should also apply to upper outer quadrant excisions.

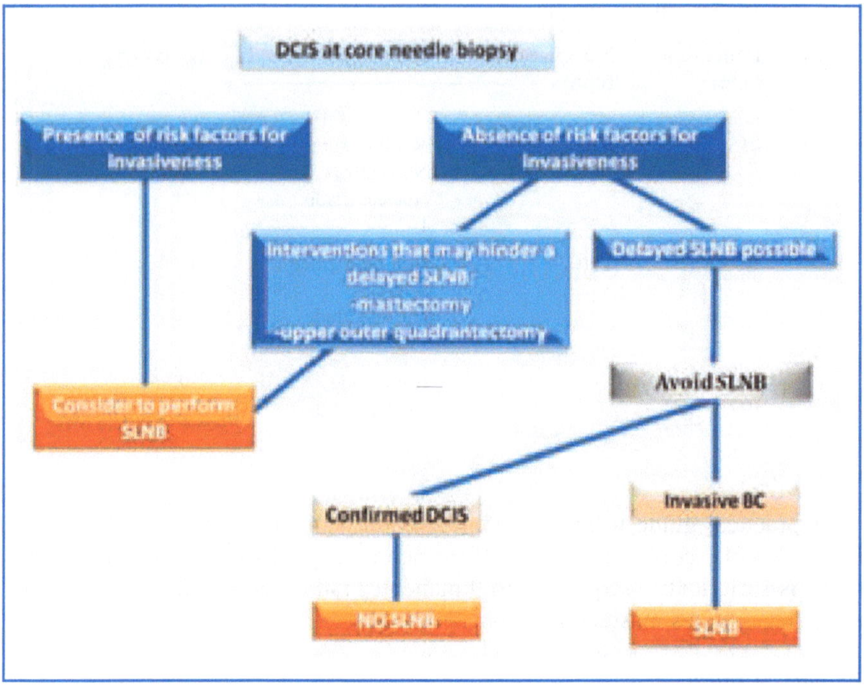

Fig. 14.2 Sentinel lymph node biopsy in ductal carcinoma *in situ*

In terms of everyday practice, the flowchart in Fig. 14.2 can be proposed as a guide for carrying out SLNB in DCIS.

14.2.1.5 Radiotherapy

The aim of local treatment of DCIS is avoidance of local recurrence, which is invasive in ≈50% of cases. To reach such a goal, RT is a crucial adjuvant support to surgical excision whenever a conservative approach is chosen.

Level-I evidence from four randomized clinical trials (NSABP B 17, EORTC 10853, SweDCIS Trial, UKCCCR Trial) suggests that RT reduces ipsilateral local recurrence by ≈50% compared with conservative resection alone. No differences were found in contralateral BC and mortality at 10 years. Whole-breast RT was the adopted modality. Results applied to all subgroups of patients. It was not possible to identify subset of patients who might avoid RT, as expressed in the VNPI. The VNPI was derived from a retrospective analysis and has not been validated (even by recent prospective analyses).

New recent modalities of RT are partial breast irradiation (PBI), also known as accelerated partial breast irradiation (APBI) and intraoperative radiation therapy (IORT), which is an intraoperative modality of PBI. Several methods using different energy sources have been described as external irradiation or as intracavitary or interstitial brachytherapy. The *rationale* for these novel methods is that local recurrence is mostly very near to the tumor bed and that recurrences "elsewhere" in the breast are <20% (<1% per year, similar to the value for contralateral tumors). Furthermore, these modalities reduce the conventional 5–7-week course of whole-breast irradiation to the same operative day or ≥4–5 postoperative days.

The primary purpose of selecting patients for APBI is to find a subgroup with a low risk of occult disease far from the lumpectomy site (or at least not too far) in an area not reached by the chosen APBI modality. Among all prospective non-randomized and randomized PBI trials with ≥4 year follow-up, none involved DCIS patients except for the American Society of Breast Surgeons MammoSite APBI trial. Therefore, PBI should be used with caution in DCIS cases outside a clinical trial. According to recommendations set by the Groupe Européen de Curiethérapie-European Society for Radiotherapy and Oncology (GEC-ESTRO), DCIS cases cannot be in low-risk groups, or be considered good candidates for PBI; instead, they should be regarded as intermediate-risk patients for PBI. Similarly, in the consensus statement provided by the American Society for Radiation Oncology (ASTRO), DCIS cases are not listed among the "suitable" cases for PBI, whereas they can be considered part of the "cautionary" group if the dimensions are <3 cm and "unsuitable" if >3 cm.

IORT is a type of PBI that uses a high, single dose irradiation as the sole or boost treatment at the resection site. It can also be used for nipple–areola treatment in case of nipple–areola-sparing mastectomy. This modality is carried out before the definitive pathology report, so thorough evaluation after the report is essential for selecting the appropriate therapy.

14.2.1.6 Systemic Therapy

Although DCIS is a local disease, individualized treatment for DCIS patients should also take into account systemic therapy. DCIS recurrences are invasive in ≈50% of cases, and a patient with a previous DCIS is a higher risk for contralateral BC. Just as RT reduces ispilateral local recurrence by ≈50%, it is well known (from randomized clinical trials) that tamoxifen reduces any breast cancer event (defined as combined ipsilateral plus contralateral breast events) by ≈30% [14] without any effect on overall survival. Therefore, it is reasonable to advise systemic treatment with tamoxifen to selected DCIS cases with hormone receptor-positivity. To identify subsets of patients who might benefit from systemic therapy, different approaches can be considered. A nomogram from Memorial Sloan–Kettering Cancer Center (MSKCC) has been proposed that considers conventional clinical and pathological parameters. Such a nomogram has not been validated from different institutions. In the near future, molecular profiling and molecular biology-based scores could potentially improve risk stratification for women with DCIS, helping to guide physicians and patients towards the correct therapeutic choice. There are ongoing trials aiming to find alternative treatments. These include aromatase inhibitors and anti-Her2 agents such as trastuzumab and lapatinib.

14.2.1.7 Follow-up

There is virtual general consensus among specialists involved in BC with regard to follow-up for DCIS patients: history-taking and physical examination every 6–12 months for 5 years and then annually, accompanied by annual mammography. Further investigations can be considered for those women treated by hormonal therapy.

14.2.2 Lobular Carcinoma In Situ (LCIS)

According to the 2003 World Health Organization (WHO) definition, non-invasive lobular carcinoma falls within the category of lobular intra-epithelial neoplasia (LIN), which comprises three identities:

- LIN 1: atypical lobular neoplasia or hyperplasia;
- LIN 2: lobular carcinoma *in situ*, classic type;
- LIN 3: lobular carcinoma *in situ* with central necrosis or pleomorphic type or with signet ring cells.

Since its first description in 1941 by Foote and Stewart, LCIS treatment has ranged from simple biopsy to bilateral mastectomy. This diversity (which in part is present today) is dependent upon whether it is considered to be a marker of increased BC for both breasts ("risk factor theory") or a real BC precursor ("precursor theory").

In a literature review spanning decades of LIN series [15], a detailed comparison of these theories was carried out. Recently, the precursor theory has gained respect after demonstration of a common lack of expression of the E-cadherin adhesion cell molecule for LIN and invasive lobular neoplasia, suggesting a possible transformation of LIN into invasive lobular BC. Moreover, BC, developed after diagnosis of LIN, is lobular in 30% of cases as compared with 16% in the general population. Usually, an ipsilateral BC develops in the same quadrant of LIN, and the rate of ipsilateral BC is slightly higher than contralateral BC (51% *vs* 41%, respectively). There are many issues favoring the isk factor theory: BC develops >10 years after a diagnosis of LIN in 50% of cases; the percentage of contralateral BC cases is not too different from ipsilateral invasive BC; the vast majority of BC, diagnosed after a LIN diagnosis, do not contain invasive lobular pathological features.

A LIN report after breast biopsy should prompt surgical local excision. Instead, some authors believe that proceeding with an excision is not necessary, but the possibility of cancer progression or of a surrounding DCIS (or even invasive BC) must be taken into account. Mastectomy (especially bilateral) is becoming outdated because LIN around an invasive BC does not have any effect on recurrence rate or survival. Thus, bilateral mastectomy can be deemed a level-V recommendation only. An important topic remains margin status. Absence of prospective randomized clinical trials and the paucity of cases in most studies limit any conclusions to be drawn. Guidelines are derived mostly from retrospective reviews and inferences from experts. Many

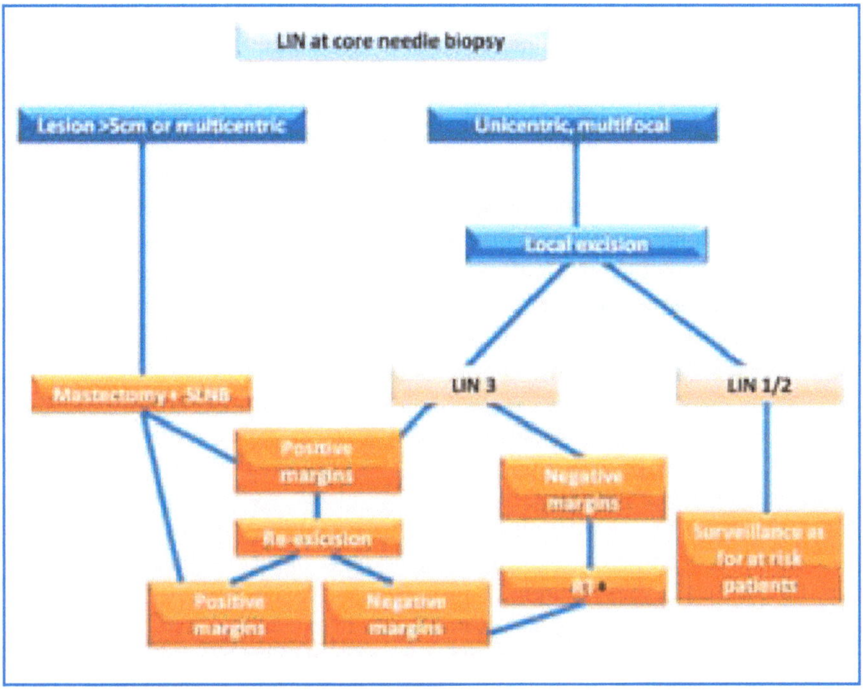

Fig. 14.3 Treatment for lobular carcinoma *in situ*. *To be evaluated case by case; LIN, lobular intra-epithelial neoplasia; SLNB, sentinel lymph-node biopsy; RT, radiotherapy

experts judge LIN 3 similar to DCIS and treat it equally.

If LCIS is interpreted to be a risk factor, a chemopreventive therapies could be proposed to patients. A National Surgical Adjuvant Breast and Bowel Project (NSABP) study showed that tamoxifen reduces the chances of development of invasive BC after LCIS in 56% of cases; the Study of Tamoxifen and Raloxifene (STAR) study showed similar results for raloxifene. The follow-up for LCIS can be planned as that for DCIS. Figure 14.3 can be proposed as a guide for LIN treatment.

14.2.3 Paget's Disease (PD)

PD of the breast was first detailed by James Paget in 1874. He described 15 women with chronic eczematous lesions of the nipple–areola skin with an associated intraductal carcinoma of the mammary gland.

PD is seen almost exclusively in women; male reports are anecdotal. The appearance of a nipple–areola chronic rash must be recognized promptly to initiate the appropriate diagnostic workup and detect underlying BC. A similar rash can be seen in the skin of external male and female genitalia, but this condition, known as extramammary PD, is not associated with breast PD in terms of pathophysiology and etiology.

The origin of PD can be traced to the superficial extension (epidermotropism) of malignant ductal epithelial cells derived from the underlying breast gland or an intraepidermal origin ("*in situ* transformation theory"), as described by Muir in 1939. Malignant cells extend from luminal lactiferous ductal epithelium and infiltrate the epidermis, causing the well-known chronic rash. Most dedicated studies have shown shared genetic changes and biomarkers between PD cells and underlying breast adenocarcinoma cells. The exact worldwide frequency of PD is not known, but ≈1–3% of BC are associated with PD and nearly 90–100% of PD have a DCIS or invasive BC in the gland beneath (either identifiable or not). If there are imaging findings of breast lesions associated with PD, these are invasive BC in 90% of cases and only 10% in DCIS whereas, for PD lesions without any other finding, a DCIS is found in ≈70% of cases in the gland beneath and invasive BC in the remaining 30% [16].

Once signs and symptoms such as rash, itch, erythema, burning and sometimes bloody nipple discharge (associated with skin thickening and nipple inversion) raise the suspicion of PD, a diagnostic workup must be started. Physical examination, MXR, ultrasound and cytology testing by nipple–areola scraping are the first step. If negative, a dermatology consultation and short-term follow-up (2 weeks) might be a sensible option. Otherwise, if treatment for a positive or suspicious lesion has to be taken, after considering further investigations such as breast MRI, the mammary gland should be evaluated. In the case of negative tests, but very suspicious physical examination, a full-thickness biopsy must be undertaken. If an associated breast lesion is identified, histologic confirmation should be completed. Confirmed BC with suspicious PD requires full-thickness skin biopsy to rule out possible associated PD.

Eventually, after the diagnostic workup, two situations can be outlined: PD with associated BC or PD without an identifiable underlying BC. The former case has to be treated according to BC stage. Surgical excision must include the nipple–areola complex (NAC) in continuity or not with the BC. Adjuvant therapies are chosen based on the parameters of BC. PD can be addressed only with the following surgical options: central quadrantectomy including NAC excision, simple mastectomy, or skin-sparing mastectomy. These options have different reconstruction options. Axillary staging with a SLB is a sensible choice if mastectomy is carried out for DCIS and conservative procedures because of the high number of invasive BC associated [15]. In case of a breast-conservation surgery, RT is indicated afterwards to provide a boost to the surgical site. As for DCIS, patients with treated PD are at a higher risk of developing any BC event in the future, which is why systemic therapy with tamoxifen is a viable option to be discussed with the patient.

14.3 Invasive Breast Cancer

According to the seventh edition of the AJCC cancer staging manual, the categories of BC detailed in Table 14.2 can be identified [1]. Please also see Figs 14.4–14.6.

Table 14.2 Categories of breast cancer as stipulated by the AJCC

pT1: Tumor 2 cm or less in greatest dimension
- **pT1mi**: Microinvasion 0.1 cm or less
- **pT1a**: More than 0.1 cm but not more than 0.5 cm
- **pT1b**: More than 0.5 cm but not more than 1 cm
- **pT1c**: More than 1 cm but not more than 2 cm

pT2: Tumor 2–5 cm across
pT3: Tumor greater than 5 cm across
pT4: Tumor of any size with direct extension to chest wall* and/or to skin (ulceration or skin nodules)
- **Pt4a**: chest wall
- **pT4b**: ulceration, ipsilateral satellite skin nodules, or skin edema (including *peau d'orange*)
- **pT4c**: 4a and 4b above
- **pT4d**: inflammatory carcinoma (diffuse, brawny induration of the skin with an erysipeloid edge, usually with no underlying mass)

Regional lymph nodes (pN)
- Axillary (ipsilateral): interpectoral (Rotter) nodes and lymph nodes along the axillary vein and its tributaries;
- Infraclavicular (subclavicular) (ipsilater);
- Internal mammary (ipsilateral);
- Supraclavicular.

Note: Intramammary lymph nodes are coded as axillary lymph nodes level I.
Note: Any other lymph node metastasis is coded as a distant metastasis (pM1) (cervical or controlateral internal mammary lymph nodes)

pNx Regional lymph node cannot be assessed
pN0 No regional lymph node metastasis
pN0(sn) No sentinel lymph node metastasis

Isolated tumor cells (ITCs)
pN0(i-) No regional lymph node metastasis histologically, negative morphological findings (E&E) for ITC
pN0(i+) No regional lymph node metastasis histologically, positive morphological findings (E&E) for ITC
pN0(mol-) No regional lymph node metastasis histologically, negative non-morphological (RT-PCR) findings for ITC
pN0(mol+) No regional lymph node metastasis histologically, positive non-morphological (RT-PCR) findings for ITC

ITCs in sentinel lymph nodes
pN0(sn)(i-)
pN0(sn)(i+)
pN0(sn)(mol-)
pN0(sn)(mol+)
pN1mic: Micrometastasis

Larger than 0.2 mm and/or more than 200 cells, but none larger than 2 mm (Fig. 14.4)
- **pN1a:** Metastasis in 1–3 axillary lymph node(s)
- **pN1b:** Internal mammary lymph nodes with microscopic or macroscopic metastasis detected by sentinel lymph node biopsy but not detected clinically

(*cont.*) →

*The chest wall includes the ribs, intercostal muscles, and serratus anterior muscle but not the pectoral muscle

Table 14.2 (*continued*)

- **pN1c**: Metastasis in 1–3 axillary lymph nodes and internal mammary lymph nodes with microscopic or macroscopic metastasis detected by sen tinel lymph node biopsy but not detected clinically
- **pN2a:** Metastasis in 4–9 ipsilateral axillary lymph nodes
- **pN2b:** Metastasis in clinically detected internal mammary lymph node(s) in the absence of axillary lymph node metastasis
- **pN3a:** Metastasis in 10 or more axillary lymph nodes or metastasis in infraclavic lar lymph nodes
- **pN3b:** Metastasis in clinically detected internal mammary lymph node(s) in the pre ence of positive axillary lymph node(s)
- **pN3c:** Metastasis in ipsilateral supraclavicular lymph node(s)

Metastasis (M)
cM0: clinically no distant metastasis
cM1: distant metastasis clinically (e.g., colon cancer with liver metastasis based on CT)
pM1: distant metastasis proven microscopically (e.g., needle biopsy)
pMX does not exist; **pM0** does not exist (except at autopsy)
If a cM1 (e.g., liver metastasis) is biopsied and is negative, it becomes cM0, not pM0
pM – distant metastasis
PUL Pulmonary
OSS Osseous
BRA Brain
LYM Lymph nodes
MAR Bone marrow
PLE Pleura
PER Peritoneum
ADR Adrenals
SKI Skin
OTH Others

Stage grouping
Combining the five categories of T for a hypothetical tumor with the three categories of N and the two categories of M results in various categories of TNM. These can be condensed into a smaller number of stages. The adopted stratification ensures (as far as possible) that each stage is fairly homogeneous with respect to survival.

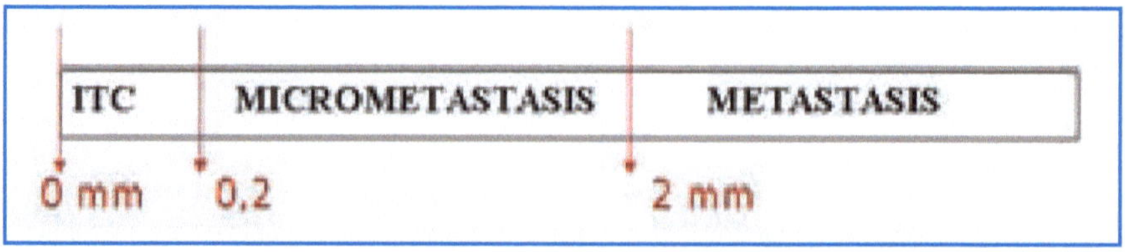

Fig. 14.4 Axillary lymph-node involvement

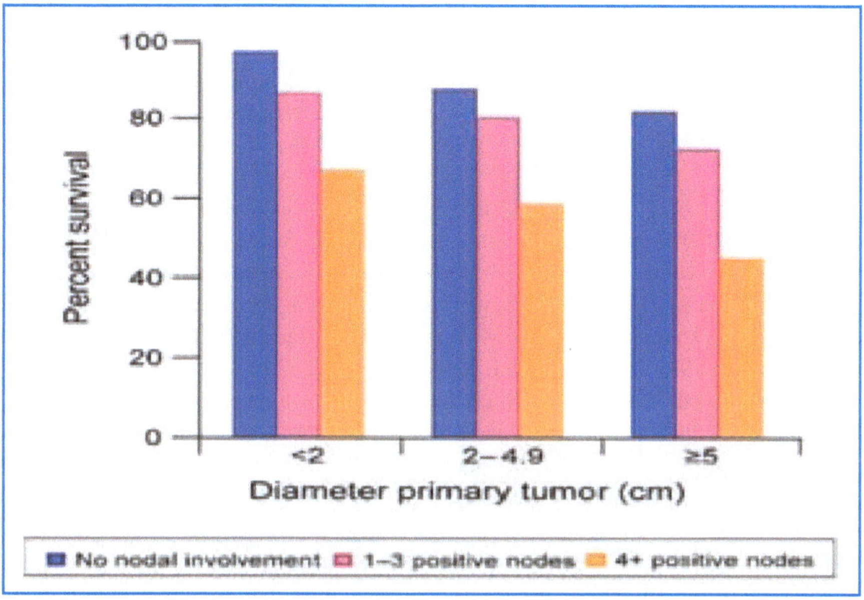

Fig. 14.5 Percentage survival at 5 years according to size of primary tumor and number of nodes involved. Material from AJCC Cancer Staging Manual (7th edition). Reproduced with permission from the AJCC

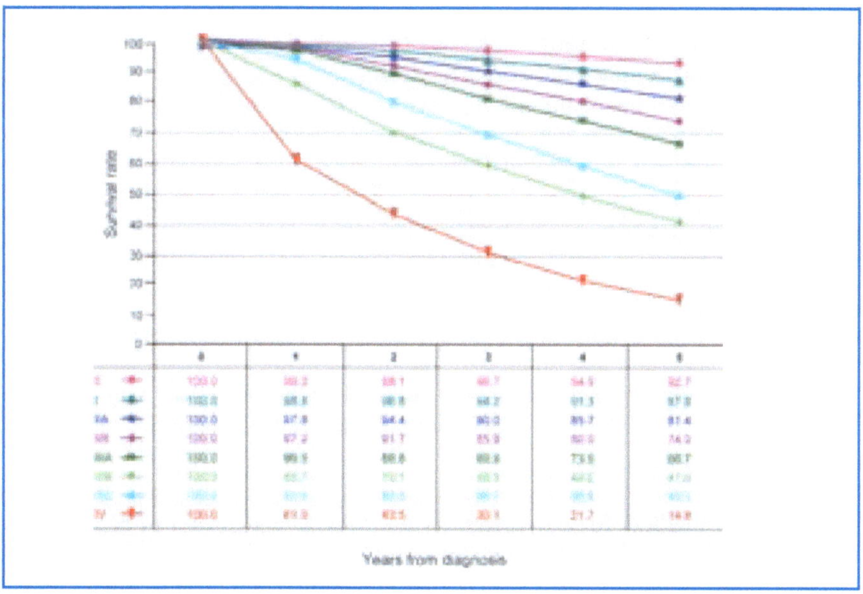

Fig. 14.6 Survival according to AJCC stage. Material from AJCC Cancer Staging Manual (7th edition). Reproduced with permission from the AJCC

14.3.1 Epidemiology

BC is the most common tumor in women; 1 out of 3 malignant tumors is a breast carcinoma (29%). These poor statistics occur in all the age groups that we have taken into consideration (0–49 years, 40%; 40–69 years, 35%; >70 years, 20%).

The geographical distribution in Italy indicates a greater incidence in the north (123/100,000 inhabitants) when compared with the center (103/100,000 inhabitants) and the south (87/100,000). These data reflect a probable different distribution of risk factors as well as an uneven implementation of breast screening. Moreover, ≈50,000 new cases are predicted in 2020 (with a percentage increase of 9.6%, and 500,000 new cases for 2030 (+15.6 %)).

The trend in mortality in 2011 showed that this was the main cause of death in females (≈12,000). For >20 years, there has been a moderate (but continuous) decreasing trend in mortality due to BC (≈1.7% per year). This is probably due to the effort to carry out early diagnosis of the disease and, undoubtedly, the consistent development in knowledge and treatment.

Finally, survival for 5 years from the diagnosis is on the increase; 81% for women affected in 1994, 87% for women affected between 2000 and 2004; specifically, 98% of those women with localized disease, 84% of those women with locoregional disease; and 27% of those patients diagnosed with and treated for diffused disease.

The reported data, alarming when viewed in terms of incidence (especially with regard to young women) is reassuring given the increase in survival. These significant considerations can be attributed to various factors:

- Diagnostic procedures and early diagnosis;
- New interpretations of the disease;
- New principles of correlated treatment.

14.3.2 Diagnosis

Technological progress has also affected diagnostic procedures. Identification of a test (mammography) to build a research network (screening) in the female population of a certain age range with the aim of achieving an early diagnosis is the main factor for the increase in survival in invasive and non-invasive cases. Conversely, there have been developments in equipment and its use in diagnostic procedures.

Mammography is the best diagnostic test to study the mammary gland. Digital methodologies such as tomosynthesis are further improvements of this methodology and refinement of obtained information.

Ultrasound is widely used and is of fundamental importance for experts. Among other developments, there are contrast agents and elastography. The latter is used to study axillary lymph nodes and, in particular, it is used by surgeons intraoperatively if localization of lesions is difficult.

In the last twenty years, MRI has been applied to the study of the breast. However, its use in diagnostic pathways is often mistakenly defined. This methodology, when staging breast tumors, can be of fundamental importance if supported by other imaging methodologies, clinical evaluation and preoperative histological findings to evaluate the type and scale of surgery, assessment of the response to medical therapy, reconstructive surgery and follow-up [16].

14.3.2.1 What to Expect from the MRI and Other Imaging Methods

1. Local staging:
   - Location and size;
   - Multifocality;
   - Multicentricity;
   - Bilaterality;
   - Assessment of the intraductal component in DCIS;
   - Assessment of infiltration in DCIS;
   - Assessment of DCIS extension and grading;
   - Assessment of borderline lesions (e.g., ADH, LCIS) for surgical indications.
2. Study of lymph-node involvement;
3. Study of the response to primary systemic therapy (timing, spatial definition of progression or reduction, modality of spatial reduction, choice of surgical approach) [17];
4. Evaluation of "possible" local relapse after QUART
5. Identification of primary occult cancer in case of axillary lymph-node metastasis (CUP syndrome) [18];
6. Study of the anatomical relationship between neoplasia and the mammary gland (skin, nipple) when planning surgery;
7. Measurement of mammary volume to design esthetic and/or reconstructive surgery (choice of implant, type, shape and size, with the availability of three-dimensional reconstruction of images);
8. Assessment of prosthetic implant (breaking, rotation of residual glands).

14.3.3 Pathology: from Morphological Data to Molecular Classification

The last 15 years have been characterized by appreciable advances in the pathological understanding of invasive BC. In particular, morphological data have been supported by the development of biomolecular assessments. Identification of the new biological aspects of invasive BC has been critical for the therapeutic approach (locoregional and systemic) (Tables 14.3 and 14.4).

Table 14.3 Histologic classification of breast cancer

- Carcinoma, NOS (not otherwise specified)
- Ductal
  intraductal (*in situ*)
  invasive with predominant intraductal component
  invasive, NOS
  comedo
  inflammatory
  medullary with lymphocytic infiltrate
  mucinous (colloid)
  papillary
  scirrhous
  tubular
  other
- Lobular
  in situ
  invasive with predominant *in situ* component
  invasive
- Nipple
  Paget's disease, NOS
  Paget's disease with intraductal carcinoma
  Paget's disease with invasive ductal carcinoma
- Other
  undifferentiated carcinoma

Table 14.4 Molecular classification of the subtypes of breast cancer

Luminal A	ER- and/or PgR-positive HER2-negative Ki-67 low (<14%)
Luminal B (1)	ER- and/or PgR-positive HER2-negative Ki-67 high
Luminal B (2)	ER- and/or PgR-positive Any Ki-67 HER2 overexpressed or amplified
Erb-B2 overexpression	HER2 overexpressed or amplified ER and PgR absent
Basal-like "Triple negative (ductal)"	ER and PgR absent HER2-negative

14.3.4 Surgery

A historical breakthrough in the surgical treatment of BC was made in the 1980s. Thanks also to the Italian School [19–21], the entire manner of treating BC has been revolutionized; "from the maximum tolerable treatment to the least effective treatment", conservative surgery as treatment for BC went beyond purely surgical facts and became a new philosophy, as well as a new way of handling and approaching patients.

The following years brought scientific confirmation and the consolidation of ideas. The conservative cycle initially focused on glandular surgery (breast-conservation therapy (BCT), and later responsible of influencing another oncological dogma–axillary lymphadenectomy–by introducing SLNB. Later it enrolled RT, which became increasingly partial breast irradiation (PBI), intra-operative or postoperative. Finally, oncoplastic surgery and conservative mastectomy, a step closer to less aggressive surgery, customized to individual cases, based on the instrumental, pathological or clinical data, and discussed and agreed with the patient. Therefore, the key points of surgical treatment are:

- Detailed study of the disease (imaging, histological and biological assessment) and of the patient;
- Choice of surgical treatment discussed and agreed with the patient;
- Local tumor control
  centering of lesion
  complete removal with free margins
  correct sending of surgical specimens to the pathologist (patient details, orientation of piece, specimen fixation);
- Esthetic (functional result).

The indications for BCT are:

- T <3 cm, N0–1a;
- No multifocality or multicentricity;
- Good esthetic results as expected;
- Easy access to RT;
- Availability of follow-up.

The absolute contraindications are:

- I and II trimesters of pregnancy;
- Multicentricity;
- Previous RT;
- Persistent positive margins after surgical treatments.

These are the "historical" indications for conservative surgery. Studies throughout these years, and the confirmations obtained through data, have led to revisiting clinical cases in which conservative surgery could be used to add innovative oncoplastic surgical methods: large tumors (T2 lesions), tumors with an extensive intraductal component, lobular histology, risk of close margins, and an unfavorable ratio between breast volume and tumor size [22–24].

The term "oncoplastic surgery" denotes integration of the principles and methods of oncological surgery with those of plastic surgery according to radical local treatment with excellent esthetic and functional outcomes [25, 26].

Oncoplastic surgery methodologies are commonly used for patients who undergo major resection of the breast gland (25–40 %), patients who in the past would undergone radical surgery. There are numerous methods that require a learning curve and may be employed collaboratively in a multidisciplinary team.

The indications for an oncoplastic approach are shown in Table 14.5.

Table 14.5 Indications for an oncoplastic approach to breast-conservation therapy

• **Oncologic**
Wide excision required;
Gain clear margin;
Poor indication for radiotherapy and/or mastectomy with reconstruction (age, large breast, comorbidity);
Patient desires to keep her breast.
• **Cosmetic**
High tumor/breast ratio (>20%);
Tumor location: central, inferior, medial;
Tumor size;
Patient desires volume reduction.

The choice of method is linked to the location, size and characteristics of the breast, the patient's requests, the need for symmetry, and previous interventions. Often, the choice is linked to the habits and knowledge of the medical team.

Oncoplastic techniques mainly consist of:

- Volume-displacement procedures: breast-conservation surgery with parenchymal remodeling based on tumor location;
- Volume-replacement procedures: breast-conservation surgery with adjacent or distant tissue transfer (latissimus dorsi flap, lateral thoracic flap).

We will not provide here a detailed description of the individual surgical methods. Instead, a personal classification of oncoplastic methods will be presented and the reader should refer to the individual cases for further information (Table 14.6).

Table 14.6 Classification of oncoplastic surgical procedures

A. Breast-conservation surgery without NAC recentralization
Local glandular flaps
B. Breast-conservation surgery with NAC recentralization
Inferior pedicle mammoplasty
Superior pedicle mammoplasty (inverted T-scar)
V or J-mammoplasty
Horizontal mammoplasty (batwing mastopexy)
Racqet technique
Grisotti flap (advancement and rotation)
Round block technique (Benelli)
C. Breast-conservation surgery and reconstruction with autologous tissues
Local flaps
Rhomboid flap
Lateral thoracic flaps
- TDAP (thoraco-dorsal artery perforator)
- Lateral thoracic flap/ Subaxillary flap
- Intercostal perforator flap
- Segmental latissimus dorsi (miniflap)

(*cont.*) →

Table 14.6 (*continued*)

Free flaps
- DIEP (deep inferior epigastric perforator)
- SIEA (superficial inferior epigastric artery)
- SGAP (superior gluteal artery perforator)
- IGAP (inferior gluteal artery perforator)
- TMG (transverse myocutaneous gracilis)
- Free TRAM (transverse rectus abdominis myocutaneous)
D. Conservative mastectomies
Skin-sparing mastectomy
Nipple-sparing mastectomy
Skin-reducing mastectomy
E. Breast-conservation surgery and reconstruction with fat trasposition

14.3.4.1 Conservative Mastectomies

Conservative mastectomies (skin-sparing mastectomy, SSM, skin-reducing mastectomy, SRM, and nipple-sparing mastectomy, NSM, are at the forefront of conservative surgery. Actually, this is the implementation of a conservative attitude in radical surgery. In reality, NSM (or NAC-sparing mastectomy) leaves behind old concepts preserving the NAC, and is thought as representing the foremost feature in oncoplastic surgery with oncological radical surgery and excellent esthetic results. It is not a new type of surgery, rather it is the revisiting of an old surgical technique with oncological purposes: the subcutaneous mastectomy. The indications for conservative mastectomies are shown in Table 14.7.

This type of surgery involves attentive and thorough assessment of the case and patient, in particular regarding:

- Lesion size, histology and location;
- Staging of the disease and anamnestic data of chemotherapy;
- Breast size and degree of ptosis;
- Comorbidities (diabetes, tobacco smoking, vascular disease);
- Physical status (ability to walk, weight, BMI);
- Characteristics of the tissue (areola, skin, muscles);
- Assessment of the contralateral breast;
- Assessment of flap donor areas;
- Environment.

The reconstruction time may be as follows:

- Single-stage with a permanent implant;
- Double-stage with expander;
- Single-stage with a permanent implant and biological (e.g., acellular dermal matrices, ADM) synthetic mesh;
- With autologous flaps;
- With fat transplantation.

Table 14.7 Indications for conservative mastectomies

A. Oncologic

- Multifocal DCIS;
- Multifocal and multicentric T1 and T2;
- T1 with extensive intraductal component (EIC)
- Margin involvement after conservative surgery;
- High tumor/breast ratio;
- Relapse post-QUART;
- Patient refuses BCT;
- Patient refusal or impossibility of radiotherapy;
- Difficulty for follow-up after conservative surgery.

B. Prophylactic

BRCA1/BRCA2 (risk reduction, 81–96%);
Opposite breast;
LCIS;
ADH?
Papillomatosis?
Phyllodes tumor?

C. Contraindications

- Tumor distance <2 cm from NAC in mammography or RM studies;
- Nipple retraction;
- Subareolar microcalcifications;
- Bleeding from the nipple;
- Skin involvement;
- T3, T4;
- Inflammatory disease;
- Paget's disease;
- N+ ??
- Distance from the nipple to the infra-mammary fold >8 cm;
- Large breast (>400 cm^3);
- Intraoperative histologic involvement of retroareolar tissue.

14.3.5 Complications

The main complications of BC surgery are listed in Table 14.8.

We must remember that breast conservation is a priority for patients with BC. Most women who undergo mastectomy could be candidates for an NSM, but the applicability of NSM must not increase the number of mastectomies.

NAC-sparing mastectomy seems to be a further step in the conservative procedure of BC treatment; it is highly difficult but difficulties can be overcome with an adequate period of training. We must highlight the necessity for a scrupulous choice of cases, careful design of surgery, which is discussed and agreed with the patient who has been informed of all difficulties (some of which are still present) regarding this innovative surgical procedure.

The results are very reassuring from an oncological viewpoint, excellent from an esthetic perspective, and preservation of the NAC enhances the reconstructive result.

Table 14.8 Main complications of breast cancer surgery

1 Minor
cyanosis/hypopigmentation of the NAC;
localized infection;
2 Major
NAC ischemia (in 30%);
NAC necrosis;
flap necrosis (more frequent if risk factors such as diabetes and smoking are present (5–8%));
seroma
bleeding/hematoma;
implant infection (2.8–15 %).
3 Late
extended and retracted scar;
nipple or skin area retraction;
bad positioning/displacement of the NAC;
changes in the sensitivity and erectile function of the nipple;
capsular retraction;
bad positioning of the implant;
rotation of the implant;
evident breast asymmetry;
cancer recurrence (4–5%).

14.4 The Problem of the Axillary Lymph Nodes

Removal of the axillary lymph nodes has always been involved in BC surgery. The *rationale* for the removal of the axillary lymph nodes lies in optimization of the locoregional blockage of the disease and, specifically, the achievement of effective staging that makes it possible to carry out a prognostic and decision-making assessment on adjuvant postoperative treatment.

For years, axillary staging was the key parameter of reference in deciding postoperative systemic treatments. Today, lymph-node data (although still relevant) form a part of a set of biopathologic elements (ER and PgR, Ki-67, HER2, grading, size of tumor, menopausal status) that determine assessment of the disease and the implications for treatment.

Up to the end of the 1990s, lymph-node status was entrusted to radical axillary dissection regardless of the characteristics (T, N) of the tumor. Thanks to mammographic screening and awareness gained by the female population, ≈80% of patients reach surgery with a small invasive tumor with a probability of lymph-node metastases amounting to ≈25%. Consequently, ≈75% of the removals of the axillary lymph nodes that used to be carried out in these cases was ineffectual.

Introduction of SLNB has taken conservative surgery a step further.SLNB is standard in procedures on axillary lymph nodes in females with invasive breast tumors [27, 28].

The SLN can be defined as the first axillary lymph node that receives lymph from the breast. Its identification is carried out with subcutaneous inoculation of albumin aggregates marked with radioactive technetium in the periareolar region. Identification of the sentinel lymph node in the axilla is 92–98% with a correlation of 97.5–100% between the SLNB and complete ALND. The rate of false negatives is 8.8% when ALND is considered to be the "gold standard".

If the sentinel lymph node is positive, there is a ≈40% chance of other lymph node metastases. The in-depth study of sentinel lymph nodes has led to the characterization of other pathological features of axillary lymph nodes besides negative or metastatic lymph nodes, such as lymph node with ITC (isolated tumor cells), micro-metastatic or metastatic.

The prognostic significance of micro-metastasis in lymph nodes is not well-defined: numerous studies have been carried out, but often using very few cases and non-homogeneous treatment. The impression (which has to be validated) is that there are no significant differences between disease-free survival and overall survival in patients who have undergone a second ALND and patients who have started the follow-up. A recent study carried out by Giuliano et al., (ACOSOG-Z0011) who hypothesized that abstention from axillary dissection should occur even in the presence of metastatic sentinel lymph nodes, has caused controversy as well as doubts and, perhaps, may encourage dangerous developments. Nevertheless, guidelines (FONCAM 2005, ASCO 2005) suggest that axillary dissection in cases of micro-metastatic and macro-metastatic cancer is warranted [29, 30]. Therefore, the action might be:

- sentinel lymph node ITC + no axillary dissection;
- sentinel lymph node with micro-metastasis: no axillary dissection?
- metastatic sentinel lymph node: axillary dissection or send to follow-up after deepening of single case features within a multidisciplinary team meeting.

14.5 Conclusions

"...the breast surgeon must be able to offer every woman with breast cancer:

- The option of preserving the breast;
- The option of undergoing conservative mastectomy;
- The correction of asymmetry or size defect;
- More and more advanced reconstructive surgical techniques..." [32].

References

1. Edge SB, Byrd DR, Compton CC (2010) (eds) AJCC Cancer Staging Manual. 7th edn. Springer, New York
2. Zanetti R, Gafà L, Panneli F et al (2002) Cancer in Italy 1993-1998: incidence data from cancer registries. Il Pensiero Scientifico Editore

3. Giorgi D, Giordano L, Ventura L et al (2010) Mammography screening in Italy: 2008 survey. Epidemiol Prev 34(5-6 Suppl 4):9-25
4. Tavassoli FA (2001) Ductal intraepithelial neoplasia of the breast. Virchows Arch 238(3):221-227
5. Livasy CA, Perou CM, Karaca G et al (2007) Identification of a basal-like subtype of breast ductal carcinoma in situ. Hum Pathol 38(2):197-204
6. Bianchi S, Vezzosi V (2008) Microinvasive carcinoma of the breast. Pathol Oncol Res 14:105-111
7. Lyons JM, Stempel M, Van Zee KJ et al (2012) Axillary node staging for microinvasive breast cancer: is it justified? Ann Surg Oncol 19:3416-3421
8. Margalit DN, Sreedhara M, Chen YH et al (2013) Microinvasive breast cancer: ER, PR, and HER-2/neu status and clinical outcomes after breast conserving therapy or mastectomy. Ann Surg Oncol 20:811-818
9. Kuhl CK, Schrading S, Bieling HB (2007) MRI for diagnosis of pure ductal carcinoma in situ: a prospective observational study. Lancet 370(9586):485-492
10. Schwartz GF, Solin LJ, Olivotto IA et al (2000) Consensus conference on the treatment of In Situ Ductal Carcinoma of the Breast. April 22-25, 1999. Cancer 88(4):946-954
11. Han JH, Molberg KH, Sarode V (2011) Predictors of Invasion and Axillary Lymph Node Metastasis in Patients with a Core Biopsy Diagnosis of Ductal Carcinoma In Situ: An Analysis of 255 Cases. Breast J 3:223-229
12. Ansari B, Ogston SA, Purdie CA et al (2008) Meta-analysis of sentinel node biopsy in ductal carcinoma in situ of the breast. Br J Surg 95:547-554
13. Meijnen P, Oldenburg HSA, Loo CE et al (2007) Risk of invasion and axillary lymph node metastasis in ductal carcinoma in situ diagnosed by core-needle biopsy. Br J Surg 94:952-956
14. Solin LJ (2012) Selecting Individualized Treatment for Patients With Ductal Carcinoma in Situ of the Breast: The Search Continues. J Clin Oncol 30(6):577-579
15. Ansquer Y, Delaney S, Santulli P et al (2010) Risk of invasive breast cancer after lobular intra-epithelial neoplasia: Review of the literature. Eur J Surg Oncol 36:604-609
16. Sukumvanich P, Bentrem DJ, Cody HS et al (2007) The Role of Sentinel Lymph Node Biopsy in Paget's Disease of the Breast. Ann Surg Oncol 14(3):1020-1023
17. Sardanelli F , Giuseppetti GM, Canavese G (2008) Indications for breast magnetic resonance imaging. Consensus document "Attualità in Senologia" Florence 2007. Radiol Med 113:1085-1095
18. Kim HJ, Im YH, Han BK et al (2007) Accuracy of MRI for estimating residual tumor size after neoadjuvant chemotherapy in locally advanced breast cancer:relation to response pattern on MRI Acta Oncologica 46: 996-1003
19. De Bresser J, De Vos B, Van der Ent F et al (2010) Breast MRI in clinically and mammographically occult breast cancer presenting with an axillary metastasis: a systematic review. EJSO 36:114-119
20. Veronesi U, Cascinelli N, Mariani L et al (2002) Twenty-year follow-up of a randomized study comparing breast-conserving surgery with radical mastectomy for early breast cancer. N Engl J Med 347:1227-32
21. Veronesi U, Salvadori B, Luini A et al (1995) Breast conservation is a safe method in patients with small cancer of the breast. Long-term results of three randomised trials on 1,973 patients. Eur J Cancer 31:1574-9
22. van Dongen JA, Voogd AC, Fentiman IS et al (2000) Long-term results of a randomized trial comparing breast-conserving therapy with mastectomy: European Organization for Research and Treatment of Cancer 10801 trial. J Natl Cancer Inst 92:1143-50
23. Freedman GM, Anderson PR, Li T et al (2009) Locoregional recurrence of triple-negative breast cancer after breast-conserving surgery and radiation. Cancer 115:946-51
24. Holland R, Connolly JL, Gelman R et al (1990) The presence of an extensive intraductal component following a limited excision correlates with prominent residual disease in the remainder of the breast. J Clin Oncol 8:113-8

25. Renton SC, Gazet JC, Ford HT et al (1996) The importance of the resection margin in conservative surgery for breast cancer. Eur J Surg Oncol 22:17-22
26. Losken A, Jones GE (2010) Oncoplastic breast-conserving surgery. In: Jones GE (ed) Bostwick's Plastic & Reconstructive surgery. Third edition. Quality Medical Publishing, St. Louis, pp 1495-1546
27. Clough KB,Kaufman GJ, Nos C (2010) Improving breast cancer surgery: a classification and quadrant per quadrant atlas for oncoplastic surgery. Ann Surg Oncol 17:1375-1391
28. Veronesi U, Paganelli G, Galimberti V et al (1997) Sentinel-node biopsy to avoid axillary dissection in breast cancer with clinically negative lymph-nodes. Lancet 349:1864-7
29. Veronesi U, Paganelli G, Viale G et al (1999) Sentinel lymph node biopsy and axillary dissection in breast cancer: results in a large series. J Natl Cancer Inst 91:368-73
30. Goldhirsch A, Wood WC, Coates AS et al (2011) Strategies for subtypes-dealing with the diversity of breast cancer: highlights of the ST Gallen International Expert Cansensus on the primary therapy of early breast cancer 2011. Ann Oncol 22:1736-47
31. Giuliano AE, Hunt KK, Ballman KV et al (2011) Axillary dissection vs no axillary dissection in women with invasive breast cancer and sentinel node metastasis. JAMA 305:569-575
32. Spear SL (2009) Partial breast reconstruction: techniques in oncoplastic surgery. Plast Reconstr Surg 124(5):1722

Pulmonary Malignancies 15

Federico Davini, Franca Melfi, Francesca Allidi
and Alfredo Mussi

15.1 Definition and Epidemiology

One century ago, a cancer diagnosis was almost always a “death sentence” but today it does not have to be. Lung cancer accounts for 12.6% of all new cancers and ≈20% of all cancer deaths. It remains one of the most common malignancies, accounting for 20% of all cancers in men and 12% of all cancers in women. The risk of lung cancer is about fourfold greater in men than in women, and this increases with age. In the European Union, the incidence of lung cancer is 7 per 100,000 for men and 3 per 100,000 for women at the age of 35 years but, in patients aged >75 years, the rates are 440 and 72 in men and women, respectivelly.

Wide geographical variations in the incidence of lung cancer have also reported, and this is primarily related to worldwide variations in smoking behavior [1]. Smoking cigarettes is by far the dominant risk factor in patients with lung cancer, accounting for 90% of lung cancers in men and ≈80% of cases in women. The relationship between smoking and lung cancer mortality was first established by Doll and Hill [2]. Occupational exposure to asbestos has also been shown to increase the risk of lung cancer, particularly with amphibolic forms of asbestos. Exposure to the following carcinogens has also been associated with an increased risk from lung cancer: radon, arsenic, beryllium, bis-choromethyl ether, cadmium, chromium, nickel, polycyclic aromatic hydrocarbons and vinyl chloride. Unlike routine early-detection tests for other neoplasms, screening for lung cancer is not recommended by any major health organization, including the American Cancer Society, the National

F. Davini (✉) · F. Melfi · F. Allidi · A. Mussi
Division of Thoracic Surgery, Cardiothoracic and Vascular Department
University of Pisa, Italy
e-mail: davinifederico@gmail.com

A. Valeri et al. (eds.), *What's New in Surgical Oncology*,
DOI: 10.1007/978-88-470-5310-6_15,

Cancer Institute, or the American Medical Association [2]. However, recently, several studies focusing on lung-cancer screening have been started in different institutions.

15.2 Presentation

Because the symptoms for lung cancer are not specific and can usually be explained by other common conditions, the disease sometimes goes undetected or is misdiagnosed. This is why the medical history of the individual—age, smoking history, family history and occupational exposure—is particularly important in diagnosing lung cancer and should always be brought to the physician's attention. The symptoms of lung cancer are varied because of very different causes: local growth, intrathoracic extension, para-neoplastic syndromes and distant spread [3].

15.2.1 Local Growth

The most common symptoms due to local disease are chronic cough with or without sputum production. Hemoptysis frequently prompts patients to visit their physician and is a presenting feature in ≤50% of cases. Chest pain is a common feature and may vary from dull, vague pain on the side of the tumor or more severe pain due to invasion into the chest wall or mediastinum. Local invasion of adjacent structures such as ribs and vertebral bodies by the tumor may also cause severe persistent pain. Recurrent focal pneumonia and segmental pneumonia suggest an obstructive lesion in the airways and should prompt further investigation. Unilateral wheezing can be a less common feature of an obstructive bronchial tumor. Stridor may occur if there is tracheal involvement.

15.2.2 Intrathoracic Extension

Extension of lung cancer to adjacent structures may also lead to symptoms and signs. Breathlessness and chest pain may be caused by pleural or pericardial involvement. The subsequent pleural or pericardial effusions may cause breathlessness and, in the case of pericardial involvement, may also lead to cardiovascular compromise. Right upper lobe tumors or adjacent mediastinal nodes may invade or externally compress the superior vena cava (SVC) and ≈10% of patients with small-cell lung cancer (SCLC) present with a relatively classical SVC syndrome. Apical tumors may also extend to involve the superior sympathetic chain, leading to a Horner's syndrome. Involvement of the and brachial plexus can cause pain in the shoulder and neck with atrophy of the small muscles of the hand. Left-sided tumors may compress the recurrent laryngeal nerve as it courses above the aortic arch, leading to a hoarse voice and left vocal cord paralysis. Direct tumor invasion or enlarged mediastinal nodes may cause esophageal compression and hence dysphagia. If the tumor damages one of the nerves that controls the diaphragm, that part of the diaphragm may become paralyzed.

15.2.3 Paraneoplastic Syndromes

Paraneoplastic syndromes are present in 10–20% of patients with lung cancers, and are usually due to the ectopic production of hormones or peptides. These patients can present with vague symptoms (e.g., tiredness, nausea, abdominal pain or confusion) or more specific symptoms (e.g., galactorrhoea). Ectopic hormone production is more common in SCLS and some of the cells show neuroendocrine characteristics. Digital clubbing with hypertrophic pulmonary osteo-arthropathy (HPOA) is considered a non-metastatic manifestation of lung cancer. Peripheral neuropathy and neurological syndromes such as Lambert–Eaton myasthenic syndrome may also be associated with lung cancer.

15.2.4 Distant Spread

A decrease of weight of >20% of baseline body weight in the preceding month is often indicative of metastatic disease. Lung cancer also frequently spreads to the adrenal glands, bone and brain. Involvement of these sites may cause localized pain. Bone metastases occur usually in the ribs, vertebrae, humeral and femoral bones. With brain metastases there may also be neurological symptoms, such as confusion, personality changes and epileptic seizures. Supraclavicular and anterior cervical lymph nodes may be involved in ≤25% of patients, and should be assessed routinely in the evaluation of lung cancer [2].

15.3 Pathology

There are many types of lung cancer, each with its own appearance, typical causes, and patterns of growth. Until more is known about the genetic origin of lung cancer cells, lung cancers are divided into two main categories based on the size and appearance of the cells: SCLC and non-small-cell lung cancer (NSCLC). Traditionally, squamous cell carcinoma has the strongest association with tobacco smoking, followed by small-cell carcinoma and adenocarcinoma. However, the association with adenocarcinoma has become stronger over time, and this histological subtype has become the most common type in many western countries. Histological subtyping (particularly the distinction between SCLC and NSCLC) is a dominant and independent prognostic indicator. With the identification of different tumor types and their presumably different disease pathways, there is hope for the development of new therapeutic strategies. The classification escribed below is based on the World Health Organisation classification of lung tumors and divides tumor groups according to their most common location on computed tomography (CT) [4].

15.3.1 SCLC

SCLC is also called "oat cell carcinoma" because the cells resemble oats under the microscope. It is the type of cancer found in ≈20–25% of people with lung cancer (almost always in smokers). SCLC usually develops in the secretory cells (neuroendocrine cells) that line the bronchial airways. Therefore, SCLC tumors can produce hormones and cause paraneoplastic syndrome (e.g., Cushing's syndrome). The cells in SCLCs divide rapidly (volume doubling time: 29 days). SCLC is a particularly aggressive form of cancer that spreads quickly and usually involves multiple tumors throughout the lung. By the time the diagnosis is made, the cancer may have spread to the lymph nodes in the center of the chest (mediastinal nodes), in the neck and above the collarbone (supraclavicular nodes), and in the abdominal cavity. It may even have spread through the bloodstream, liver, lungs, brain, and bones.

15.3.2 NSCLC

NSCLC includes several forms. Some grow as quickly as SCLC, but the usual doubling time is 30–180 days. Hence, NSCLC is more often confined to the chest at the time of the diagnosis [5].

15.3.3 Pre-invasive Lesions: Squamous Dysplasia and Carcinoma In Situ

Squamous dysplasia and carcinoma *in situ* are defined as precursor abnormalities for squamous cell carcinoma that may occur as single or multifocal lesions existing as foci of isolated disease or accompany invasive carcinoma. Another lesion worthy of mention is atypical adenomatoid hyperplasia (AAH): it is a localized peripheral lesion (usually measuring <5 mm in diameter), characterized by the proliferation of atypical cells lining the alveoli, generally in the absence of underlying interstitial inflammation or fibrosis.

15.3.4 Squamous Carcinoma

Squamous carcinomas usually present as hilar, perihilar or mediastinal masses with or without lung collapse and mediastinal shift. Squamous carcinoma is the most common cell type to show cavitation, more frequent in elderly men who smoke or who have smoked.

15.3.5 Large Cell Carcinoma

Large cell carcinoma (10% of all lung cancers) is defined as a malignant epithelial neoplasm lacking the cytological features of small cell carcinoma and glandular or squamous differentiation. Most tumors are peripheral, with the notable exception of the basaloid form.

15.3.6 Adenocarcinoma

Adenocarcinoma begins in the smaller airways and the alveoli. It affects non-smokers most frequently, but is on the increase among smokers. Adenocarcinoma presents as peripheral nodules measuring <4 cm in diameter. On CT, "solid" nodules, ground-glass opacities and combined solid/ground-glass opacities are all recognized patterns.

One distinct type of adenocarcinoma is bronchoalveolar carcinoma, which causes mucus-producing cells to proliferate on the walls of alveoli. Unlike other adenocarcinomas, it usually involves multiple tumors. It grows slowly, with a dividing time of ≥180 days. A solid peripheral nodule is by far the most common, but central or endobronchial tumors also occur. Adenocarcinomas can preferentially invade and disseminate along the pleura, thus mimicking the features of malignant pleural mesothelioma.

15.3.7 Adenosquamous Carcinoma

Adenosquamous carcinoma is defined as carcinoma showing squamous and glandular differentiation with each component comprising ≥10% of the tumor. These tumors appear to have a dismal prognosis, with an overall 5-year survival rate of ≈20%.

15.3.8 Sarcomatoid Carcinoma

Sarcomatoid carcinoma is rare, but can present as central or peripheral nodules. It is a malignant epithelial neoplasm that has undergone divergent mesenchymal differentiation and has a worse prognosis than other non-small-cell carcinomas.

15.3.9 Combined Small-Cell Carcinoma

Combined small-cell carcinoma is a small-cell component seen together with any non-small-cell cancer, most commonly adenocarcinoma, squamous cell carcinoma or large cell carcinoma. Direct tumor spread is often seen as submucosal extension and intralymphatic spread.

15.3.10 Endobronchial Tumours (Carcinoid, Typical and Atypical)

Carcinoid tumors are defined as epithelial tumours showing a particular growth pattern that suggests neuroendocrine differentiation. Carcinoid tumors are divided into two types: "typical" carcinoid (in which there are <2 mitoses per 10 high-power field (HPF) and no evidence of necrosis) and "atypical" carcinoid (containing >2 mitoses per 10 HPF and/or foci of necrosis). Although the common perception is that carcinoid tumors are endobronchial lesions, typical carcinoids may be found at any site in the lungs, and atypical carcinoids are more commonly found in the periphery. Half of all carcinoids are incidental findings. Carcinoid tumors have traditionally been regarded to be benign lesions. However, 10–15% of typical carcinoids metastasize to regional lymph nodes at presentation and ≤10% may eventually metastasize to distant sites such as the liver and bone. Fortunately, typical carcinoids are associated with an excellent prognosis (10-year survival rate: 82–95%). In stark contrast, atypical carcinoids have a significantly worse 10-year survival (35–59%) [6].

15.3.11 Salivary Gland-Like Tumors

Salivary gland-like tumors comprise mucoepidermoid, adenoid cystic and epithelial–myoepithelial carcinomas. They are rare and usually present with a prominent endobronchial component. There is no documented link with smoking and, overall, they follow an indolent course with multiple local recurrences before metastases occur. The only exception is with high-grade mucoepidermoid carcinoma, which tends to behave similarly to other non-small-cell carcinomas.

15.4 Diagnosis

Because the early symptoms of lung cancer can be so different from one person to the next and can be explained by other, more common, conditions, lung cancer usually goes unnoticed. The diagnosis of lung cancer is a multistep process. It starts with a physical examination. If cancer is suspected, additional tests are employed to confirm the diagnosis, including non-invasive (imaging) and invasive procedures (biopsy).

15.4.1 Imaging

A chest radiograph is the most common, simple imaging study done if a lung disease is suspected. It helps to dectect the tumor and abnormal widening of the mediastinum (which may suggest a tumor or lymphoadenopathy). A radiograph may also show signs of pneumonia by detecting fluid around the lungs, or even bone abnormalities. The use of CT (also called computed axial tomography (CAT)) provides more detail than a radiograph. Unlike radiographs and CT, which detect body structures, positron emission tomography (PET) highlights areas where sugar metabolism is high. Because rapidly growing cells—such as cancer cells—take up sugar more quickly than other cells, the areas highlighted by PET could very possibly be tumoral. Several studies have shown that PET can detect metastases that other standard procedures had missed, and can determine the stage of the cancer, avoiding the need for more invasive procedures [7]. To ascertain if the cancer has spread to other areas, it is extremely important to define the best treatment option. New equipment can carry out CT scan and PET simultaneously, providing more information more quickly [2].

15.4.2 Biopsy

Imaging methods reveal the location and other features of a tumor, but it is necessary to carry out a biopsy to determine with certainty that the tumor is cancer. Depending on the size and location of the tumor, the physician will choose the most appropriate of the following methods.

Flexible bronchoscopy allows the physician to see the inside of the bronchi and take samples of tissue and sputum to confirm lung cancer and determine its type. This test is recommended if CT has shown a suspicious mass in the central part of the lungs. Fine-needle aspiration is used mainly to study peripheral tumors located closer to the chest wall. Using CT or ultrasound to locate the suspect area, the surgeon or radiologist inserts a very thin, hollow needle between two ribs into the lung, sucking some of the cells into a syringe attached to the needle. Mediastinoscopy consists of insertion of a mediastinoscope through a small incision made at the base of the neck just above the breastbone. By biopsy forceps, the surgeon can collect tissue samples from lymph nodes to check for cancer and simultaneosuly assess nodal involvement to better define the disease stage. If the tumor is near the surface of the lung, a thoracoscopy can be used to carry out an excisional biopsy of the lung or nodal sampling. Unfortunately, thoracoscopic localization of small and central nodules into the lung may be difficult. A few localization methods have been described: preoperative (vital or blue dye, fluoroscopy-aided, needle wire) or intrathoracoscopic (finger palpation, intrathoracoscopic ultrasound, radio-guided surgery). Patients with pulmonary nodules smaller than 1 cm and/or deeper than 1 cm below the visceral pleura undergo CT-guided injection of a solution composed of 0.2 mL (99)Tc-labeled human serum albumin microspheres and 0.1 ml non-ionic contrast into the nodule. During the thoracoscopic procedure, a collimated probe connected to a gamma ray detector is introduced to image the lung surface. The area of major radioactivity, which matches with the area of the nodule, is resected [8]. Once lung cancer has been confirmed, the next step is to determine which type of lung cancer it is, which grade it is, and which stage it has reached. This information is a very important part of the diagnosis because it will guide the choice of treatments.

15.4.3 Staging

Staging is the process of determining how far a cancer has spread. Stage I is early cancer: in this stage, cancer is found only within the lung. Stage IV is the most advanced stage: the tumor has metastasized to other parts of the body. Staging is determined by imaging and biopsies. The stage of the disease is the most important indicator of the prognosis. Uniform criteria for reporting the findings of clinical and/or pathological evaluation are important in the initial management of patients with NSCLC. The staging system is based on three factors: the size and location of the tumor (T), the extent of lymph-node involvement (N) and presence or absence of metastases (M). The treatment of choice for NSCLC in the absence of disseminated disease is resection. The primary aim of staging is thus to determine if a tumor can be completely removed by surgery; clear surgical margins in resection specimens and the absence of tumor cells in resected lymph nodes being the prime determinants of local recurrence and survival.

For the purposes of staging, lung cancer is divided into NSCLC and SCLC types, reflecting the significant differences in natural history and the response to therapy. The International Staging System for NSCLC stratifies disease extent in terms of prognosis and is based on the TNM grading of the primary tumor, regional nodes and distant metastases which was revised very recently. Resection is indicated for early stage (I, II, selected IIIA) disease, whereas chemotherapy and radiotherapy are used for more advanced disease. The mainstay of surgical therapy remains anatomic lobectomy with complete mediastinal lymph-node dissection, provided the patient can physically tolerate this procedure. Recent developments in the care of patients with resectable lung cancer include adoption of adjuvant chemotherapy for patients with completely resected stage II–III disease, the importance of resection in the multimodal therapy regimen for stage IIIA NSCLC, as well as the use of induction chemoradiotherapy for tumors of the superior sulcus. With increasing use of low-dose screening CT for individuals thought to be at high risk for the development of lung cancer, the discovery of much smaller tumors is increasing in frequency, and further studies are necessary to establish the standard of care for these lesions [9].

15.5 New Developments in Thoracic Surgery

15.5.1 Robotic Surgery

In the past two decades, there has been a revolutionary transition in surgical methods and technology with minimally invasive approaches. Many advantages have been obtained by using video-assisted thoracic surgery (VATS): less pain and trauma, shorter hospitalization, better cosmetic results. In thoracic surgery, compared with conventional thoracotomic procedures, few studies have suggested improvements in earlier discharge from hospital, in postoperative pain control, lower levels of perioperative inflammatory cytokines, lower complication rates, and earlier return to normal activities. Moreover, limitations of VATS lobectomy remain due to impaired vision, restricted manoeuverability of instruments, poor ergonomics for the surgeon, and unstable camera platforms. Some of the more prominent limitations involve the mechanical and technical nature of the equipment, such as two-dimensional (2D) imaging, unsteady camera platforms and limited manouverability of instruments due to the rigid shaft axis fixed to the thorax by the trocar. This implies an unnatural surgical feel with hands, and misaligned and fixed instrument tips inside the patient together with inverted movements. Robotic-assisted minimally invasive surgery represents an extraordinary technological advance for a wide range of procedures traditionally requiring open surgery. By enabling surgeons to undertake complex procedures through small incisions, the surgeon's hand movements are scaled and filtered to eliminate hand tremor, which are then translated into micro-movements of the proprietary instruments. These improved ergonomic conditions and instrument mobility at distal articulations seem beneficial in thoracic procedures.

Different types of robotic devices are used, but the da Vinci™ Robotic System represents the only complete surgical system applied in a wide range of surgical procedures. Robotic pulmonary lobectomy was first carried out in 2002. Subsequently, other centers confirmed that this method is feasible and safe (even though technical differences from various centers have been reported [10, 11]).

15.5.1.1 Robot Features

Surgical Robot System (Master–Slave Manipulator)

The da Vinci Robotic System is the only complete surgical robot system that can overcome some of the limitations of conventional minimally invasive surgery (Fig. 15.1). The da Vinci System is a sophisticated robotic platform designed to expand the surgeon's capabilities and, for the first time, offer a minimally invasive option for major surgery. Small incisions are used to introduce miniaturized wrist instruments and a high-definition three-dimensional (3D) camera. Seated comfortably at the da Vinci console, the surgeon views a magnified, high-resolution 3D image of the surgical site. Simultaneously,

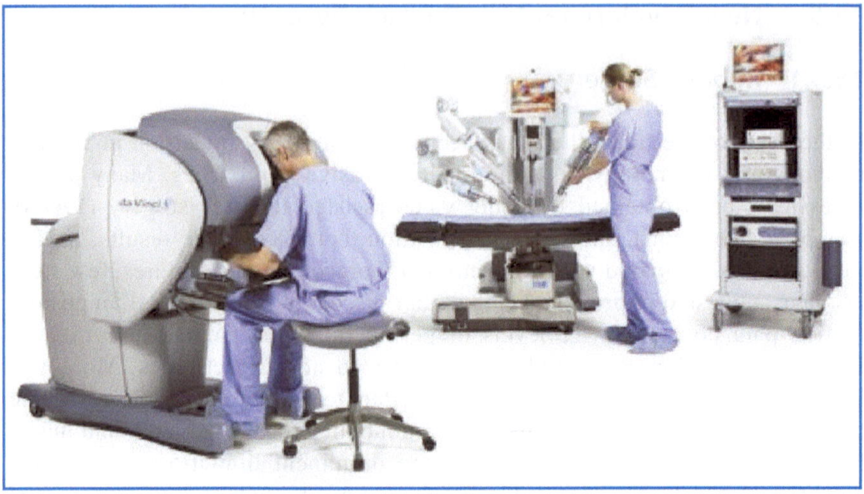

Fig. 15.1 The da VinciTM robotic system (courtesy of Surgical Intuitive, Inc., Sunnyvale, CA, USA)

state-of-the-art robotic and computer technologies scale, filter and seamlessly translate the surgeon's hand movements into precise micro-movements of the da Vinci instruments. This system comprises three main parts:

- **Surgeon console** is controlled by the surgeon. It is connected to a surgical manipulator with three instrument arms and a central arm to guide the endoscope. Two master handles at the surgeon's console are manipulated by the user. The position and orientation of the surgeon's hands on the handles trigger highly sensitive motion sensors which transfer the surgeon's movements to the tip of the instrument at a remote location.
- **Surgical cart** (of which three arms directly carry out the procedures) provides three degrees of freedom (pitch, yaw, insertion). Attached to the robot arm is the surgical instrument, the tip of which is provided by a mechanical cable-driven wrist (EndoWrist®). This adds four more degrees of freedom (internal pitch, internal yaw, rotation and grip).
- **Vision system**: The computer system which controls the entire system resides in the surgeon console. The surgical instruments with EndoWrist move like human hands by artificial articulation, and visualization through a high-quality 3D endoscope is optimal. This system provides surgeons with intuitive translation of the movement of the instrument handle to the tip, thereby eliminating the: mirror-image effect; scaling; tremor filtering; and coaxial alignment of the eyes, hand and tooltip image. An internal articulated endoscopic wrist provides an additional three degrees of freedom.

Instruments

EndoWrist instruments are designed to provide surgeons with natural dexterity and a full range of motion for precise operation through tiny incisions. *EndoWrist* instruments provide enhanced dexterity thanks to a great range of motion that allows precision and control. The features of the instruments are: seven degrees of freedom, 90° of articulation, i*ntuitive* motion and fingertip control, motion scaling and tremor reduction (Fig. 15.2).

Dual-console surgical system

The newly refined da Vinci Si Surgical System includes a dual console used for training and collaboration. During a dual-console operation, each surgeon sits at his/her individual console and can see the same high-definition images of the anatomy from the 3D endoscope (flexible tube with a camera and light at the tip). If the dual console is used for training, control over instruments can be readily and quickly exchanged during surgery. Hence, the tutor surgeon can handover control of the instruments to the resident at any time. This enables a see-and-repeat model of instruction designed to accelerate the learning curve. For collaborative surgery with the dual console, two surgeons can operate in concert. While one surgeon undertakes the primary tasks of the procedure, the second surgeon can assist with another task (e.g., retraction) (Fig. 15.3).

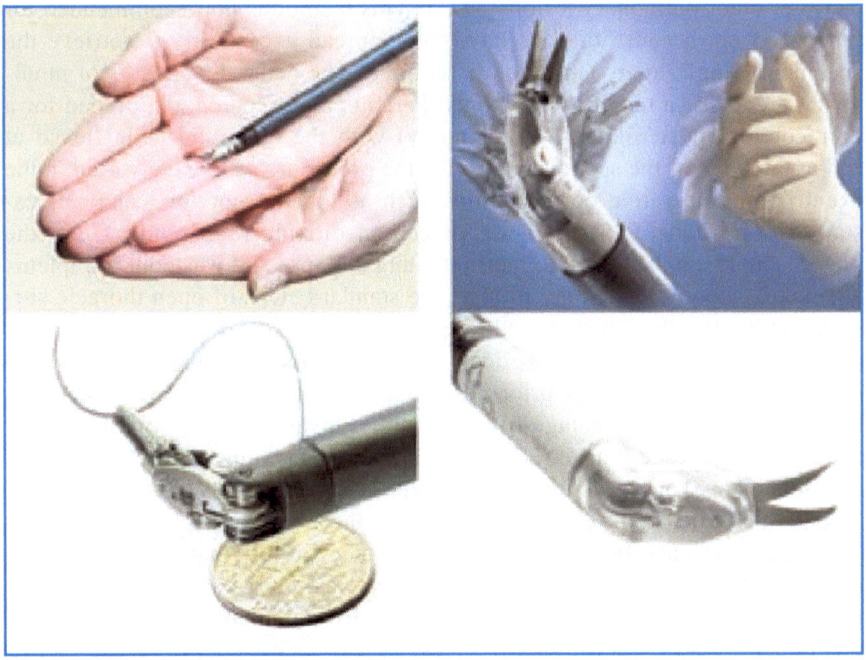

Fig. 15.2 EndoWrist (courtesy of Surgical Intuitive, Inc., Sunnyvale, CA, USA)

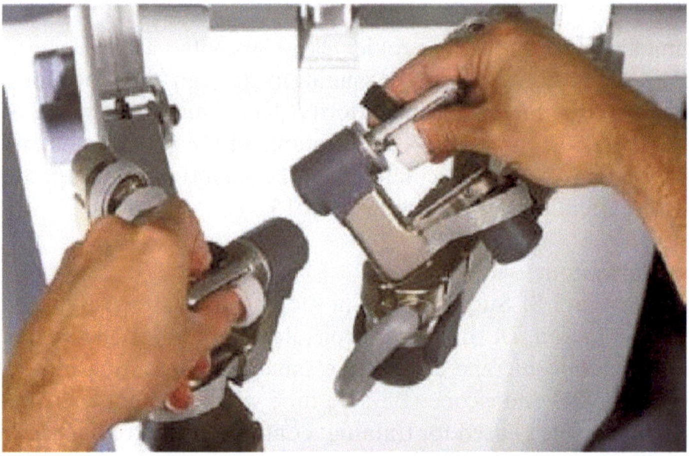

Fig. 15.3 The da Vinci dual-console surgical system (Master Handles) (courtesy of Surgical Intuitive, Inc., Sunnyvale, CA, USA)

Procedures

Currently, the indications for robotic lobectomy are strictly defined: patients must be in clinical stage I with a negative mediastinoscopy and without evidence of other pulmonary lesions on CT. This method is not recommended for tumors >4 cm because the ribs have to be spread excessively to retrieve the specimen. Single-lung ventilation is required. The general standards of monitoring are as for a major thoracotomy. Patients are prepared and draped for a thoracotomy (posterolateral thoracotomy) with the operating table flexed at 30° at the level of the scapula tip so that the procedure can be converted in the event of intraoperative complications such as bleeding or for technical reasons. Insufflation of low-pressure of carbon dioxide (5–8 mmHg) into the pleural cavity can be useful to facilitate lung collapse and wash out intrapleural smoke. Robotic lobectomy follows the standard steps of open thoracic surgery and implies the isolation and resection of the vascular and bronchial hilar elements. Usually, the artery is dealt with before the vein and eventually the bronchus is transacted, but priorities are not set strictly. Robotic technology has added certain advantages in minimally invasive thoracic surgery for anatomic lung resection (especially pulmonary lobectomy). Minimally invasive lobectomy for early-stage lung cancer is entering daily clinical practice. In part it is due to the detection of lung cancer at smaller sizes thanks to screening programs. In part it is due to advances in minimally invasive technology, with the development of robotic systems. Only a few robotic lobectomies have been carried out. Consequently, few surgeons have experience in this field.

Although this method is evolving and larger series are required, some studies have demonstrated that robotic procedures may have advantages over conventional approaches. In 2002, we reported the encouraging results of pulmonary lobectomies undertaken with robotic technology [12]. Subsequently, other authors reported their experiences with the da Vinci robotic system, mainly for right lower lobectomies. These very first experiences showed robotic surgery to be feasible and safe, but with this type of approach increased operating times were noted with respect to conventional surgery. Especially in thoracic surgery, this new method offers clear benefits for the treatment of mediastinal lesions and lung cancer, particularly lobectomy in stage-I NSCLC [13].

15.5.2 Radiofrequency Ablation (RFA)

About one-fifth of patients with resectable NSCLC are unsuitable for surgery. RFA offers an alternative minimally invasive option [14]. An electrode connected to an RFA generator is placed directly into the target tissue. When an electric current (in the frequency of radio waves, 460–480 kHz) is applied, tissue heating results from resistive energy loss as electrons agitate ionic molecules in tissue as they move toward the reference electrodes. The goal is to heat tissue to 60–100°C because this temperature is considered to be lethal to the target tissue [15]. RFA of lung tumors is a relatively safe procedure with low mortality and excellent tolerance in terms of respiratory function. The most common periprocedural complication is pneumothorax, and occurs in ≤60% of ablation sessions. Most cases of pneumothorax do not require treatment (4% to 12% of procedures require chest tube drainage). Small reactive pleural effusions and parenchyma hemorrhage can also occur. Surgery remains the standard therapy, but RFA is becoming a valid tool in specific scenarios as single treatment as well as in combination with other treatments, such as radiotherapy.

References

1. Bunn PA, Kato H, Mulshine JL (2006) Textbook of Prevention and Detection of Early Lung Cancer. Wiley, pp 1-9
2. Desai SR et al (2007) Lung Cancer. Cambridge University Press, 1-11
3. Carmen F (2007) Deadly disease and epidemics: Lung Cancer. Infobase Publishing 5:61-70
4. Weitberg A, Klastersky J (2002) Cancer of the lung. From Molecular Biology to Treatment Guidelines 2:35-80
5. Heine H (2008) Textbook of lung cancer (Second edition). Informa Healthcare, pp 61-73
6. Davini F, Gonfiotti A, Comin C et al (2009) Typical and atypical carcinoid tumours: 20-year experience with 89 patients. J Cardiovasc Surg 50:807-11
7. Singh D, Miles K (2012) Multiparametric PET/CT in oncology. Cancer Imaging 12:336-44
8. Davini F, Gonfiotti A, Vaggelli L et al (2006) Thoracoscopic localization techniques for patients with solitary pulmonary nodule: radioguided surgery versus hookwire localization. J Cardiovasc Surg 47:355-9

9. Rami-Porta R, Crowley JJ, Goldstraw P (2009) The revised TNM staging system for lung cancer. Ann Thorac Cardiovasc Surg 15:4-9
10. Melfi FMA et al (2005) Multimedia Manual of Cardiothoracic Surgery. Video Robotic Lobectomy. doi: 10.1510/mmcts.2004.000448
11. Bodner J, Wykypiel H, Wetscher G, Schmid T (2004) First experiences with the da VinciTM operating robot in thoracic surgery. Eur J Cardiothorac Surg 25:844-851
12. Melfi F, Menconi F, Mariani M, Angeletti A (2002) Early experience with robotic technology for thoracoscopic surgery Eur J Cardiothorac Surg 21:864-868
13. Park BJ, Melfi F, Mussi A et al (2012) Robotic lobectomy for non-small cell lung cancer (NSCLC). Long-term oncologic results. J Thorac Cardiovascular 143:383-9
14. Ambrogi MC, Fanucchi O, Cioni R et al (2011) Long-term results of radiofrequency ablation treatment of stage I non-small cell lung cancer: a prospective intention-to-treat study. J Thorac Oncol 6:2044-51
15. Dupuy DE, Shulman M (2010) Current status of thermal ablation treatments for lung malignancies. Semin Intervent Radiol 27:268-75

Surgical Emergencies in Cancer Patients 16

Ferdinando Agresta, Nereo Vettoretto,
Gian Luca Baiocchi and Fabio Cesare Campanile

16.1 Obstruction

The debut of a previously unknown abdominal malignancy as an intestinal obstruction is a common event in each surgical practice. Similarly, surgeons are asked to evaluate possible surgical options for the treatment of malignant bowel obstructions (MBOs) secondary to known abdominal secondary localizations or to peritoneal carcinosis: this can be one of the most challenging aspects of advanced cancer care. The main cause might be due to obstruction at various levels: proximal or distal small bowel, right or left colon, or the rectum.

The bowel obstruction might be complete (thereby requiring emergency treatment) or incomplete. The main causes of abdominal metastatic disease are attributed to ovarian cancer (5% to 51%) and to gastrointestinal cancer (10% to 28%). Diffuse peritoneal carcinomatosis remains the more common presentation, but 10% of cases might be due to a single secondary neoplasm. For non-gastrointestinal tumors, the most frequent are metastases from breast cancer and melanoma [1]. The prognosis is poor and expected survival does not generally exceed 3 months. Obstruction is not always purely mechanical: in fact, extramural involvement is the pre-eminent etiology, and dysmotility

F. Agresta (✉)
Local Healthcare Unit ULSS 19 – Veneto, Adria, Italy
e-mail: fagresta@libero.it

N. Vettoretto
Laparoscopic Surgical Unit, M.Mellini Hospital, Chiari (Brescia), Italy

G.L. Baiocchi
Medical and Surgical Scineces, University of Brescia, Italy

F.C. Campanile
Division of General Surgery, Andosilla Hospital, Civita Castellana (Viterbo), Italy

A. Valeri et al. (eds.), *What's New in Surgical Oncology*,
DOI: 10.1007/978-88-470-5310-6_16, © Springer-Verlag Italia 2013

disorders due to mesenterial infiltration, bowel muscle or the celiac and enteric plexus might be classified as "functional obstruction", and might benefit most from medical therapy [2]. Alas, ≤50% of small-bowel obstructions might be caused by adhesions and thus be non-malignant [2]. We will not examine proximal obstructions (duodenal or gastric) because the clinical aspects are quite different and the obstructive symptoms configure a different pathological entity, being mostly due to cholangiocarcinoma, pancreatic carcinoma and gastric carcinoma [3]. The diagnosis and treatment of this condition has changed in recent years due to the (i) amelioration of diagnostic radiology, endoscopy and laparoscopy; (ii) introduction of new medications, devices; (iii) propagation of minimally invasive radical or palliative surgery. We will delve into the most recent acquisitions in these fields.

16.1.1 Clinical Aspects

The site of obstruction determines the signs and symptoms patients will experience. Proximal obstructions cause more severe nausea and vomiting, early pain and anorexia, whereas more distal localizations cause abdominal distension, late pain and impaired stool passage, with an increased risk of ischemic complications or perforation. Most MBOs are progressive and incomplete, with worsening nausea, vomiting, pain and obstipation [4].

16.1.2 Imaging

Plain radiography of the abdomen can prove unreliable but remains an important initial imaging as well as for the follow-up in response to treatment [5]. Contrast radiographs (with oral idrosoluble contrast) might be useful in incomplete or multiple obstructions, as well as for its prognostic value for the need for surgery [6]. The diagnostic mainstay remains computed tomography (CT) for its high specificity and sensitivity (100–94%) for determining the causes and possible complications [5]. Magnetic resonance imaging (MRI) has not yet gained a significant role in the diagnosis of MBOs [5].

16.1.3 Decision-making

"When the sun can set on an unoperated bowel obstruction" is the significant title of an article inquiring the decision plan for an MBO that concludes "...especially when the sun is setting for the patient" [7]. This common (but difficult) problem remains a challenge for the above-mentioned reasons. An English report highlights the excessive numbers of "inappropriate and aggressive operations performed on frail or terminally ill patients" [8]. In fact, the goals of treatment must be clear to the physician, patients and to their families.

The surgical approach is affected by high mortality (5–32%), morbidity (42%) and re-obstruction rates (10–50%) [9]. Quality of life (QoL) must be a primary goal and, because the prognosis is not necessarily changed, all the treatment options must be evaluated, with particular attention to minimally invasive treatments as they become indicated [9]. Some factors might influence the prognosis and the decision for palliation treatment. For example, one of the most important predictors of the success of surgery is the absence of ascites [10]. Other variables influence the prognosis, and clinical scores for the selection of patients have been published: the Krebs–Goplerud index is one of the more commonly used, and it determines age, nutritional status, tumor extension, ascites, and previous chemotherapy or radiation as prognostic variables [10]. Alas, its index of improvement is controversial because survival must necessarily be joined by QoL, which includes the ability to tolerate oral food, restoration of normal bowel habits, return home, recurrent obstructions, social acceptance and self-esteem.

16.1.4 Role of Medications

Medical therapy can palliate symptoms effectively for most patients [2]. Colicky and continuous pain can benefit from the concomitant use of opioids (e.g., morphine, hydromorphone and fentanyl in various routes of administration) together with non-opioid drugs (e.g., ketorolac) to prevent segmental contractions caused by opioid-related stimulation of the circular smooth muscle and a functional ileus. Reduction of nausea and vomiting can be accomplished with phenotiazines, haloperidol, anticholinergics, octreotide, metoclopramide and olanzepine. Corticosteroids play an important (but unknown) part in the resolution of obstruction by acting centrally against vomiting, reducing edema and preventing pain, being capable of improving bowel symptoms in 60% of patients taking high doses (with minimal side effects if used for 4–5 days) [9]. Combination therapy with these drugs is beneficial. Nasogastric tubes can be useful measures, but only for short periods. Total parenteral nutrition (TPN) has failed to improve outcome, survival, performance status nor QoL [11]. Chemotherapy can provide some success in newly diagnosed cancers but it has no role for previously treated tumors that evolve into MBOs [12].

16.1.5 Role of Endoscopy

The relief of symptoms in patients with MBO, poor performance status, and short life expectancy can be obtained with placement of a percutaneous endoscopic gastrostomy (PEG), to serve as a venting device. Especially in patients with neoplastic ascites, PEG is associated with a lower morbidity and increased survival compared with an open surgical approach [13]. Compelling evidence shows a relief of nausea and vomiting in 80–90% of these patients and restoration of partial oral intake [13]. Some studies show a non-surgical role in bowel obstruction for "endoscopic long-tube decompression" which comprises the passage of a proximal obstruction with an endoscopically placed tube, and seems successful for shortening spontaneous resolution in ≤90% of treated cases [13].

An increasing role is to be assumed by colonic stenting in cases of colonic obstruction. The procedure involves the insertion of a self-expanding metallic stent *via* endoscopy with the help of fluoroscopy and under sedation. The indication is appropriate for a single colonic obstruction at the level of the left colon: the transverse colon, flexures and the rectum are not amenable to stenting in consideration of the high rate of failure, displacement and stent migration, tenesmus and incontinence [14]. Deaths due to stenting are <1%, migration occurs in 10% of cases, bleeding in 5% and perforation in 4%, especially if preceded by balloon dilatation. Tumor ingrowth, overgrowth or fecal impaction cause recurrent obstruction in 10% of patients, who can be re-treated with a stent-over-stent procedure or with neodymium-doped yttrium aluminum garnet (nd:YAG) laser endoluminal therapy [14]. Meta-analyzed data have shown lower rates of mortality, complications and long-term need for stomas when compared with emergency surgery, with the implication of fewer resources in terms of bed stay and intensive care facilities. This procedure may serve also as a "bridge to surgery" in case of complete obstruction. No difference in survival has been found between stent and subsequent resection *vs* emergency bowel resection. Moreover, the subsequent minimally invasive approach is facilitated in comparison with *d'embleé* resection [15].

16.1.6 Role of Surgery

The main role of surgical intervention is accomplishing complete resection of an obstructive tumor with a negative margin. With the exception of ovarian cancer (in which debulking and tumor mass reduction) is beneficial together with chemotherapy, incomplete resection is of scarce benefit for survival, but might present advantages only as a palliative procedure; resection might not necessarily entail restoration of bowel continuity. Otherwise, side-to-side intestinal bypasses or diverting stomas are the preferred procedures [9]. Increasing interest has been aroused after the studies of Sugarbaker and colleagues, who advocated a very aggressive approach to surgical palliation which involved extensive debulking, peritonectomy and hyperthermic intraperitoneal chemotherapy (HIPEC) [16]. Success is more likely in cases of low-grade tumors such as pseudomixoma peritonei, and the difficulty of the procedure (>10 h, >1000 mL of blood loss, 55% morbidity and 7% mortality) suggests its application in clinical trials and specialized environments with accurate patient selection done in high-volume centers. Factors which are very likely to influence the final outcome are the peritoneal cancer index (PCI), the number of visceral resections, and performance status.

Initial determination of the PCI may be optimized by the accurate use of exploratory laparoscopy [17]. The propagation of minimally invasive surgery and its role in the treatment of small bowel obstruction does not exclude impending importance in the treatment of MBO. In fact, the better outcome of laparoscopy in terms of postoperative pain, complications, hospital stay, and wound infections might be particularly attractive in the cancer patient. An increasing number of reports regarding laparoscopic procedures in MBO and including emergency colectomies, internal bypass, diverting ostomies and ileal resections, have been completed. Indeed, emergency laparoscopic surgery (especially for MBO) is challenging and requires experienced surgeons and an adequate hospital environment [18–19].

16.2 Gastrointestinal (GI) Bleeding

GI bleeding in patients with known cancer can be a severe emergency problem with a wide variety of etiologies. It can also be the sentinel event in the discovery of a primary or metastatic cancer lesion to the GI tract. Locating the site of bleeding is essential to its treatment and management.

16.2.1 Upper Gastrointestinal Bleeding (UGIB)

UGIB is defined as hemorrhage from a site proximal to the ligament of Treitz. It can be due to peptic ulcer disease, variceal disease, or more obscure cancer-related etiologies. There are a wide variety of cancers that may metastasize to the stomach, proximal duodenum, or regional lymph nodes which can then erode the lumen, leading to blood loss. The mortality rate of UGIB in cancer patients is ≈7% [20].

16.2.1.1 Non-interventional Measures

The stability of a blood clot in an acid environment is low. Acid-suppressing drugs therefore have the potential to optimize clot formation and reduce the risk of re-bleeding. It is crucial that the pH does not fall below 6, and this can be practically achieved only by continuous infusion of a proton pump inhibitor (PPI). There is no evidence regarding the efficacy of gastric acid-suppressing drugs in controlling bleeding in patients with GI malignancy. However, patients receiving palliative care have multiple risk factors for peptic ulceration, and therefore they should be treated with a PPI in case of bleeding [21]. Somatostatin and its analog octreotide are theoretically attractive because they reduce mesenteric (splanchnic) arterial flow and suppress secretion of gastric acid and pepsin. They also suppress angiogenesis and activate platelet aggregation *in vitro*. Possible side effects include hypoglycemia, thrombocytopenia, heart block and severe liver failure in those with cirrhosis and heart failure. Nevertheless, there is weak evidence supporting the use of somatostatin or octreotide in upper GI hemorrhage. The main evidence for benefit is again if bleeding is due to peptic ulcer disease. There is some evidence in case reports of the successful use of octreotide in patients undergoing palliative care, where more invasive interventions are not appropriate [22]. Pressins work in variceal bleeding because they cause systemic vasoconstriction (which increases blood pressure) and they also reduce flow/pressure in the portal vein due to splanchnic arteriolar constriction. Case report evidence supports the use of vasopressin in cancer patients with UGIB, but the best evidence supports its use in variceal bleeding. Its use is limited in the palliative setting by the need for intravenous administration and potentially serious side effects [23]. Tranexamic acid appears to be effective in reducing re-bleeding as well as the need for repeat endoscopy and blood transfusion in patients with acute UGIB. However, many of the studies about its use have excluded patients with cancer as a cause of bleeding, so efficacy in the palliative setting is not known [22].

16.2.1.2 Interventional Measures

Endoscopy not only offers the opportunity to diagnose the cause of bleeding accurately, it can also provide a means for therapeutic intervention to stop active bleeding or reduce the risk of re-bleeding. This approach has been studied and described if peptic ulcer disease is the cause of bleeding. Major endoscopic predictors of persistent or recurrent bleeding include active bleeding during endoscopy (90% recurrence), a visible vessel in the ulcer base (50% recurrence), or an adherent clot (25% recurrence). If the ulcer has a clean base, there is a low risk of recurrent bleeding (5% recurrence). Various methods have been used to control bleeding, including thermal coagulation, injection therapy, and endoscopically placed hemostatic clips [24]. These methods also can be easily combined. If medical and endoscopic treatments fail, surgery or interventional embolotherapy are the options. For this latter procedure, the typical candidate patient presents with the following: (i) massive bleeding (transfusion requirement of ≥4 U blood over 24 h) or hemodynamic compromise (systolic blood pressure <100 mmHg and heart rate >100 beats per minute or clinical shock), (ii) endoscopy-refractory acute bleeding, (iii) recurrent bleeding after surgery. In general, the more hemodynamically unstable a patient is, the greater is the chance of identifying the source of bleeding. There are no absolute contraindications because angiography and embolization may be needed as lifesaving procedures. For patients with severe reactions to iodinated contrast media, alternative contrast agents such as carbon dioxide can be used. Relative contraindications include renal insufficiency, contrast allergy, and uncorrectable coagulopathy. There is an increased risk of gastric or duodenal infarction after embolotherapy in patients with previous extensive surgery or radiotherapy. If the rate of bleeding is massive, surgery may be preferable to angiography because angiography may not be able to control the bleeding as quickly as surgery [25]. Distinct from patients without known cancer, patients with gastric cancer may benefit from acute surgery to control hemorrhage and may not be amenable to endoscopic intervention. Despite the improvement in mortality rate with surgery, curative resection is relatively uncommon, and postoperative complications are common [26].

16.2.2 Lower Gastrointestinal Bleeding (LGIB)

Rectal bleeding can be due to the cancer or to co-existing disease (e.g., inflammatory bowel disease (IBD), gut pathogens causing bloody diarrhea, angiodysplasia, diverticular disease, polyps, or rectal fissure/haemorrhoids). Management of rectal bleeding should be directed at treating the underlying cause (if appropriate). Radiotherapy can cause or exacerbate rectal bleeding. Radiation proctitis can occur after any form of pelvic radiotherapy, especially after prostatic and cervical treatment. Acute proctitis is usually self-limiting and can last ≤3 months. A chronic form can present months or years after the radiation exposure (median time, 8–12 months) and is the result of obliterative endarteritis and submucosal fibrosis and the formation of new vessels. There can be associated non-healing mucosal ulceration. The incidence is not known because there are no clearly defined diagnostic criteria. It usually presents with rectal bleeding (among other symptoms) which can range from mild to life-threatening. Tissue biopsy may be inconclusive and the diagnosis may have to be made by excluding any comorbidity and recurrent tumors [27]. As with UGIB, endoscopic evaluation is the key to the definitive diagnosis of LGIB in most patients. Though specific therapy is more limited than in UGIBs, colonoscopy usually localizes and diagnoses the cause of bleeding expeditiously. Biopsies can be obtained, and non-cancer-related bleeding excluded. There are risks in the emergency department related to emergency endoscopy, which include poor visualization due to lack of extensive bowel cleansing and the potential adverse events associated with procedural sedation. Rapid bowel cleansing can be obtained in 2 h by administering a large volume of polyethylene glycol solution, but the optimal timing of colonoscopy is controversial. Overall, complication rates are low (1–2%), but fluid overload, perforation and subsequent sepsis can occur. A randomized controlled trial of urgent *vs* routine colonoscopy in patients with apparent LGIBs demonstrated that urgent colonoscopy improved detection of the source of bleeding but did not reduce mortality, hospital stay, transfusion requirements, need for surgery, or re-bleeding episodes. Although colonoscopy appears to be the primary evaluation and potential therapeutic modality for LGIB, only 12% to 27% of patients have a lesion treatable by endoscopic therapy as compared with 51% of patients with UGIB [28].

16.2.2.1 Radionuclide Imaging

Other modalities for the diagnosis are considered when colonoscopy is negative or the source of bleeding is suspected to be in the small bowel. Radionuclide imaging is more sensitive than angiography because it requires a lower bleeding rate but is less specific. There are two modalities available, each with different strengths and limitations.

First is 99m-technetium sulfur colloid, which is rapidly cleared from the intravascular space so the scan is made shortly after injection. Its uptake in the spleen, liver, and bone marrow may obscure the GI source. The second is 99m-technetium pertechnate-labeled red blood cells, which need to be imaged in the first 30 min and then every few hours up to 24 h to pick up intermittent bleeding. A comparison of the two methods found similar detection rates for LGIB. These methods localize only an area of the abdomen, and there are a significant number of false-positive findings that may lead to unnecessary interventions. Patients with a negative scan are likely to have negative arteriograms [29].

16.2.2.2 Multidetector Helical CT

Multidetector helical CT requires active bleeding for good localization. It has been found to have a sensitivity and specificity of 90% and 99%, respectively, in the setting of massive bleeding compared with angiography as the "gold standard" [30].

16.2.2.3 Angiography

Mesenteric angiography requires ongoing blood loss of 1–1.5 mL/min for good visualization of the bleeding source. Angiography offers therapeutic options to control bleeding that other modalities do not, including vasoconstriction with vasopressin or microembolization with various substances. Frequently, bleeding due to cancer is not easily amenable to embolization, but this can be considered if the patient is a poor candidate for surgery. A significant number of patients with negative angiograms still require surgery, and there is a significant complication rate associated with intestinal and lower extremity ischemia, arterial dissection, renal failure due to contrast infusion, and catheter-site infections [31].

Emergency surgery may be indicated for the complications of colorectal cancer, including hemorrhage. Emergency surgery has a high mortality and morbidity, but outcomes have improved gradually with better supportive care. Better outcomes are found with more accurate preoperative localization, resulting in a lower re-bleeding rate. Surgery for patients with LGIB has defined risks and must take into account comorbidities [32].

16.2.3 Perforation

The perforation of a malignant GI neoplasm is a rare and serious event, with high immediate morbidity and mortality as well as poor long-term survival. Several retrospective series have investigated the perforations of gastric, small intestine and colorectal tumors in relation to pathological features, clinical pictures and prognostic factors [33–35]. Few studies have considered a control group of patients with non-perforated cancer of the same stage [33, 36], whereas no study has prospectively compared different treatment strategies, which are therefore based more on common sense and clinical experience than on scientific evidence.

Like all parietal lesions of the GI tract, tumors can cause a perforation in many ways. The most obvious is the mechanism inherent to the parietal infiltration, but it is also possible that a stenosing tumor causes relaxation of the upstream bowel section. The prevalence of perforations of tumors of the digestive tract is not known, but several retrospective series have compared the number of patients undergoing urgent surgery for perforated tumors with that of patients treated for uncomplicated cancer, estimating the prevalence to be 4–9% for gastric and 5% for colorectal cancers [33–36].

16.2.3.1 Presentation

The presentation does not differ substantially from those of perforations from benign disease. Older patients are more frequently involved, sometimes with a history of global wasting, vomiting and other occlusive symptoms, chronic pain and bleeding. Typical signs and symptoms of peritonitis such as constant and fixed abdominal pain, abdominal tenderness and septic shock in its various stages may be present. The diagnosis is made upon free air in upright chest or abdominal radiographs, and completed with abdominal CT, even without intravenous contrast medium, looking for confirmation of free air and estimation of the perforation site. In the absence of subdiaphragmatic free air, the clinical picture of hypogastric and/or right or left iliac fossa peritonitis is normally studied with abdominal CT to exclude pericolic air bubbles, which is indicative of buffered perforation. With specific reference to the perforations for malignancy, carrying out thoraco-abdominal CT with intravenous contrast medium would allow an increase in the rate of cases coming to the operating room with a suspicion of malignancy as well as to obtain complete and systemic staging of the disease (upon which a correct therapeutic indication should be based). Indeed, it is commonly reported in clinical series that the lack of information about the hematogenous extent of the disease (lungs, bones and also the liver if the surgeon does not have the equipment and specific experience for adequate intraoperative liver ultrasonography) adversely affects the therapeutic strategy. This is because in most cases of advanced cancer it is logical to assume synchronous hematogenous metastases (which would render useless a locally curative intervention) with particular regard to the extension of the lymphadenectomy [33–36]. In cases of free air and diffuse peritonitis, the surgical strategy is dependent upon the associated peritonitis and from the suspicion of the malignant nature of the perforation. For colonic-buffered perforations with localized peritonitis, a conservative strategy (based on fasting and antibiotic therapy) has recently gained consent to bring the patient to an elective intervention after colonic cleansing and reduction of local inflammatory phenomena, which allows to hypothesize a resection and direct anastomosis instead of the more common and invasive Hartman procedure [34]. In this specific case, there are often the conditions for a morphological study of the large bowel aimed to obtain information about the degree of eventually associated occlusion (hence the urgency of the intervention) and the extension of diverticular disease, which is commonly supposed to be the cause of perforation (hence the extent of colonic resection). The best way to obtain this information would be CT colonography. However, due to the need to blow air into the colon, it must be postponed at least 1 month after the acute event and made only in cases of optimal clinical evolution, with resumption of flatus and feeding.

16.2.3.2 CT Colonography

CT colonography can elicit the diagnostic dilemma of malignant instead of diverticular disease, but sometimes the condition of an inflammatory pseudotumor does not allow discrimination between these two entities. In such cases, colonoscopy with biopsy, even though potentially dangerous, can bring a therapeutic strategy rational for the illness [34–38].

16.2.3.3 Laparoscopic Approach

Once the decision to undergo surgery has been made, the choice of approach is correlated with localization of the presumed site of perforation. The laparoscopic approach to gastro-duodenal peptic ulcer perforations has been practised for many years, although a recent meta-analysis raised some doubts about the superiority of this approach as opposed to laparotomy [19]. In the case of jejunal-, ileal- and colonic-free perforations, the laparoscopic approach can elicit rare cases of diverticular perforations with purulent generalized peritonitis (Hinchey stage 3), in which a first surgical step of peritoneal washing and drainage is proposed [19]. The laparoscopic approach is likely to make harder the recognition or suspicion of malignancy at gastric and colonic levels, which can have a negative impact on outcome.

The first problem that arises intraoperatively is recognizing the malignant nature of the perforation. The gastric (instead of duodenal) ulcer localization, a parietal mass, regional pathological nodes and metastases are the only elements to realize the suspicion. From a theoretical viewpoint, carrying out a correct oncologic surgical procedure in gastric and in small and large bowel perforations (gastrectomy instead of suture, removal of at ≥15 lymph nodes for gastric cancer, and vascular ligation with removal of ≥12 nodes for colorectal cancer [37]), is rational only if the histological nature of the disease and staging of hematogenous metastases are known. However, even in those cases in which an intraoperative histopathological examination is available, the general condition of the patient has more influence on decision-making; aggressive surgery can be done only within hemodynamic stability and absence of advanced local sepsis. In all other cases (i.e., malignancy not confirmed, incomplete staging, patient in shock, severe peritoneal inflammation), the task of the surgeon is to practice an intervention that solves the acute phase and to refer to a second step completion of the surgical procedure according to the rules of oncologic surgery. Accordingly, in addition to the obvious and abundant washing of the abdominal cavity (associated with the placement of multiple drains), one must carry out a simple suture in the stomach (enlarging the parietal suture until healthy tissue), resection with direct anastomosis in the small bowel, and resection with a fecal transit diversion in the large bowel [19, 34–40].

Almost all series agree in defining that the postoperative prognosis in malignant perforation cases is poor: the 30-day mortality varies from 14% to 40.5% [34–38]. The causes of death are obviously related to sepsis, to which, however, certainly contributes a general cachexia, which justifies marked worsening of survival rates compared with perforation for benign diseases. Among the prognostic factors significantly correlated with postoperative mortality are advanced age, higher ASA grade, higher CR POSSUM score, degree of peritonitis [34–35] and a period between perforation and surgery >24 h. Data relating to long-term survival are less dramatic because not all perforated cancers are of advanced stage [38–39]. If patients with colorectal cancer treated radically are considered separately, the prognosis for cancer is not so different from that of patients with the same stage undergoing elective surgery, with 1-year survival of 55%, 2-year survival of 47% [36] and 5-year survival ranging from 14% [38] to 28% [36] and 54% [37], and overall mean survival time for stage II, III, and IV of 63.7, 38.1, and 13.8 months, respectively [39]. The same applies to perforated gastric cancer: the median survival time was 17.3 months [33], not different from that of a group of patients matched for cancer stage who underwent elective surgery. In the few reported cases in which long-term survival after non-radical local surgery (local enlargement and simple suture) of malignant gastric ulcer was analyzed, the results were acceptable only if the tumor was at a very initial stage [40]. In another small series of 6 patients treated with local resection, however, the survival rate was only 52.8±52.9 days [41].

References

1. Mercadante S (2009) Intestinal dysfunction and obstruction. In: Walsh D (ed) Palliative Medicine. Saunders/Elsevier, Philadelphia, pp 1267–1275
2. Ripamonti C, Twycross R, Baines M et al (2001) Working Group of the European Association for Palliative Care. Clinical-practice recommendations for the management of bowel obstruction in patients with end-stage cancer. Support Care Cancer 9:223–233
3. Baron TH (2009) Interventional palliative strategies for malignant bowel obstruction. Curr Oncol Rep 11:293–297
4. Helyer L, Easson AM (2008) Surgical approaches to malignant bowel obstruction. J Support Oncol 6:105-13
5. Maglinte DD, Howard TJ, Lillemoe KD, Sandrasegaran K Rex DK (2008) Small-bowel obstruction: state-of-the-art imaging and its role in clinical management. Clin Gastroenterol Hepatol 6:130–139
6. Abbas S, Bissett IP, Parry BR (2007) Oral water soluble contrast for the management of adhesive small bowel obstruction. Cochrane Database Syst Rev CD004651
7. Krouse RS, McCahill L, Easson AM, Dunn GP (2002) When the sun can set on an unoperated bowel obstruction: management of malignant bowel obstruction. J Am Coll Surg 195:117-28

8. Report of the National Confidential Enquiry into Perioperative Deaths 1996/1997. NCEPOD
9. Cirocchi R, Trastulli S, Abraha I et al (2012) Non-resection versus resection for an asymptomatic primary tumour in patients with unresectable stage IV colorectal cancer. Cochrane Database Syst Rev 15:CD008997
10. Higashi H, Shida H, Ban K et al (2003) Factors affecting successful palliative surgery for malignant bowel obstruction due to peritoneal dissemination from colorectal cancer. Jpn J Clin Oncol 33:357-9
11. Hoda D, Jatoi A, Burnes J, Loprinzi C, Kelly D (2005). Should patients with advanced, incurable cancers ever be sent home with total parenteral nutrition? A single institution's 20-year experience. Cancer 103:863–868
12. Doyle C, Crump M, Pinitilie M, Pza AM (2001)Does palliative chemotherapy palliate? Evaluation of expectations, outcomes, and costs in women receiving chemotherapy for advanced ovarian cancer. J Clin Oncol 19:1266–1274
13. Soriano A, Davis MP (2011) Malignant bowel obstruction: individualized treatment near the end of life. Cleveland Clin J Med 78(3):197-206
14. Turner J, Cummin T, Bennett A, Swift G, Green J (2008) Stents and stentability: treatment for malignant bowel obstruction. Br J Hosp Med (Lond) 69:676–680
15. Cheung HY, Chung CC, Tsang WW et al (2009) Endolaparoscopic approach vs conventional open surgery in the treatment of obstructing left-sided colon cancer: a randomized controlled trial. Arch Surg 144:1127-32
16. Averbach AM, Sugarbaker PH (1995) Recurrent intraabdominal cancer with intestinal obstruction. Internat Surg 80:141–146
17. Valle M, Federici O, Garofalo A (2012) Patient selection for cytoreductive surgery and hyperthermic intraperitoneal chemotherapy, and role of laparoscopy in diagnosis, staging, and treatment. Surg Oncol Clin N Am 21:515-31
18. Chen FM, Yin TC, Fan WC et al (2012)Laparoscopic management for acute malignant colonic obstruction. Surg Laparosc Endosc Percutan Tech 22:210-4
19. Agresta F, Ansaloni L, Baiocchi GL et al (2012) Laparoscopic approach to acute abdomen from the Consensus Development Conference of the SICE, ACOI, SIC, SICUT, SICOP, EAES. Surg Endosc 26:2134-64
20. Periera J, Phan T (2004) Management of bleeding in patients with advanced cancer. Oncologist 9:561-570
21. Wee E (2011) Management of nonvariceal upper gastrointestinal bleeding. J Postgrad Med 57:161-7
22. Wu JC, Sung JJ (2011) Pharmacologic therapy for nonvariceal upper gastrointestinal bleeding. Gastrointest Endosc Clin N Am 21:671-9
23. D'Amico G, Pagliaro L, Pietrosi G, Tarantino I (2010) Emergency sclerotherapy versus vasoactive drugs for bleeding oesophageal varices in cirrhotic patients. Cochrane Database Syst Rev 17:CD002233
24. Chung IK (2012) How can we maximize skills for non-variceal upper gastrointestinal bleeding: injection, clipping, burning, or others? Clin Endosc 45(3):230-4
25. Jairath V, Kahan BC, Logan RF et al (2012) National audit of the use of surgery and radiological embolization after failed endoscopic haemostasis for non-variceal upper gastrointestinal bleeding. Br J Surg 99(12):1672-80
26. Lee HJ, Park do J, Yang HK, Lee KU, Choe KJ (2006) Outcome after emergency surgery in gastric cancer patients with free perforation or severe bleeding. Dig Surg 23:217-23
27. Hreinsson JP, Gumundsson S, Kalaitzakis E, Björnsson ES (2013) Lower gastrointestinal bleeding: incidence, etiology, and outcomes in a population-based setting. Eur J Gastroenterol Hepatol 25:37-43
28. Strate LL, Naumann CR (2010) The role of colonoscopy and radiological procedures in the management of acute lower intestinal bleeding. Clin Gastroenterol Hepatol 8(4):333-343
29. Currie GM, Kiat H; Wheat JM (2011) Scintigraphic evaluation of acute lower gastrointestinal hemorrhage: current status and future directions. J Clin Gastroenterol 45(2):92-99

30. Geffroy Y, Rodallec MH, Boulay-Coletta I et al (2011) Multidetector CT angiography in acute gastrointestinal bleeding: why, when, and how. Radiographics 31(3):35-46
31. Millward SF (2008) ACR Appropriateness Criteria on treatment of acute non variceal gastrointestinal tract bleeding. J Am Coll Radiol 5:550-554
32. Czymek R, Kempf A, Roblick UJ et al (2008) Surgical treatment concepts for acute lower gastrointestinal bleeding. J Gastrointest Surg 12(12):2212-20
33. Shih CH, Yu MC, Chao TC et al (2010) Outcome of perforated gastric cancer: twenty years experience of one institute. Hepatogastroenterology. 57:1320-4
34. Anwar MA, D'Souza F, Coulter R et al (2006) Outcome of acutely perforated colorectal cancers: experience of a single district general hospital. Surg Oncol 15:91-96
35. Tan KK, Bang SL, Ho CK (2012) Surgery for perforated small bowel malignancy: a single institution's experience over 4 years. Surgeon 10:6-8
36. Abdelrazeq AS, Scott N, Thorn C et al (2008) The impact of spontaneous tumour perforation on outcome following colon cancer surgery. Colorectal Dis 10:775-80
37. Zielinski MD, Merchea A, Heller SF, You YN (2011) Emergency management of perforated colon cancers: how aggressive should we be? J Gastrointest Surg 15:2232-2238
38. Khan S, Pawlak SE, Eggenberger JC et al (2011) Acute colonic perforation associated with colorectal cancer. Am Surg 67:261-4
39. Tan KK, Hong CC, Zhang J et al (2010) Surgery for perforated colorectal malignancy in an Asian population: an institution's experience over 5 years. Int J Colorectal Dis 25(8):989-95
40. Jwo SC, Chien RN, Chao TC et al (2005) Clinicopathological features, surgical management, and disease outcome of perforated gastric cancer. J Surg Oncol 91:219-25
41. Kotan C, Sumer A, Baser M et al (2008) An analysis of 13 patients with perforated gastric carcinoma: A surgeon's nightmare? World J Emerg Surg 10:3-17

Cancers of Unknown Origin

17

Fabio Cesare Campanile, Gian Luca Baiocchi,
Nereo Vettoretto and Ferdinando Agresta

Cancers of unknown primary origin (CUP), or occult primary tumors, are malignancies, documented in a metastatic localization, without an identified primary origin. This malignant syndrome accounts for approximately 3–5% [1,2] of all cancer diagnosis. An estimated 31,000 patients have been diagnosed with an occult primary tumor during 2001 in the USA [3]. An analysis of the Swedish Family-Cancer Database demonstrated that incidence of CUP was between 6.00 and 6.98 cases per 100,000 from 1987 to 2008 [4]. Herein we report new developments in the diagnosis and treatment of CUP.

17.1 Introduction

The definition of cancers of unknown primary origin (CUP) varies among authors because a uniform set of inclusion and exclusion criteria is not available. Almost one-third of advanced tumors is diagnosed after its metastases have been discovered. In some of those cases, the organ site of the primary lesion becomes evident shortly thereafter, upon completion of a first set of clinical, pathological and imaging evaluations; those patients should be treated accordingly to a specific protocol. An extensive diagnostic workup deter-

F. C. Campanile (✉)
Division of General Surgery, Andosilla Hospital, Civita Castellana (Viterbo), Italy
e-mail: campanile@surgical.net

G. L. Baiocchi
Medical and Surgical Scineces, University of Brescia, Italy

N. Vettoretto
Laparoscopic Surgical Unit, M.Mellini Hospital, Chiari (Brescia), Italy

F. Agresta
Local Healthcare Unit ULSS 19 – Veneto, Adria, Italy

A. Valeri et al. (eds.), *What's New in Surgical Oncology*,
DOI: 10.1007/978-88-470-5310-6_17, © Springer-Verlag Italia 2013

mines the origin of some of those neoplasms; however, it is estimated that a primary site is eventually found in <30% of patients who present initially with an occult primary tumor. In 20% to 50% of cases, the primary tumor is not identified even after *post mortem* examination [5,6].

Guidelines [7] set by the UK National Institute of Health and Clinical Excellence (NICE) in 2010 provide some practical definitions related to the stage of the workup. A metastatic malignancy without an obvious primary site, before comprehensive investigation, is called a "malignancy of undefined primary" (MUO). If a careful review of histological specimens (or cytological specimens for pleural effusions or ascites) can then exclude non-epithelial tumors (melanoma, sarcoma, lymphoma, germ cell) and a selected initial screen of investigations (complete history and physical examination, routine laboratory tests, chest radiograph, routine imaging and endoscopy guided by signs, symptoms or laboratory abnormalities) cannot identify the primary source, the tumor is defined as a "provisional carcinoma of unknown primary" ("provisional CUP"). Only after specialist review and further appropriate specialized investigations, the lesion should be defined as metastasis of an occult primary tumor and termed "confirmed carcinoma of unknown primary" ("confirmed CUP").

The classification described above constitutes a straightforward and practical framework. However, it cannot account for the lack of consensus about the basic tests required in the initial diagnostic phase, and for the extreme complexity and variability of the "specialized investigations" available today.

In fact, many technological advances have been proposed as an aid in the diagnosis of CUPs, and several of them have been introduced in clinical practice. An initially confirmed CUP can be attributed to a putative origin by a more sophisticated level of diagnosis, even without anatomical localization of the original tumor. Typically, the quest for a primary origin of an occult lesion may include positron emission tomography-computed tomography (PET-CT), immunohistochemistry (IHC), assessment of serum markers and gene-expression profiling essays. Interestingly, research on this topic has focused on the relationship between the metastatic lesion and the original tissue, but is far from being established if thorough identification of the histological origin translates into a better outcome [8]. Recent research shows that cancers originating from the same tissue or organ do not necessarily respond to therapy in the same manner, and specific genetic factors can influence the response to treatment. This is particularly true for CUPs (with the exception of the most favorable subsets), which seem to behave more aggressively than metastatic tumors whose origin is known.

17.2 Recent Technological Developments that Aid Diagnoses

A comprehensive coverage of the diagnostics for CUPs is beyond the scope of this chapter, which focuses on the role of surgery. Technological advances in the diagnosis of CUPs are among the most important achievements in recent research on this topic. Their impact on outcome has yet to be demonstrated, but their potential influence on the knowledge of tumor biology (and even therapy) should not be underestimated. New biological and pathological features (including IHC profiling and gene expression-based assays) could be integrated, in the future, in algorithms to better define subsets of patients who could benefit from specific treatments, targeted to the identified tissue of origin, or even addressing the genomic abnormalities responsible for a certain behavior of the tumor itself. All this body of knowledge will certainly have an impact on the role of surgery in the treatment of these situations.

17.2.1 Immunohistochemistry

In general, hematoxylin and eosin staining can be used to determine the diagnosis, but the role of IHC has been increasing in recent years. Most guidelines consider at least a limited IHC study to be necessary for the diagnosis of CUP to exclude a non-epithelial origin of the lesion and to determine the origin of a carcinoma. IHC can accurately predict the origin of ≈35–40% metastatic cancers [9]. We cannot examine all the suggested IHC stains, but screening panels including cytokeratins (CK-7, CK-20), thyroid transcription factor-1 (TTF-1) and breast/ovarian markers are taken into consideration in most guidelines. Some authors have identified a new favorable subset of patients called "adenocarcinoma with colon cancer profile" that have a specific pattern of keratins and tumor-specific antigens (CK20+, CK7−, CDX2+). This subset responds to colon cancer-specific combination chemotherapy regimens with a median survival of 20–24 months [10]. Even if experiences on the surgical treatment of this subset have not been published, a role for hepatectomy in selected patients showing this IHC pattern can be foreseen.

17.2.2 Molecular Profiling

Different organ tissues show different patterns of gene expression, with some genes showing greater expression in one organ than another. The specific pattern of gene expression constitutes a "signature" of that tissue. Neoplasms share some of the patterns of the original tissue. Cell type-specific differential gene expression profiles have been used to develop assays that can provide additional information for the classification of tumors, including unknown primary cancers. The accuracy of the classification of these assays is >80% [11]. Multiple gene signatures for the prediction of primary sites have been generated, and there are several commercial tests available using this technology. All of them can be used to identify accurately types and subtypes of cancer on specimens with extremely low numbers of neoplastic cells. The ability to detect tumor signatures on particularly small specimens is extremely relevant for reducing the invasiveness of the diagnostic phase. A molecular profile consistent with six primary sites (lung, breast, colon, ovary, pancreas, and prostate) has been found, evaluating the expression of a 10-gene panel [12], and 10 cancer types could be distinguished by a second panel using 495 predictive genes [13]. Even though validation of this method to predict the origin of a CUP has not been established, its potential role in typing an otherwise "orphan" tumor (and even in determining specific drug response signatures) is enormous.

17.2.3 Advances in Imaging Methods

The widespread availability of complex (but highly effective) technologies such as computed tomography (CT) and magnetic resonance imaging (MRI) means that these imaging modalities are included in most diagnostic protocols for CUPs. The same definition of "putative CUP" cannot be obtained from a chest and abdominal multislice spiral CT, and MRI is often used in the diagnosis of occult tumors of the breast, head or neck.

The need to localize exceptionally small tumors, however, has prompted considerable interest in 18-F-fluorodeoxyglucose-positron emission tomography (18-FDG-PET), especially if combined with CT (PET-CT). CUPs are supposedly too small to be detected in the initial investigation phase, which generally includes CT. The ability of PET-CT to provide functional and metabolic information, along with the imaging, makes this technology particularly useful [14]. A recent meta-analysis demonstrated the excellent sensitivity and specificity of PET-CT in the localization of the primary tumor of an occult metastasis [15]. However, FDG remains a rather non-specific agent that can also accumulate in non-neoplastic tissues. Several other radiotracers are being evaluated for use in PET-CT to enhance its specificity [16,17]. Clinical use of tracers aimed at specific molecular tumor targets and the use of PET-MRI could induce substantial changes to the approach to these tumors.

17.3 Overview of Surgical Treatment

It could be argued that the role of surgery is extremely limited in a disease that, by definition, is already diffuse at diagnosis and whose biology is probably more aggressive for its early metastatic potential. However, such heterogeneous conditions can be divided into subsets with relatively homogeneous clinicopathological features. Most patients have aggressive disseminated disease that is relatively resistant to chemotherapy and with little curative potential, but 15–20% of subjects belong to subsets with a more favorable prognosis for whom a better outcome can be achieved [18].

Examining this topic under an evidence-based prospective is very difficult. Obtaining a series large enough to achieve a solid level of evidence for each of the significant subsets is not easy in such a heterogeneous group of conditions. Moreover, as research advances and our ability to determine the origin of the tumor increases, more lesions become associated with their putative primary origin, sometimes even if their diagnosis is likely but, in fact, uncertain. These lesions are often studied within a specific group of tumors and excluded from the CUP series (which are left only with unidentified cases). The same technological progress does not allow consideration of series collected over a long timespan because it is extremely likely that the diagnostic methods used in the most recent cases were not available for patients enrolled just few years earlier, making the group inhomogeneous. This is probably the only situation in which the passing of time does not help in accruing larger and more significant series and obtaining a better level of evidence.

Even with the limitations mentioned above, several organizations have recently issued guidelines for the diagnosis and management of CUPs [7, 19-21] using different methodologies.

A complete and detailed overview of all the diagnostic and multidisciplinary treatments of CUPS lies outside the scope of this chapter. Complete diagnostic and therapeutic algorithms can be found in the guidelines mentioned above. There is no question, however, that identification of potentially treatable anatomoclinical entities, in which it is possible to obtain long-term disease control with appropriate multidisciplinary management, has been one of the most relevant scientific achievements in this matter. Surgery plays a pivotal role for some of these subsets. We will examine the treatment of these subsets but not discuss those with minimal surgical interest.

17.3.1 Women with Papillary Adenocarcinoma of the Peritoneal Cavity

Ascitic fluid is a common manifestation of CUP. Cytology is sometimes sufficient to provide the diagnosis. In other cases, imaging can show definite peritoneal or omental implants that can be subjected to percutaneous ultrasound-guided biopsy. Diffuse peritoneal disease, without bulk localizations and a negative cytological diagnosis, require diagnostic laparoscopy and biopsy.

Peritoneal carcinomatosis, with papillary serous histology (serous papillary carcinoma), is considered to be consistent with ovarian histology even in the absence of ovarian involvement and, as such, is treated. Serum levels of cancer antigen Ca125 is elevated in ≈80% of cases. The origin of this type of tumor (and also of the "ovarian" cancer) is incompletely understood, and several theories have been proposed based on morphological, immunohistochemical and molecular findings [22]. Clinical reports seem to suggest that ovarian cancer and serous papillary carcinoma behave as distinct (although similar) entities [23]. As ovarian carcinoma, this condition is highly sensitive to platinum-based chemotherapy, and all guidelines agree that it should be treated as FIGO stage III ovarian cancer, with aggressive surgical cytoreduction followed by platinum-based postoperative chemotherapy. This indication is based on the analogy with ovarian cancer and to the fact that the outcome after cytoreduction and chemotherapy is similar to that obtained in the stage-III and -IV ovarian cancer [24].

17.3.2 Women with Adenocarcinoma Involving Only Axillary Lymph Nodes

Occult breast cancer should be suspected in all women with axillary lymph-node adenocarcinoma. After a thorough physical examination, a mammography is required. Estrogen and progesterone receptors should be obtained as well as HER2 status. If physical examination and mammography do not identify a primary breast cancer, ultrasound and MRI of the breast should be done; PET should also be taken into consideration. MRI can be used to identify a primary breast cancer in ≤75% of cases [25]. The prognosis and treatment in this situation is similar to that of stage-II breast cancer and requires locoregional treatment with surgery and radiotherapy according to the protocols adopted for that stage. If a breast lesion is identified, it should follow the treatment protocol for the appropriate stage. If not, axillary lymph-node dissection should be offered (as in breast cancer, the number of positive nodes is related to the prognosis). With respect to breast treatment, "mastectomy or radiotherapy" is recommended by the European Society of Medical Oncology (ESMO) Clinical Practice Guidelines 2011, which are based on expert consensus. The French National Federation of Cancer Centres (FNCLCC) evidence-based guidelines did not find evidence of the need to treat the breast in the absence of an identified primary lesion and, if MRI of the breast is negative, suggest not to offer locoregional treatment apart from axillary dissection. There is little evidence to support the superiority of local breast treatment (surgery or radiation) over watchful waiting if a primary lesion cannot be found. Primary cancer is often not found even in mastectomy specimens, and observational series have shown contradictory results about the advantages of local treatment with regard to treatment [26-28]. Aside from breast cancer, many other adenocarcinomas can present with axillary lymph-nodes metastases (including lung, pancreas, thyroid, stomach, uterus and colon) and this possibility should not be overlooked.

17.3.3 Squamous Cell Carcinoma Involving Cervical Lymph Nodes

Cervical lymph-node metastasis of a squamous cell carcinoma of an unknown primary tumor is believed to originate from the upper respiratory/digestive tract and is considered to be a highly curable disease [29]. The diagnosis is based upon a mass in the neck, and fine needle aspiration (FNA) is considered appropriate to obtain the necessary pathological diagnosis. Core or open biopsies should not be undertaken unless the patient is in the operating room, ready to undergo surgery if malignancy is confirmed [30]. The workup should include direct examination of the pharyngeal structures along with endoscopic and bioptic assessment of the nasopharynx, oropharynx, hypopharynx, larynx, and upper esophagus. Contrast multislice spiral CT and/or MRI are routinely added to abdominal and thoracic imaging. 18F-FDG-PET and PET-CT have shown high sensitivity for the detection of the origin of cervical lymph-node metastases, and their early use is recommended as a diagnostic tool that is additional to conventional workup in this subset of CUPs [31-33]. Ipsilateral tonsil biopsy or tonsillectomy can be used to detect a primary tumor not identified previously in ≈25% of patients. Human papillomavirus (HPV)-16 and Epstein–Barr Virus (EBV) testing can be useful. An HPV-positive test suggests a tonsil or base of the tongue localization of the primary tumor.

If the primary tumor is not identified despite extensive workup, lymph-node dissection should be offered followed by radiotherapy or chemoradiotherapy. Unresectable tumors can be treated with induction chemotherapy with a platinum-based combination or chemoradiotherapy. These recommendations, confirmed by ESMO Clinical Practice Guidelines and by the FNCLCC, are based on weak evidence. In the 2012 NCCN Guidelines, it is specified that, if most of the panel members agreed with the course of action described above, others believed that a neck dissection may be recommended after treatment with one of the following options: (i) chemoradiotherapy, (ii) primary radiotherapy, (iii) induction chemotherapy followed by chemoradiotherapy or radiotherapy. If a neck dissection is the initial treatment, it can be followed by a wide variety of adjuvant treatments based on the stage and level of node involvement. Evidence is limited to observational studies, but a systematic review failed to show a significant difference in the outcome between surgery plus chemoradiotherapy and chemoradiotherapy alone [34].

17.3.4 Isolated Inguinal Adenopathy (Squamous Carcinoma)

This uncommon subset is not always considered in the main guidelines on CUPs. ESMO Clinical Practice Guidelines does not include it. The FNCLCC examined the need for proctoscopy and colposcopy to rule out genital or anal neoplasia but included its treatment among those not belonging to a specific anatomoclinical entity if the tests fail to discover a primary tumor. A tumor in this location may arise from the skin of the lower limb or the trunk, or from genital/anal locations. An attempt at curative treatment is based on the hypothesis that the original tumor may have regressed spontaneously or can be eradicated by treatment for metastatic disease. Therefore, NCCN and NICE maintain a recommendation for inguinal lymphadenectomy followed by radiotherapy, if indicated. Evidence on this particular topic is extremely poor[7]. An article published in 1987 by Guarischi [35] supported lymph-node dissection or radiotherapy is the only available study to compare treatments, and its conclusions showed that only radiotherapy is a valid alternative to surgery in the management of this disease. However, there is no evidence that surgery or radiotherapy have a positive impact on survival if the origin of the tumor cannot be demonstrated.

17.3.5 Patients with a Single, Small, Potentially Resectable Tumor

Solitary metastasis from unknown primary (or limited, potentially resectable, metastatic disease) can be found in various sites (liver, lung, brain, adrenal, bone). Other occult metastatic lesions should be assessed in this group of patients, and PET is appropriate for this purpose. An unusual primary tumor of a parenchymal organ can also be mistaken for a metastasis (and *vice versa*) and this possibility should be taken into consideration before planning treatment [36-38]. Occasionally, long-term survival is reported after resection of the liver, brain and spine metastasis [39-41], and a primary tumor can be discovered later during follow-up [42]. Stereotactic radiosurgery is an option for brain lesions [43]. A systematic review about the treatment of solitary brain metastasis from occult tumors [44] could not prove that surgery, in addition to radiotherapy, confers a survival advantage over radiotherapy alone. However, a more recent revision of the literature, including also secondary lesions from known tumors, suggests that the treatment of brain metastases should be aggressive and independent of the primary site because of the satisfactory results obtained. This recommendation applies also to occult tumors [45]. Evidence in favor of surgical resection of lung, bone or skin metastasis of unknown primary is lacking.

References

1. Abbruzzese JL, Abbruzzese MC, Hess KR et al (1994) Unknown primary carcinoma: natural history and prognostic factors in 657 consecutive patients. J Clin Oncol 12(8):1272-1280
2. Pavlidis N, Briasoulis E, Hainsworth J et al (2003) Diagnostic and therapeutic management of cancer of an unknown primary. Eur J Cancer 39:1990-2005
3. Siegel R, Naishadham D, Jemal A (2012) Cancer statistics, 2012. CA Cancer J Clin 62:10-29
4. Bevier M, Sundquist J, Hemminki K. (2012) Incidence of cancer of unknown primary in Sweden: analysis by location of metastasis. Eur J Cancer Prev 21(6):596-601
5. Blaszyk H, Hartmann A, Bjornsson J (2003) Cancer of unknown primary: clinicopathologic correlations. APMIS. 111(12):1089-94
6. Hillen HF (2000) Unknown primary tumours. Postgrad Med J 76(901):690-693
7. NICE - National Collaborating Centre for Cancer (2010) Diagnosis and management of metastatic malignant disease of unknown primary origin Full Guideline July 2010. http://www.nice.org.uk/nicemedia/live/13044/49864/49864.pdf (Accessed 3 November 2012)
8. Pentheroudakis G, Greco FA, Pavlidis N (2009) Molecular assignment of tissue of origin in cancer of unknown primary may not predict response to therapy or outcome: a systematic literature review. Cancer Treat Rev 35(3):221-7
9. Greco FA, Oien K, Erlander M et al (2012) Cancer of unknown primary: progress in the search for improved and rapid diagnosis leading toward superior patient outcomes Ann Oncol 23(2):298-304

10. Varadhachary GR, Raber MN, Matamoros A et al (2008) Carcinoma of unknown primary with a colon-cancer profile – changing paradigm and emerging definitions. Lancet Oncol 9:596-599. doi:10.1016/S1470-2045(08)70151-7
11. Stella GM, Senetta R, Cassenti A et al (2012) Cancers of unknown primary origin: current perspectives and future therapeutic strategies. J Transl Med 10:12. doi: 10.1186/1479-5876-10-12
12. Varadhachary GR, Talantov D, Raber MN et al (2008) Molecular profiling of carcinoma of unknown primary and correlation with clinical evaluation. J Clin Oncol 26:4442-4448
13. Horlings HM, Van Laar R, Kerst J-M et al (2008) Gene expression profiling to identify the histogenetic origin of metastatic adenocarcinomas of unknown primary. J Clin Oncol 26:4435-4441
14. Fletcher JW, Djulbegovic B, Soares HP et al (2008) Recommendations on the use of 18F-FDG PET in oncology. J Nucl Med 49(3):480-508
15. Kwee TC, Kwee RM (2009) Combined FDG-PET/CT for the detection of unknown primary tumors: systematic review and metaanalysis. Eur Radiol 19(3):731-744
16. Kumar R, Dhanpathi H, Basu S et al (2008) Oncologic PET tracers beyond [(18)F]FDG and the novel quantitative approaches in PET imaging. Q J Nucl Med Mol Imaging 52(1):50-65
17. Smith G, Carroll L, Aboagye EO (2012) New Frontiers in the Design and Synthesis of Imaging Probes for PET Oncology: Current Challenges and Future Directions. Mol Imaging Biol, Sep 5 [Epub ahead of print]
18. Pavlidis N (2012) Optimal therapeutic management of patients with distinct clinicopathological cancer of unknown primary subsets Ann Oncol 23:x282-x285
19. Bugat R, Bataillard A, Lesimple T et al (2003) FNCLCC. Summary of the Standards, Options and Recommendations for the management of patients with carcinoma of unknown primary site (2002). Br J Cancer 89:S59-66
20. Fizazi K, Greco FA, Pavlidis N et al (2011) Cancers of unknown primary site: ESMO Clinical Practice Guidelines for diagnosis, treatment and follow-up Ann Oncol 22:vi64-vi68
21. National Comprehensive Cancer Network (2012) NCCN Clinical Practice Guidelines in Oncology. Occult Primary (Cancer of Unknown Primary [CUP]) http://www.nccn.org/professionals/physician_gls/pdf/occult.pdf (Accessed 3 November 2012)
22. Li J, Fadare O, Xiang L et al (2012) Ovarian serous carcinoma: recent concepts on its origin and carcinogenesis. J Hematol Oncol 9:8
23. Pentheroudakis G, Pavlidis N (2010) Serous papillary peritoneal carcinoma: unknown primary tumour, ovarian cancer counterpart or a distinct entity? A systematic review. Crit Rev Oncol Hematol 75(1):27-42
24. Ben-Baruch G, Sivan E, Moran O et al (1996) Primary peritoneal serous papillary carcinoma: a study of 25 cases and comparison with stage III-IV ovarian papillary serous carcinoma. Gynecol Oncol 60(3):393-6
25. de Bresser J, de Vos B, van der Ent F et al (2010) Breast MRI in clinically and mammographically occult breast cancer presenting with an axillary metastasis: a systematic review. Eur J Surg Oncol 36(2):114-9
26. Vlastos G, Jean ME, Mirza AN et al (2001) Feasibility of breast preservation in the treatment of occult primary carcinoma presenting with axillary metastases. Ann Surg Oncol 8(5):425-31
27. Walker GV, Smith GL, Perkins GH et al (2010) Population-based analysis of occult primary breast cancer with axillary lymph node metastasis. Cancer 116(17):4000-6
28. Wang X, Zhao Y, Cao X (2010) Clinical benefits of mastectomy on treatment of occult breast carcinoma presenting axillary metastases. Breast J 16(1):32-7
29. Pavlidis N, Pentheroudakis G, Plataniotis G (2009) Cervical lymph node metastases of squamous cell carcinoma from an unknown primary site: a favourable prognosis subset of patients with CUP. Clin Transl Oncol 11(6):340-8
30. National Comprehensive Cancer Network (2012) NCCN Clinical Practice Guidelines in Oncology. Head and Neck Cancers. http://www.nccn.org/professionals/physician_gls/pdf/head-and-neck.pdf (Accessed 3 November 2012)

31. Johansen J, Buus S, Loft A et al (2008) Prospective study of 18FDG-PET in the detection and management of patients with lymph node metastases to the neck from an unknown primary tumor. Results from the DAHANCA-13 study. Head Neck 30(4):471-8
32. Al-Ibraheem A, Buck A, Krause BJ et al (2009) Clinical Applications of FDG PET and PET/CT in Head and Neck Cancer. J Oncol 2009:208725
33. Kwee TC, Kwee RM (2009) Combined FDG-PET/CT for the detection of unknown primary tumors: systematic review and meta-analysis. Eur Radiol 19(3):731–744
34. Balaker AE, Abemayor E, Elashoff D, et al (2012) Cancer of unknown primary: does treatment modality make a difference? Laryngoscope 122(6):1279-82
35. Guarischi A, Keane TJ, Elhakim T (1987) Metastatic inguinal nodes from an unknown primary neoplasm. A review of 56 cases. Cancer 59(3):572-7.
36. Campos S, Davey P, Hird A et al (2009) Brain metastasis from an unknown primary, or primary brain tumour? A diagnostic dilemma. Curr Oncol 16(1):62-6
37. Beckers F, Ludwig C, Cerinza J et al (2009) Der pulmonale Rundherd bei maligner Grunderkrankung - nicht zwingend eine Metastase des Primärtumors. Pneumologie 63(12):693-696
38. Savage NM, Alleyne CH, Vender JR et al (2011) Dural-based metastatic carcinomas mimicking primary CNS neoplasia: report of 7 cases emphasizing the role of timely surgery and accurate pathologic evaluation. Int J Clin Exp Pathol 4(5):530-40
39. Adam R, Chiche L, Aloia T et al (2006) Hepatic Resection for Noncolorectal Nonendocrine Liver Metastases. Annals of Surgery 244(4):524-535
40. Nieder, C, Spanne, O, Mehta, MP et al (2011) Presentation, patterns of care, and survival in patients with brain metastases. Cancer 117:2505–2512
41. Aizenberg MR, Fox BD, Suki D et al (2012) Surgical management of unknown primary tumors metastatic to the spine. J Neurosurg Spine 16(1):86-92
42. Ozeki Y, Abe Y, Kita H et al (2011) A case of primary lung cancer lesion demonstrated by F-18 FDG positron emission tomography/computed tomography (PET/CT) one year after the detection of metastatic brain tumor. Oncol Lett 2(4):621-623
43. Niranjan A, Kano H, Khan A et al (2010) Radiosurgery for brain metastases from unknown primary cancers. Int J Radiat Oncol Biol Phys 77(5):1457-62
44. Hart MG, Grant R, Walker M et al (2007) Surgical resection and whole brain radiation therapy versus whole brain radiation therapy alone for single brain metastases. Cochrane Database of Systematic Reviews 2007, Issue 2
45. Kyritsis AP, Markoula S, Levin VA (2012) A systematic approach to the management of patients with brain metastases of known or unknown primary site. Cancer Chemother Pharmacol 69(1):1-13

Index

Printed in May 2013

MIX
Papier aus verantwortungsvollen Quellen
Paper from responsible sources
FSC® C105338

If you have any concerns about our products,
you can contact us on
ProductSafety@springernature.com

In case Publisher is established outside the EU,
the EU authorized representative is:
Springer Nature Customer Service Center GmbH
Europaplatz 3, 69115 Heidelberg, Germany

Printed by Libri Plureos GmbH
in Hamburg, Germany